Nursing: a knowledge base for practice

SECOND EDITION

Nursing: a knowledge base for practice

SECOND EDITION

Edited by

Abigayl Perry

Medical Sociologist, Department of Human Science and Medical Ethics,
St Bartholomew's and the Royal London Medical School, London, UK

A member of the Hodder Headline Group
LONDON • NEW YORK • SYDNEY • AUCKLAND

First published in Great Britain in 1997 by
Arnold, a member of the Hodder Headline Group,
338 Euston Road, London NW1 3BH

Whilst the advice and information in this book is believed to be true and accurate at the date of
going to press, neither the author(s) nor the publisher can accept any legal responsibility or
liability for any errors or omissions that may be made.

British Library Cataloguing in Publication Data
A catalogue record for this book is available from the British Library

Library of Congress Cataloging-in-Publication Data
A catalog record for this book is available from the Library of Congress

ISBN 0 340 63188 0

Typeset in 10/12pt Palatino by Saxon Graphics Ltd, Derby
Printed and bound in Great Britain by J W Arrowsmith Ltd, Bristol

Contents

List of contributors

Paul Barber PhD, MSc, RNMS, RMN, RGN
Director, Human Potential Resource Group, Department of Educational Studies, University of Surrey, Surrey

Jennifer Boore OBE, PhD, FRCN, RNT, RM, RGN
Professor of Nursing, School of Health Sciences, University of Ulster, Northern Ireland

E. Jane Chapman MSocSci, BSc Hons, Dip Risk Management, RGN
Clinical Risk Manager, Northwick Park and St Mark's NHS Trust (Harrow) and Chair, Association of Litigation and Risk Managers (ALARM), London

Andrzej Kuczmierczyk PhD, MSc, BA, Cert Psychology, AFBPS
Senior Lecturer, Health Psychology and Director, Health Psychology Postgraduate Training, Department of Psychology, City University, London

Sue McBean MSc Health Ed, BSc Hons, Dip N Ed, NDN Cert, RHV, RGN
Lecturer in Nursing, School of Health Sciences, University of Ulster, Northern Ireland

Kim Manley MNurs., PGCEA, BA, Dip Nurs., RCNT, RGN
Lecturer in Nursing, RCN Institute, Royal College of Nursing, London and formerly Project Leader/Clinical Nurse Specialist, ITU Nursing Development Unit, Chelsea and Westminster Hospital, London

Alan Myles MA Ed, Dip Ed, RNT, RGN
Head of Education Development, RCN Institute, Royal College of Nursing, London

Abigayl Perry MSc Econ, Cert FE, BSc Hons Soc, RGN
Medical Sociologist, Department of Human Science and Medical Ethics, St Bartholomew's and the Royal London Medical School, University of London, London

Jane Robinson PhD, MA, MIPM, HVT, RHV, ONC, RGN
Professor and Head of Department, Nursing and Midwifery Studies, University of Nottingham, Nottingham

Mary Watkins PhD, M Nurs., RMN, RGN
Head of Institute of Health Studies, Faculty of Human Sciences, University of Plymouth, Plymouth

Mary Watts PhD, MA, BSc, Cert Psychology, Dip Counselling, RNT, RMN, RGN
Senior Lecturer in Health and Counselling Psychology and Co-director, Centre for Counselling Psychology, Department of Psychology, City University, London

Preface to the second edition

The popularity of this book since it was first published in 1991 has led to a new, revised edition. The basic structure of ten chapters or specialisms remains the same as in the previous edition. In three of the chapters (Chapters 2, 6 and 8) only the references cited have been updated where appropriate. Elsewhere, the material has been amended to reflect current emphases (Chapter 1). More substantial revisions have been carried out in the areas of health promotion (Chapter 3), the biological sciences (Chapter 4) psychology (Chapter 5), sociology (Chapter 7), education (Chapter 9) and nursing theory (Chapter 10).

This book is an educational text, organised primarily in accordance with the demands of nursing students and practitioners. It is also a scholarly work in that it aims to explore debates in the various disciplines as critiques of contemporary processes such as nursing, therapeutics and health. Several examples of original work in this volume are relevant to a wider student readership in the specialism of health care.

Abigayl Perry

Introduction

This book is intended as a text for a range of students which addresses the main concerns of nursing. It reflects the direction that nursing knowledge has taken over the past decade in terms of higher education and academic research. The chapter sequence has been altered in this edition, mainly in response to the critical feedback received from reviewers and readers. I hope that relationships and shared themes among the various subjects have been made more explicit. For example, the biological sciences (Chapter 4) have established links with psychology (Chapter 5) in the study of sensory data and individual and environmental adaptation.

Collectively, the authors articulate an array of issues and disciplinary interests relevant to the social practice of nursing. Each chapter is capable of standing alone, while also contributing to the book's structure in applied science. The overall emphasis is theoretical/comparative, in order to incorporate the experiences of different practitioners. We have not, therefore, lost sight of either the reality facing those in various branches of nursing, or the ethical and political problems arising from health care arrangements.

Nursing practice is informed by different disciplines within the biological, behavioural and social sciences. The subjects selected here represent a defensible core for an explicit nursing knowledge base, even though a national advanced curriculum has not yet been established. All knowledge bases are narrow but very deep (specialised) – they have to be so in order to penetrate the complex structures, human and/or social bodies, which they attempt to reveal and explain. The authors of this textbook provide in-depth frameworks for the training in logical analysis, the development and construction of formal arguments about debatable issues, and the ability to search the literature for factual information that is useful to practice. These academic skills are not only necessary to pass examinations; they are essential components of professional accountability. They enable us to review the 'tools' (knowledge and experience) not only of our own 'trade', but also of others. Theory is not, therefore, just an academic subject, and as academics are aware, it should not be sustained independent of research, that is, engagement with social issues. Taken together, these elements constitute what is known as methodology – a means whereby professionals measure and test what they do in the light of public scrutiny. These themes and issues are relevant to nursing practitioners in intensive care, mental health or midwifery, as well as to diploma, degree and graduate students and their teachers.

This is a resource book, not a novel; it can be read, to some extent, in an order other than the chapter sequence published. The first and last chapters have deliberate connections. Both investigate the constituents of nursing knowledge, but from differing disciplines and degrees of application. In Chapter 1, Mary Watkins uses a social action perspective to report on well-known definitions of nursing and nursing knowledge. The knowledge that nurses use is clearly identified and discussed in terms of current and future standards of care. The principles which inform these qualities, derived from the parent discipline of philosophy or, more explicitly, the philosophy of science, are examined in some detail by Kim Manley in Chapter 10. The general purpose here, as in the other chapters, is to encourage nurses to think about what they do in terms of their knowledge base, from the viewpoints of relevant disciplines.

In Chapter 1, Mary Watkins locates the processes of value clarification and the relationship between theoretical and practical knowledge in a variety of social settings. Different standards of nursing knowledge, from the intuitive to the professional, are analysed in terms of specific nursing teams and patient outcomes. Readers will appreciate the author's account of her participatory research in night hospital care for the elderly (Mental Health Unit), which appears as an appendix to the chapter.

In Chapter 2, Jane Chapman clarifies the fundamental purpose of nursing research, that is, its function in evaluating honestly the relationships between practices and patient outcomes. The author skilfully uses a questioning approach to guide the reader through different dimensions of the 'application problem'. This example will have a direct appeal to those new to the area.

Chapter 3 provides a cogent analysis of the varied and often contradictory definitions of 'health' in current usage, and the subsequent problems this implies for implementing health promotion models. Sue McBean maps out this complex territory for us, taking considerable care to identify the source material. The principal aim is to integrate the diverse strands of theoretical debates and practical, social issues in health promotion into a structure which people can use.

In Chapter 4, Jennifer Boore applies her expertise to the selection and maintenance of the biological sciences in nursing. Four key concepts that are prevalent in nursing theories (person, environment, health and nursing) are used to construct a framework relevant to practices. Homeostasis, age-related bodily changes, genetic characteristics, stress and immunity are clearly linked throughout the discussion to the aims of providing care and promoting health. These themes are seen to be common to the behavioural sciences, to which we now turn.

In Chapter 5, Mary Watts and Andrzej Kuczmierczyk identify specific theories and research findings in psychology which are significant to the enhancement of nursing practices. Relevant topics under discussion include learned helplessness in patients, stress adaptation and the psychological risk factors associated with heart disease. Drawing upon research with student psychiatric and general nurses, the authors analyse the attitudes and basic assumptions, often implicit, which have a bearing on the interpersonal activity of nursing and therapeutic relationships generally.

Caring as a therapeutic relationship is the subject of Chapter 6, in which Paul Barber provides an intimate account of his experiences as a hospital patient, paralleled by professional insights into the nurse–patient relationship. Through the processes of social psychology we truly enter the world as felt and experienced by those on the receiving end of surgical treatment regimes. In addition, the section entitled 'On the clinical environment: the need for research-minded care' is a valuable learning resource for novice and expert researchers alike.

Chapter 7 (sociology) and Chapter 8 (politics) are structuralist accounts of power relations in nursing and health organisation. In Chapter 7, Abigayl Perry presents a sociologist's view of organised nursing with special reference to the explanatory concepts of class, ideology and gender. Many of the issues raised in this chapter are expanded and developed in Jane Robinson's analysis of politics in nursing, which follows in Chapter 8. Starting with a definition of sexual politics, the author examines the hidden face of power in society apart from its recognised form in organised politics. The problem of powerlessness which many feminist theorists have struggled with is seen to have a bearing on the way in which nurses have been overlooked in government health policies.

In Chapter 9, Alan Myles focuses on developments in curriculum design in response to the most significant policy change in late twentieth-century nursing. The nature of the affiliation between colleges of nursing and midwifery and higher education is examined in terms of the modular system. The relative merits of modular courses are discussed in terms of principles and objectives (educational philosophy), schemes of study, teaching methods and student accreditation. Examples of curriculum development and value clarification exercises for pre- and post-registration courses are provided throughout the chapter in order to illustrate this process in action.

Finally, in Chapter 10, Kim Manley discusses the abstract philosophical principles which inform all professional practices, including nursing. The generation of knowledge is explored and applied in the study of nursing as a science and an art. Using a multi-faceted approach, the author attempts to explain some quite complex philosophical ideas, which are then related to levels of theory. The work on levels of theory is developed in the application to nursing theories. Through the development and application of knowledge, nurses are seen to be truly accountable practitioners.

I am taking this opportunity to thank Helen Thomas, librarian in the RCN library, for her help in checking the references cited in this volume.

Abigayl Perry

Nursing knowledge in nursing practice

1

Mary Watkins

Definitions of knowledge and nursing

Knowledge is defined in several ways, including 'the range of information, perception or understanding enjoyed by an individual or group' and 'the fact or condition of knowing something through experience or association' (Longman, 1984). These two definitions seem particularly pertinent to nursing, as together they embrace the concepts of 'a group having knowledge', that knowledge can be developed 'through experience' and that having knowledge can be 'enjoyable'! Nursing is more difficult to define, especially if one turns to nursing textbooks where complex explanations of nursing include the following:

> Nursing is a process of human interactions between nurse and client whereby each perceives the other and the situation and, through communication, they set goals, explore means, and agree on means to achieve goals.
>
> (King, 1981, p. 144)

> Nursing is a science and the application of knowledge from that science to the practice of nursing.
>
> (Andrews and Roy, 1986, p. 8)

> Nursing ... as a learned profession is both a science and an art. A science may be defined as an organised body of abstract knowledge arrived at by scientific research and logical analysis. The art of nursing is the imaginative and creative use of this knowledge in human service.
>
> (Rogers, 1989, p. 182)

At first glance all three of the above explanations may seem wordy and irrelevant to the practising nurse, who is inclined to see nurse theorist's work as 'out of touch' with the clinical nurse's role (Miller, 1985a). Yet on close examination all of the definitions have useful insights to offer, namely that nursing involves individual perception and communication between nurse and client (King, 1981), the application of knowledge in practice (Andrews and Roy, 1986) and the imaginative use of knowledge to assist others (Rogers, 1983). Different concepts of nursing are present in Henderson's (1969) definition, which states:

> Nursing is primarily assisting the individual (sick or well) in the performance of those activities contributing to health or its recovery that he would perform unaided if he had the necessary strength, will or knowledge.
>
> (Henderson, 1969, p. 4)

Likewise, it is the unique contribution of nursing to help the individual to be independent as soon as possible. The main advantage of Henderson's (1969) definition, when compared to the others referred to here, is that it is easily understandable. This quality, together with the fact that the role of the nurse and the aim of nursing (i.e. to help people to gain independence) are clearly identified, is presumably the reason for its adoption by the International Council of Nurses. It is interesting to note, however, that the universally accepted definition does not allude to the need for nurses to have a sound *knowledge base* from which to plan imaginative individualised nursing care.

Knowledge for practice?

It could be argued that it is irrelevant whether or not 'knowledge' is referred to in the International Council of Nurses' definition of nursing, yet the inclusion does seem to be important to many nurses, especially to nurse theorists, and the argument for its inclusion is not just an academic one. The United Kingdom Central Council for Nursing, Midwifery and Health Visiting (UKCC) Code of Conduct (1992) states that nurses 'shall act at all times in such a manner as to safeguard and promote the interests of individual patients and clients', while Rule 18 of the Nurses, Midwives and Health Visitors Act (Statutory Instrument, 1983) places a responsibility on first-level nurses to assess, plan, implement and evaluate care. McFarlane (1977) believes that it is impossible for nurses to make decisions regarding the prescriptions of nursing care and ways of safeguarding patients without having a sound understanding of theory on which to base those decisions.

While there is clearly evidence to suggest that nurses require knowledge for practice, questions need to be asked, e.g. 'what knowledge do they require?' and 'what characteristics do nurses need to select and apply relevant knowledge?'

The knowledgeable practitioner

The aims of Diploma programmes which prepare nurses for initial registration in the UK (see Chapters 3 and 9) are designed to enable students to become *knowledgeable doers* in practice. The effective knowledgeable doer is presumably a reflective decision-maker who uses relevant theory to underpin practice. Such nurses require a clear understanding of nursing, health, people and the effects of society, the environment and the politics of health care from which to problem-solve. In order to practise effectively, nurses today and in the future will need to have an understanding of theory from the social sciences (see Chapters 5 to 8), including sociology and psychology, as well as biology (see Chapter 4), in addition to specific nursing knowledge (UKCC, 1986; see Chapters 2 and 10).

There is an implication that the use of knowledge from these sciences is new; in fact, nurse theorists have developed conceptual frameworks for practice over the last century which have incorporated similar knowledge. Several nurse academics have suggested that it is necessary to be explicit about the nature of man, nursing, health and society in order to depict nursing as an entity (Stevens, 1984).

Nightingale (1859) reported the importance of clean air, rest, quiet and good food for patients, while more recently nurse theorists have described the need to encourage *patient independence* (Henderson, 1969; Orem, 1985) and to extend patients' *coping abilities* through teaching, counselling (Peplau, 1952) or altering those stimuli which are known to contribute to disability (Roy, 1984). Most clinical nurses incorporate knowledge that is related to the concepts described by these theorists into practice.

For example, a nurse on a medical ward will ensure that a patient who has just been diagnosed as suffering from diabetes understands the nature of diabetes, the need for an appropriate diet and regular mealtimes, the effects of prolonged exercise, the signs of hypo- or hyperglycaemia, the actions to take in the event of hypo- or hyperglycaemia commencing and, if necessary, how to self-administer insulin prior to discharge. Such a nurse will apply knowledge concerning teaching, health promotion, counselling, diabetes, the pancreas, diet and the nature of anxiety, in order to help the patient to extend his or her own ability to cope with the actual and potential problems of diabetes. When planning the best form of intervention for this kind of patient, the nurse will also consider their social circumstances, financial position and family support. If relevant, the nurse will then assist the patient in applying for financial help, or in teaching other family members about the disease. Many nurses reading this paragraph may feel that what is written is just common sense. That is precisely where nurses have denigrated their own knowledge in the past, frequently implying that nursing is common sense rather than recognising it as a complex human task which involves the application of theory in practice (Benner, 1984; Kitson, 1993; Stevens, 1984).

Present practice – knowledge and ritual?

Accepting the hypothesis that nurses do underpin much of their practice with knowledge, do they, as has been reported, also resort to *ritual* (Chapman, 1983; Menzies, 1960)? There is little doubt that nursing is a stressful occupation in which relatively young people come into contact with the horrifying realities of disease, disability and death. Psychological theory suggests that humans try to avoid stress by utilising defence mechanisms to protect themselves from reality (Hilgard *et al.*, 1975). It is hardly surprising, therefore, that Menzies (1960) reports nurses using rituals to distance themselves from the reality of human suffering. A more recent work hypothesises that some of the rituals which Menzies described as *a defence against anxiety* are, in fact, concerned with conveying social meaning (Chapman, 1983). Chapman (1983) cites Max Weber, who described four types of actions: *traditional* actions or those determined by habit; *zweckrational* or purposive rational actions which involve assessing the probable results of a given act, based on empirical evidence; *vertrational* actions, where the means and ends of an action are based on a systematic set of ideas and beliefs which are not empirically proven; and *affective* actions which are carried out under emotive impulses. The last mentioned action roughly equates with Menzies' observations, but the other three involve different interpretations of ritual. Taking temperatures may be a zweckrational action when the result will influence care, but to some extent it becomes a non-rational ritual or traditional action when the patient is well. Alternatively, it may be that taking a temperature at this time is perceived by the nurse as a reassuring measure to the patient (a vertrational action).

Both authors infer that ritual actions in nursing inhibit the delivery of psychosocial patient care (see Chapter 6), yet any solution designed to enhance practice will clearly be dependent upon which interpretation of the defined problem, sociological (Chapman, 1983) or psychoanalytic (Menzies, 1960), is accepted.

At least two interpretations of ritual actions in nursing can be made, and it is probable that they both contain truth, yet neither can be proven in the empirical scientific sense. This is because social science theory is developmentally in its infancy (Jacox, 1974). Chapman (1976) suggests that this is doubly so for nursing, which is such a new discipline in the academic sense. The complexity of relating nursing actions to client outcomes is also a factor which may have prevented the rapid development of nursing knowledge relating to effectiveness as opposed to descriptions (Bloch, 1977; Closs and Tierney, 1993; Donabedian, 1966; Kitson *et al.*, 1990).

It is only by accepting a level of uncertainty in nursing knowledge and relevant theory from the social and behavioural sciences that nursing is likely to develop and grow. The clinical nurse can be respected for her cynicism about nursing theory if her desire is to have concrete prescriptive theory from which to practise. In the absence of being told by nurse theorists what is right and therefore how to act, clinical nurses must have the ability to be reflective decision-makers who are prepared to choose the 'best' option when delivering care, rather than the 'correct' one. The 'best' option today may well not be the best one tomorrow. For example, in the early 1970s, I, along with many other nurses, used egg white and oxygen to treat superficial pressure sores. This action worked, and I asked a senior sister how this occurred. She gave me a complex description which involved oxygenation of the tissues combined with the protein in albumin. I remained convinced of this action for some years, until I read Norton et al.'s (1975) work on pressure sores. It was difficult to change my practice in the light of this (to me) new knowledge, because I had incorporated a set of actions to prevent and treat pressure sores into my repertoire based, it seems now, on ritual rather than on theory! Imagine, then, my horror on subsequently finding a patient, who did not score highly enough on the Norton scale to warrant preventative care, developing a sore. It took some time for me to 'problem-solve' how this had happened. The patient was on steroids, and no calculation was made for this on the Norton scale, yet the patient's skin was papery thin. The penny dropped, and I now consider steroids when using the tool. However, the point of revealing my inadequacies is to note the following:

- steroids were not commonly given to elderly people when Norton undertook her work, and the pressure area assessment tool was valid and reliable when produced;
- advances in medical care and the use of steroids reduced the reliability of a nursing instrument;
- I ignored the evidence of papery thin skin, and just used the scale;
- nurses need to update their knowledge continually, in order to adapt patient assessment prescriptions for care as necessary;
- I had begun to use Norton's scale in a ritualistic manner, rather than in a thoughtful proactive one.

Clearly, tomorrow's individual accountable practitioner needs constantly to evaluate practice, to read research, to judge the relevance of research and to instigate useful findings into practice if the decisions he or she makes about care are to be based on a sound level of theory (McFarlane, 1977) and reduce unnecessary ritual. If nurses have the common objective of enhancing client care through the application of knowledge as suggested in the code of conduct (United Kingdom Central Council for Nursing, Midwifery and Health Visiting, 1992), it is necessary to have formal methods of evaluating the efficiency and effectiveness of nursing care.

Evaluating nursing care

Bailey and Claus (1975) believe that if evaluation of nursing is to be effective, it should be conducted in accordance with accepted and proven principles.

The American Medical Association (American Medical Association, 1982) has developed a mode of quality assurance which is widely used and proven in practice. It is cyclical in nature, demonstrating that the quality assurance process involves not only identification of standards and evaluation of care given, but also striving to enhance nursing care by changing standards as necessary (see Figure 1.1).

Standard setting

The first step in the development of standards involves *value clarification* (American Medical Association, 1982) and defining nursing (Van Maanen, 1984; Wright, 1984). At this stage, the use of a *nursing model* may help nurses to define their values and beliefs about nursing (Wright, 1984). The purposes and values of nursing will vary according to the practice setting of care delivery, and the selection or development of an appropriate model will be dependent on these factors. For example, psychiatric nurses involved in caring for clients suffering from clinical depression may value the concept of nursing being an *interpersonal process* through which clients develop and grow (Peplau, 1952), while nurses involved with clients who have a learning difficulty may wish to adopt the values of Orem (1985), whose model emphasises the need to motivate and educate people to achieve their maximum *ability to self-care*. Well-recognised models are sometimes considered to

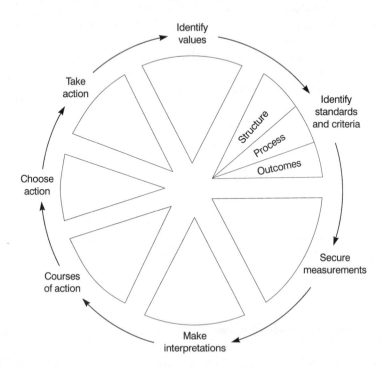

Figure 1.1 American Nurses' Association Quality Assurance Cycle (American Nurses' Association, 1977)

be restricted, and for this reason Wright (1990) describes the development of a model designed specifically for care of elderly people, while Watkins (1988) has adapted two models, namely the *activities of living* model (Roper *et al.*, 1980) and a *stress adaptation* model (Zarit *et al.*, 1985; see Chapter 4), to encompass the care of elderly people who are primarily supported at home by carers. These latter models embrace the values of small nursing teams involved with care. Although this can be regarded as a strength, because models developed in this way tend to be client-group specific, they can also be less useful in terms of value clarification for nursing in a broader sense. Mega-models such as Roy's (1984) stress adaptation model and Roper *et al.*'s (1980) activities of living model, have been shown to be applicable in many nursing settings, and may, therefore, be more useful in terms of value clarification where quality assurance standards are to be agreed upon across several types of nursing within one hospital or community care setting.

Having identified professional nursing values, the second stage of value clarification commences (Kitson *et al.*, 1990). This is a complex procedure because nurses must attempt to reach a consensus between the values of the nursing profession, the public, government, general managers and other health care workers. Lang and Clinton (1984) acknowledge that this can be especially difficult when cost containment of a service conflicts with professional values. A simple example of such a situation would be when the nursing team of a surgical day-patient unit values having time to communicate with patients on a one-to-one basis, which can be costly in terms of nursing time, while management favours fast throughput of patients and cost containment of the nursing budget. If nurses are to be able to debate these kinds of issues with health care professionals and politicians, and to present their case for consideration, it is vital that they apply knowledge from the study of ethics and relevant nursing research (Department of Health, Nursing Division, 1989). Once a group of nurses has completed the formidable task of defining values of care which are consistent with both their professional values and the constraints of their working environment, the remaining steps of the quality assurance cycle are relatively simple.

The next stage is to develop standards and criteria with which to assess nursing (Wright, 1984). It is suggested that the terms can be used interchangeably, but in fact a standard evolves from a criterion (Bloch, 1980). 'A criterion is the value-free name of a variable believed or known to be a relative indicator of the quality of patient care' (Bloch, 1977, p.22). Thus a nurse may decide that one criterion for measuring nursing is the level of knowledge that a patient possesses about the side-effects of the medication he is taking. With this criterion established, an acceptable standard can be set, against which nursing performance can be compared. A standard can be defined as the desired and achievable level (or range of performance) corresponding to a criterion, against which performance is compared (Bloch, 1977; Kitson *et al.*, 1990; Wright, 1984). Crow (1981) noted that the term 'standards of care' is often used synonymously with effectiveness, although this is not necessarily true. A 'good' standard of terminal nursing care can be achieved, yet the patient outcome will still be death. Thus measures which indicate a *quality of life* standard for patients must be developed, as well as more traditional *outcome measures*.

Three types of standard will emerge, namely those of structure, process and outcome. *Structural standards* involve factors within the new system such as staffing, styles of supervision, organisational, environmental, and physical resources (Bloch, 1977; Lang and Clinton, 1984; Smith-Marker, 1988). *Process standards* involve defining the activities expected of nurses when caregiving, which will include, among other processes, methods of assessment, planning, implementation and evaluation of care delivery. *Outcome standards* are concerned with changes in the patient's health status, feelings, knowledge and satisfaction; thus the standard referring to patient knowledge is an outcome standard. Standards will, of necessity, vary to some extent between different nursing teams, and if, as Hockey (1979) suggests, most evaluation takes place within the boundaries of one hospital or health care centre, standard setting may best be done at a local level. Several authors note the need for standard setting groups to consist of experts in their own clinical fields who have access to and who examine relevant literature to ensure that standards are based on the best available scientific knowledge (Crow, 1981; Kitson *et al.*, 1990; Wright, 1984).

Whenever possible, nurses should incorporate research-based knowledge into their standards (see Chapter 2). For example, Hayward's (1975) research demonstrated the need for trained staff to have sufficient time to explain the nature of post-operative pain pre-operatively in order to reduce this type of pain. Thus the number of trained staff on a surgical ward (structural standard) needs to reflect such research (Bloch, 1980), and the process standards need to incorporate the action of pre-operative preparation. Unfortunately, the extent of nursing knowledge available today is insufficient to ensure that all nursing standards can incorporate empirically developed theory in this way. However, in the long term, accurate quality assurance programmes may demonstrate new relationships between nursing processes and patient outcomes which could in turn provide theory on which to base development of future standards (Henney, 1984; Thomas and Bond, 1995). The recent development of the 'Cochrane Collaboration' database (a compilation of health care clinical effectiveness data), may assist nurses in identifying appropriate practice based on outcome (Cochrane Library, 1997).

The study of process–outcome

Bloch (1975) believes that it is possible to establish new nursing theory by observing the relationships between current nursing practice and patient outcomes, and suggests that this is the most important evaluative work for nurses. As relationships between variables are found and acknowledged, *grounded theory* which has a clear basis in practice should emerge (Pursey, 1996). This kind of research is very exciting in that it may reveal and explain some of the nursing practices which have evolved through experience without previously having been subjected to scientific scrutiny. Although it is difficult to measure 'nursing effectiveness', there is an increasing amount of research being published which has examined the relationship between particular interventions, the use of specific products and the skill mix of nursing teams to patient outcomes (Barker, 1992; Carr-Hill *et al.*, 1992; Curran, 1992; Thomas and Bond, 1995). The importance of these types of studies cannot be overemphasised in an environment where it is necessary for nurses to prove the value of nursing (Royal College of Nursing, 1992).

Research by Benner (1984) has attempted to uncover the knowledge embedded in clinical nursing practice by systematic observation and interpretation not only by the researcher but also by clinical nurses themselves (see Chapter 10). In order to understand the study it is necessary to acknowledge that there are differences between practical and theoretical knowledge. She refers to the work of Kuhn (1970) and Polanyi (1958), who observe that *knowing that* and *knowing how* are two different kinds of knowledge, the former being the scientific or theoretical knowledge which is established by identifying the relationships between variables, whereas 'knowing how' is practical knowledge which 'may elude such scientific formulations' (Benner, 1984, p. 2).

Benner (1984) uses the *Drefus model of skill acquisition* to explain the development of the clinician nursing expert. This model outlines five stages of performance – those of novice, advanced beginner, and competent, proficient and expert practitioner. Novices must be given rules for behaviour to guide their performance due to the fact that they have no experience, yet those very rules legitimate against success because the rules do not 'tell them the most relevant task to perform in a given situation' (Benner, 1984, p. 20). For example, a novice nurse may be taking a patient's temperature and fail to observe that the patient's situation is changing rapidly, their skin becoming cold and clammy, their pulse weak and thready and their respiration slow and shallow. Conversely, the expert nurse operates from a deep understanding of a total situation and, taking a holistic view and presumably using a *gestalt*, makes an accurate assessment and intervenes – in this situation giving oxygen and alerting the cardiac team, all within a matter of seconds. Ways in which nurses move from being novices to experts are outlined by Benner (1984), although she is unable to explain in a prescriptive manner the step-by-step process whereby 'knowing how' develops. She suggests that nurses accrue clinical knowledge and lose track of what they have learned, although they recognise that their clinical judgement becomes more refined and acute 'over time'. It is probable that, as individual clinical nurses observe that a certain action works in terms of patient outcome, they begin to incorporate that action into their repertoire. In this way, expertise is developed but not always adequately understood or explained. It is this lack of explanation which often makes 'knowing how' undervalued compared to the scientifically developed 'knowing that' knowledge.

One way of increasing the respectability of clinical nursing knowledge would be to study the relationships between acknowledged expertise and patient outcome. If it could be demonstrated that the experienced expert nurse positively affects patient outcome through the use of skilled nursing, imagine the power of the 'know-how' theory. The fact that one could not fully interpret the 'know-how' would be of secondary importance if the practical knowledge could be found to be cost-effective in terms of patient care. A recent study by the University of York, which examined skill mix and the effectiveness of nursing care, illustrates the value of qualified nurses in practice (Carr-Hill *et al.*, 1992). This study used QUALPACS to assess the quality of nursing care and a range of outcome measures. Both outcomes and quality of care were more highly rated in relation to the seniority and qualifications of individual nurses. This study did not attempt to examine the 'know-how' of nurses, which may have been important in that Benner (1984) warns researchers to remember that some of the richness of 'know-how' theory could be lost by trying to break it down into subsets of knowledge and examine it in a reductionist fashion. Benner (1984) reminds us that nursing is essentially a rich humanistic practice which lends itself to synthesis rather than to analysis. This interpretative approach (see Chapter 6) relies on an understanding of the context of any situation in which particular actions occur. It is demonstrated that, by such interpretation, the concepts and principles underlying practical knowledge can frequently be extrapolated and the expertise which is based on experience can be at least partly explained. Benner (1984) suggests that some nursing actions may, as Chapman (1983) postulates in her category of vertrational actions, be based on systematic sets of ideas which are not yet empirically proven. Benner (1984) has shown that the 'know-how' of clinical nursing can be partly explained. The next stage of research in this area needs to examine the relationships between 'know-how' knowledge and patient outcome. As described, the York skill mix study chose not to examine 'know-how' knowledge in any detail, although other researchers are beginning to focus on these issues, particularly at the Institute of Nursing in Oxford (Titchen and Binnie, 1993).

An experimental research design approach can also be used to identify differences in terms of patient outcome between two nursing structures or processes intended for similar patient care situations. However, it is sometimes difficult from an ethical perspective to deny *control groups* a specific nursing action which is currently accepted practice, in order to compare their outcomes with those of patients who receive the same action (see Chapter 7). Yet when it is believed that a new type of nursing action may be superior to current practice there is rarely an ethical problem, and an 'experimental' process–outcome design can be used. For example, the use of this method by Miller (1985b) demonstrated experimentally that individualised nursing care was more effective in terms of preventing nurse-induced patient dependence in elderly people than was task allocation. Similar approaches have been used in several studies where single variables could be controlled, although the results cannot necessarily be explained in an empirical fashion because of the complexity of human nature (Patel *et al.*, 1985).

Clearly, the case for process–outcome research in practical nursing knowledge development is strong (Benner, 1984; Bloch, 1975), yet until recently little of this kind of work has been undertaken in either general nursing (Goodman, 1989) or psychiatric nursing (Davis, 1981). The reluctance to evaluate currently practised nursing actions may be due to several factors, including lack of finance, education and, perhaps more importantly, the fear of finding out how ineffectual some actions may actually be in terms of patient outcome. In many respects the path of process–outcome research could be bumpy for investigators who need to accept that the results will reveal the weaknesses of nursing actions as well as their strengths. However, the rewards of process–outcome research are likely to outweigh the disadvantages in that by its very nature this kind of research brings clinicians and theorists closer together, which can only help to dispel the current gap between the two groups' philosophies (Miller, 1985b). Similarly, it is through the development of 'know-how' knowledge that nurses may begin not only to understand the complexity of their practice, but also to *enjoy* possessing knowledge which is developed from experience.

Interdependence of nursing clinicians, educators, managers and researchers

The topics of quality assurance and process–outcome research demonstrate the interdependence of the four groups of nurses alluded to (clinicians, educators, managers and researchers). In particular, clinicians require the theory developed by researchers to identify suitable standards of care, while in turn researchers need to develop theory from practice if 'know-how' knowledge is to be understood. Benner's (1984) work has clear implications for nurse education in that she suggests that knowledge is gained from experience and therefore curricula need to reflect this, with sufficient time being allocated to gaining practical experience during training.

The two processes of quality assurance and process–outcome research are symbiotic in that they feed one another in order to enhance practice and produce new theory. Inevitably, therefore, standards of care will need to be adapted as the results of quality assurance programmes are produced and new knowledge is developed. Nurse managers have an essential part to play in ensuring that relevant change in practice is both resourced and implemented when quality assurance programmes demonstrate new ways of enhancing care.

Nurse managers, clinicians and researchers need to work together to help to develop suitable standards for care which are based on sound theory. This may involve altering and adapting recognised quality assurance tools, such as Monitor (Goldstone *et al.*, 1982) and QUALPACS (Wandelt and Stewart, 1975), if new research demonstrates the need to update their validity. The validity of such broad tools must inevitably be questioned when it is recognised that nursing values will vary within different practice settings. For this reason, the recent development of specialist editions of Monitor for psychiatry and paediatrics must be applauded (Goldstone and Doggett, 1990).

Communication between nurse clinicians, managers and researchers needs to be open so that, in addition to researchers informing clinicians and managers about theory development, the latter two groups can commission research to investigate particular problems or questions concerning structure, process and outcome standard-setting as necessary. Figure 1.2 demonstrates how this has been achieved in the Mental Health Unit at West Lambeth Health Authority, London (Watkins, 1989). In this instance, a nurse researcher identified the need for night hospital care for elderly confused people following a process–outcome study of the existing provision of care.

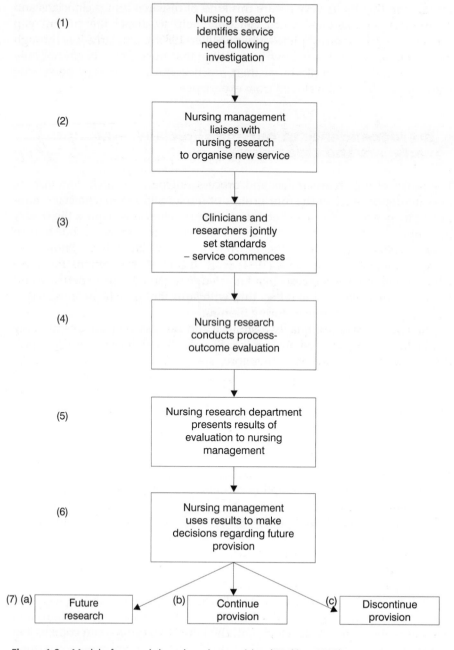

Figure 1.2   Model of research-based service provision (Watkins, 1989)

Nurse management wished to know whether night hospital nursing care would actually work in terms of patient and carer outcome. As a result, a research study was commissioned, with money for the project being provided from both research trust and nursing budgets. Structure and process standards for care were set jointly by the research leader, managers and clinicians, as can be seen in Appendix 1.1. These standards were based on relevant theoretical knowledge and elements of 'know-how' practical expertise.

Patient outcomes were being measured using a *dependency tool* (Morrison, 1983) designed to identify changes in elderly patients' behaviour, and by asking carers to give their opinions of the effectiveness of the service. The results demonstrated the value of the service in terms of carer and patient outcome, so that managers were able to make decisions with regard to future care provision. It is part of the Mental Health Unit's philosophy (see Appendix 1.1) that care provision should be based on clients' perceptions of value, as well as professional opinions, and for this reason the research design was considered to be pertinent.

While it is accepted that nurses from all fields of the profession have to work closely together in order to monitor and improve standards of care through the use and development of knowledge, their paths will sometimes be disparate. This is because nurse managers, practitioners, educators and researchers inevitably have differing motivations for and goals of nursing knowledge.

Knowledge for practice

'All clinical practice should be founded on up-to-date information and research findings; practitioners should be encouraged to identify the needs and opportunities for research presented by their work' (Department of Health, Nursing Division, 1989). This statement, extracted from the recent report entitled, *A Strategy for Nursing*, reinforces the fact that clinical nurses require not only a sound theoretical base from which to practise, but also an understanding of the research process in order to identify areas for future investigation. The same report acknowledges the necessity of setting achievable standards of nursing care based on relevant research findings, as discussed previously. The additional targets state that practising nurses should be accountable for care delivery, encourage primary nursing and use health education. They should also consider the views of consumers, contribute to the work of ethical committees, computerise procedures where possible, be trained in the use of information technology and develop the role of specialist practitioners. These targets, developed by senior members of the profession following extensive consultation with nurses at all levels, embrace quite clearly the objectives for knowledge in the practice area.

All of the goals outlined here involve enhancing patient care through the application of knowledge in practice, which must surely be the ultimate goal of knowledge for practising nurses and all health care professionals (McFarlane, 1977; National Health Service Executive, 1994). What is important is the breadth and depth of knowledge which clinical nurses will be required to have if the strategy for nursing targets is to be achieved. In particular, the level of knowledge required in order to be truly accountable is indicated in the United Kingdom Central Council for Nursing, Midwifery and Health Visiting (1989) paper outlining ethical aspects of professional practice. This paper acknowledges the need for collaboration between all health care workers as well as with patients and their relatives when considering the best method of provision or improvement of services. Therefore, clinical nurses require not only a sound knowledge base from which to practise, but also the skills necessary to communicate research-based findings and 'know-how' knowledge to other professional groups when decisions concerning client care are made within multidisciplinary teams.

The nursing strategy document (Department of Health, Nursing Division, 1989) highlights the need for clinicians to indicate areas of practice which require further investigation, and also encourages the use of *primary nursing*. The advantages of primary nursing have been demonstrated over short periods of time, with both nurses and patients reporting satisfaction with the system (Sellick *et al.*, 1983). It has also been shown to be cost-effective (Marram, 1976), yet this method of care delivery requires great commitment on behalf of the nurse, as it demands close involvement with individual patients (Pearson, 1988), which can be stressful (Menzies, 1960). Further work needs to be undertaken to establish the extent to which primary nursing can be conducted with long-term clients without causing the adverse effects of burn-out in nurses. This kind of research is very time-consuming in that a longitudinal study is the only way of establishing sound results. However, if clinical nurses are to be accountable not only for the care that they deliver but also for their own health promotion, they must be provided with sufficient knowledge from which to decide upon appropriate methods of care delivery for long-term as well as short-term clients. There are several other areas for investigation, but perhaps Bloch (1975) is correct in believing that the most vital work for clinical nurses, in terms of theory development, is to discover the relationships between current nursing actions and patient outcome. Nursing actions in this context could include not only 'nursing processes' but also the 'structural standards' currently employed in terms of staffing, skill mix and the environment of care delivery. The results of structure-outcome and process–outcome evaluation studies should produce useful theory which clinical nurses could then employ in practice.

The literature suggests that clinical nurses need to use theory in order to problem-solve the 'best' way of delivering care, yet it must be recognised that many research findings have not, as yet, been fully incorporated into practice (Miller, 1985a). There is a debate as to whose responsibility this may be. Some suggest that the situation has arisen because nurses do not read and evaluate published research (Wells, 1980), while others imply that it has arisen because nurse researchers fail to explain their findings fully in a clear, concise manner (Hockey, 1987). There is little to be gained from arguing who is really responsible for the problem but much could be gained from finding methods of ensuring that current knowledge is incorporated into practice in addition to developing new practice-based theory.

Knowledge for education

The Committee on Nursing (1972), usually referred to as the Briggs' Report, stated that nurse educationalists should incorporate research findings into their teaching. This seems doubly pertinent today, when it is clear that knowledge is not always used by clinical nurses. If 'education is today's great enabler' (Department of Health, Nursing Division, 1989, p. 23), then nurse education must use knowledge derived from adult education theories to assist nurses in developing the skills of critical thinking, decision-making and the delivery of individualised patient care. This implies that nurse educators must themselves possess those skills at a high level, in addition to teaching skills and a sound academic background (Department of Health, Nursing Division, 1989; United Kingdom Central Council for Nursing, Midwifery and Health Visiting, 1986).

The main objective for knowledge in nurse education is to facilitate the development of able practitioners in all spheres of nursing, at both basic and advanced levels of practice. This is a complex task when one considers that Benner (1984) acknowledges the difficulty of explaining how nurses move through various levels of competency from novice to expert. One way of enhancing nursing education is outlined by Dolan (1984), who believes that the use of a 'preceptor system' and 'clinical judgement seminars' is useful in developing 'know-how' knowledge among both undergraduate and post-graduate student nurses. If nurse educators are to work in this way, there is clearly a need for them to be clinically credible in the area of practice which they teach (Department of Health, Nursing Division, 1989). In other words, they too must be able to apply knowledge in practice.

Theory derived from the social sciences needs to be incorporated into the curriculum (United Kingdom Central Council for Nursing, Midwifery and Health Visiting, 1986) in order to ensure that nurses have a sound theoretical base from which to practise. The increase in time made available within the new Diploma in Nursing programmes (Project 2000) should allow curriculum time to be allocated to these subjects. The ultimate goal for knowledge from a nurse teacher's perspective must be to develop a curriculum which allows both basic and advanced nursing students to become 'knowledgeable doers' who are reflective decision-makers. It may be useful for nurse educators to remember Merlin's adage, in *The Sword in the Stone*, that 'Education is experience and the essence of experience is self-reliance' (White, 1939). Thus curriculum planning should be orientated towards developing self-reliant nurses who enjoy using theory, read research findings and are willing and able to be accountable for care (see Chapter 2).

Knowledge for management

Nurse managers require knowledge derived from the study of leadership, organisations and management if they are to provide *managerial leadership* in addition to the theory necessary for *professional leadership*. The Department of

Health, Nursing Division (1989) details the complex role of today's nurse manager, identifying some nine targets for manpower planning and seven targets for leadership and management. The manpower planning goals indicate the need for nurse managers to conduct skill-mix exercises, to find methods for encouraging practitioners taking a career break to re-enter nursing, and to use systematic methods to ensure that staff appointed to posts have the relevant skills for such jobs. Nurse managers are also expected to 'encourage and enable practitioners to function at their highest level of ability' (Department of Health, Nursing Division, 1989, p.39), and it is suggested that personal appraisal systems should be used to achieve this objective.

It is clear that nurse managers are required to apply managerial theory in practice in order to ensure that appropriate structural standards, in terms of staff, are agreed upon and employed in the clinical area. In addition, they need to be able to conduct *managerial processes* aimed at developing individual nurses and care assistants to their maximum potential (Vaughan and Pillmoor, 1989).

Since its inception, the National Health Service (NHS) has consumed steadily increasing levels of resources, and it now uses approximately 6 per cent of our gross national product (Patel *et al.*, 1985). It is hardly surprising, therefore, that there is an increasing emphasis on resource management and auditing in health care within the system (Department of Health, 1991). Nurse managers require an understanding of and the ability to measure care in terms of both efficiency and effectiveness (Butler and Vaile, 1984), so that the policies, practices and procedures agreed upon within a nursing team meet the objectives of the organisation within which that team operates. The current demographic changes in society will result in a shortage of nursing manpower in the future. Nurse managers need to use information technology to assist nurses in their work, particularly where this can be demonstrated to be cost-effective. For example, computerisation of care plans could save nursing time (Sovie, 1989). There may be other advantages in this approach, e.g. meta-analysis studies of the nursing process outcome revealed that patients who receive research-based nursing interventions can expect significantly better outcomes than those who receive standard nursing care (Heater *et al.*, 1988). If research-based interventions were programmed into a computer, this could aid clinical nurses in their practice, since up-to-date care plans would be available as a response to the identification of patients' problems. Clearly the nurse manager has a vital role both in agreeing research-based standards with staff and in providing the resources in terms of structure to ensure that those standards can be achieved.

The alteration of skill mix and introduction of information technology are just two examples of change which nurse managers may be expected to facilitate. Change is both disturbing and exciting, and often causes emotional responses in those expected to change. The skilled nurse manager will prepare staff for, and assist them in, the process of introducing change for applying relevant change theory (Bailey and Claus, 1975). Change should not be introduced for its own sake, but only if it is believed that it will be innovative in terms of improving performance. Enhancing performance through the use of quality assurance programmes, the application of research and the development of staff are the main tasks of nurse managers (National Health Service Executive, 1993). Their ultimate goal, in terms of the application of knowledge, seems therefore to involve balancing the efficiency and effectiveness of nursing care. As nurses well know, faster throughput does not necessarily mean 'better care'. Alternatively, 'better care' for a few may not be just if others are left to suffer without any access to nursing care. If nurse managers apply knowledge developed from both managerial and professional studies, it may soon be possible to identify the most cost-effective methods of nursing care delivery.

Knowledge for research

This chapter has discussed at some length the advantages of process–outcome research, and has indicated that this may well be the most important work for both researchers and clinicians (Bloch, 1975). However, it is vital to acknowledge that theory must be developed both inductively and deductively (see Chapter 10) if nursing is to develop in an academic sense. The advantages of nursing developing in this way should include both an improvement in patient care through the application of research-based theory (Heater et al., 1988) and an enhancement of the quality of research undertaken (Treece and Treece, 1982). Most theory produced by researchers is questionable and subject to change (McFarlane, 1977), and nurse theorists must explain to those to whom they give research results that theories are generally open to conjecture (Rines and Montag, 1976). It is by explaining the differences between *descriptive* and *explanatory* theory to all nurses in the profession that researchers can help nurses to choose how best to select and apply theory. Descriptive theory looks at a phenomenon and identifies its major elements or events. It involves a basic level of conceptualisation including:

- factor-isolating theories which classify and label; and
- factor-relating theories which depict and relate a single factor to another (Dickoff and James, 1968; Stevens, 1984).

Explanatory theories include situation-relating theory, which is predictive in nature, and situation-producing theories, which have the status of a law or principle (McFarlane, 1977). 'The test of explanatory theory is whether it holds true of a prediction of future interactions of the same constituents in that phenomenon' (Stevens, 1984, p.4).

While researchers should seek to develop explanatory theory wherever possible, this cannot always be achieved in the complex human world of nursing, where each individual is another variable! It is essential that this concept is one that all nurses comprehend in order that it can be accepted that an individual patient may react differently to other patients in response to a certain 'nursing action'. A wide spectrum of research methods, including experimental designs, case studies, action research and surveys, needs to be employed by researchers to ensure that eclectic new theory is developed (Treece and Treece, 1982).

The debate about *qualitative* vs. *quantitative* research approaches continues, and has been well outlined by Leddy and Pepper (1989), who suggest that it is essential for nursing to use both domains (see Chapters 2 and 10). In future, nurse researchers need to remember that there is a danger that nursing research could become too introspective, that much nursing activity is complementary to, and interdependent with, medicine and other relevant disciplines, and that the development of multiprofessional research needs more attention (Goodman, 1989; National Health Service Executive, 1993). Although many nurse theorists are criticised for being removed from practice (Miller, 1985b), this may sometimes be essential. If nursing is to develop and grow, it requires an academic body of nurses who take time out to have ideas and to be imaginative, for it is from the imagination that truly exciting theories are sometimes developed. For example, it is very difficult to believe that at one point we knew absolutely nothing about aeroplanes, insulin and psychoanalysis, yet it was by man's imaginative thought that these things were developed. It is interesting to note that 50 years ago the terms computer, megabyte, nuclear energy, echocardiograph and allograft were unknown. It was due to research that theories concerning these phenomena were developed, and it is vital that nursing encourages and values original thinkers today. It is currently fashionable to criticise Rogers' 'unitary fields of nursing theory', yet one cannot help but wonder whether in 100 years from now we will look back on her new words 'integrality' and 'helicy' (Rogers, 1989), understand their meaning and, more importantly perhaps, realise that the role of the nurse may encompass therapeutic touch and the moving of magnetic fields around a patient's body in order to improve patient health status. It certainly seems essential to acknowledge that visionary thought has its place in nursing and that nurse researchers should be allowed and expected to develop and investigate radical ideas.

Chapman (1989) outlines the aims for nursing research over the next 25 years, and these include the need to maintain high-quality work, use multiple methods, increase replication studies and improve dissemination of results, in addition to increasing the application of theory in practice. These aims are challenging but clearly essential if it is accepted that changes in nursing cannot occur without the use of theories, principles and concepts (Rines and Montag, 1976). Nursing researchers, it seems, have a duty not only to analyse current practice but also to develop new theories which will provide the building blocks for change within the profession.

The value and effectiveness of nursing

The Royal College of Nursing (1992) produced a collection of reflective insights into nursing practice which, it is argued, illustrate the value of skilled nursing practice in certain areas. The introduction to this document states that it is essential that nurses 'demonstrate that they are cost-effective', and that they must be able to show that they 'bring particular skills which make a tangible, measurable difference to the quality of care received by patients' (Royal College of Nursing, 1992, p.1). The document illustrates that, by providing a variety of single case studies which replicate the value of interpersonal work between nurses and patients, the 'artistic' nature of nursing can be validated (Royal College of Nursing, 1992).

It is essential to 'demonstrate the value of nursing in terms of its effect on patients' (Thomas and Bond, 1995, p. 143). The only way to achieve this objective is to develop and apply knowledge both to and from practice. A recent review of the effectiveness of nursing illustrated an increasing number of research projects examining effectiveness, the majority of which have been published during the last 5 years (Thomas and Bond, 1995). The conclusions of this review were that a variety of methods had been used to measure nursing effectiveness with differing types of client, and that in some instances the study designs had not been so rigorous as may have been appropriate. Recommendations for future work included the suggestion that there should be more multicentre studies, rather than small independent studies from particular settings. The use of multicentre studies would, it is argued, improve the extent to which findings could be generalised (Thomas and Bond, 1995). It is vital that multicentred and multiprofessional collaborative studies are developed if health care knowledge is to increase substantially and inform the development of appropriate services (National Health Service Executive, 1993).

Conclusion

The way forward for knowledge in nursing must be both to *value* and to *enjoy* developing and applying theory. There is a need to recognise the vast body of experience and expertise within clinical nursing teams, and to try to identify the relationships within the 'know-how' of nursing (Benner, 1984). In addition, more traditional theory derived from scientific investigation, commonly referred to as 'know-that' knowledge, needs to be both applied and developed. It has been argued that nurse researchers, managers and educators have interdependent roles in developing quality patient care through the use of quality assurance cycles and the study of process–outcome research. This is because nursing is perceived as a practice discipline, and therefore any theory of nursing or theory applied to nursing must be intimately related to practice (McFarlane, 1977).

A theory–practice gap exists, and it is evident that clinicians do not readily use theory in practice. When attempting to disseminate findings, researchers must avoid the Jargon Induced Drivel Syndrome (JIDS) from which many suffer, and write up their results in a manner that is readily understood by most colleagues, if their aim is to encourage others to use the findings in practice (Chapman, 1989; Miller, 1985b). It is vital that nursing knowledge is applied in practice, because research demonstrates that this can positively affect patient outcome (Hayward, 1975; Heater *et al.*, 1988; Miller, 1985b). The ultimate objective for nursing knowledge must therefore be the enhancement of care through the application of knowledge. If nursing is to develop and grow, then new concepts and theories must be produced so that changes can occur (National Health Service Executive, 1993; Rines and Montag, 1976). Researchers must be encouraged not only to investigate present practice, but also to test imaginative ideas in order that the development of new theory is not restrictive in the sense of rejecting originality of thought.

Although nurse managers, researchers, clinicians and educators have a common purpose in improving care through the use of knowledge, the paths that they follow to achieve this end will inevitably differ due to varying motivations. Orem (1985) describes three levels of objectives for care: short-term, intermediate and long-term. It may be useful to conceptualise the long-term goal for nursing knowledge as enhancement of care delivery, with each of the four groups of nurses described having differing short-term and intermediate goals in order to achieve the ultimate goal. The intermediate goals for each group are outlined in Table 1.1.

Table. 1.1   Intermediate goals to achieve long-term goal enhancement of care through application of theory

Education	Enabling basic and advanced nurses to develop the skills of critical thinking, analysis of research, decision-making and the application of theory in practice
Research	To have original thoughts and to test some of these ideas in practice, respond to requests from clinicians to investigate problems, and produce and disseminate theory for application and standard-setting
Management	Provide adequate resources to achieve agreed standards of care and facilitate quality assurance progress, and develop staff to their maximum potential. Conduct manpower-planning exercises to ensure relevant skill mix. Commission research as appropriate. Minimise stress of change through the use of appropriate principles
Clinicians	Apply theory in practice using the skills outlined in education goals, conduct quality assurance cycles and introduce change into practice as appropriate

It is interesting to note that each group has highly complex objectives to achieve, but that they are in fact all interdependent because the ultimate aim is to identify the value of nursing in terms of efficiency and effectiveness through the development and application of knowledge. Indeed Baroness Warnock (1986) wrote that 'if we can't follow knowledge where it leads us, we are unlikely to be able to lead ourselves or others'. It is postulated that if nurses do follow knowledge we will become truly accountable practitioners who work in partnership in care with patients in order to maximise their health status. This could just be enjoyable.

References

American Medical Association 1982 *The American health care system*. Chicago: American Medical Association.

American Nurses' Association 1977 *Guidelines for review of nursing care at the local level*. Kansas City: American Nurses' Association.

Andrews, H. A. and Roy, C. 1986 *Essentials of the Roy adaptation model*. New York: Appleton-Century-Crofts.

Bailey, J. T. and Claus, K. E. 1975 *Decision-making in nursing: tools for change*. St Louis: Mosby.

Barker, W. 1992 Health visiting: action research in a controlled environment. *International Journal of Nursing Studies* **29**, 251–9.

Benner, P. (ed.) 1984 *From novice to expert*. Menlo Park: Addison Wesley.

Bloch, D. 1975 Evaluation of nursing care in terms of process and outcome: issues in research and quality assurance. *Nursing Research* **24**, 256–63.

Bloch, D. 1977 Criteria, standards, norms: crucial terms in quality assurance. *Journal of Nursing Administration* **7**, 20–30.

Bloch, D. 1980 Interrelated issues in evaluation and evaluation research: a researcher's perspective. *Nursing Research* **29**, 69–73.

Butler, J. R. and Vaile, M. S. B. 1984 *Health and health services: an introduction to health care in Britain*. London: Routledge and Kegan Paul.

Carr-Hill, R., Dixon, P., Gibbs, J. *et al.* 1992 *Skill mix and the effectiveness of nursing care*. York: Centre for Health Economics, University of York.

Chapman, C. 1976 The use of sociological theories and models in nursing. *Journal of Advanced Nursing* **1**, 111–27.

Chapman, C. 1989 Research for action: the way forward. *Senior Nurse* **9**, 16–18.

Chapman, G. E. 1983 Ritual and rational action in hospitals. *Journal of Advanced Nursing* **8**, 13–20.

Closs, S. J. and Tierney, A. J. 1993 The complexities of using a structure, process and outcome framework: the case of an evaluation of discharge planning for elderly patients. *Journal of Advanced Nursing* **18**, 1279–87.

Cochrane Library 1997 Cochrane Collaboration database. Oxford: Cochrane Library. (Database available at the time of writing, from the Cochrane Library, PO Box 696, Oxford OX2 7YX.)

Committee on Nursing 1972 *Report*. London: HMSO.

Crow, R. A. 1981 Research and the standards of nursing care: what is the relationship? *Journal of Advanced Nursing* **6**, 491–6.

Curran, E. 1992 A programme to audit the use of urinary catheters. *Journal of Clinical Nursing* **1**, 329–34.

Davis, B. D. 1981 The training and assessment of social skills in nursing: the patient profile interview. *Nursing Times* **77**, 649–51.

Department of Health, Nursing Division 1989 *A strategy for nursing: a report of the steering committee*. London: Department of Health.

Department of Health 1991 *Framework of audit for nursing services*. London: NHS Management Executive.

Dickoff, J. and James, P. 1968 A theory of theories: a position paper. *Nursing Research* **17**, 197–203.

Dolan, K. 1984 Building bridges between education and practice. In Benner, P. (ed.), *From novice to expert*. Menlo Park: Addison Wesley, 275–84.

Donabedian, A. 1966 Evaluating the quality of medical care. *Millbank Memorial Fund Quarterly* **44**, 166–206.

Goldstone, L. A. and Doggett, D. P. 1990 *Psychiatric nursing monitor: an audit of the quality of nursing care in psychiatric wards.* Loughton: Gale Centre Publications.

Goldstone, L., Ball, J. A. and Collier, M. 1982 *Monitor: an index of the quality of nursing care for acute medical and surgical wards.* Newcastle upon Tyne: Newcastle Polytechnic Products.

Goodman, C. 1989 Nursing research: growth and development. In Jolley, M. and Allan, P. (eds), *Current issues in nursing.* London: Chapman and Hall, 95–114.

Hayward, J. 1975 *Information: a prescription against pain.* London: Royal College of Nursing.

Heater, B. S., Becker, A. M. and Olson, R. K. 1988 Nursing interventions and patient outcomes: a meta-analysis of studies. *Nursing Research* **37**, 303–7.

Henderson, V. 1969 *Basic principles of nursing care.* Basel: Karger.

Henney, C. R. 1984 The use of computers for improvement and measurement of nursing care. In Willis, L. D. and Linwood, M. E. (eds), *Measuring the quality of care.* Recent Advances in Nursing 10. Edinburgh: Churchill Livingstone, 171–91.

Hilgard, E. R., Atkinson, R. C. and Atkinson, R. L. 1975 *Introduction to psychology,* 6th edn. New York: Harcourt-Brace-Jovanovich.

Hockey, L. 1979 Collaborative research and its implementation in nursing. In European Nurse Researchers, (ed.), *Collaborative research and its implementation in nursing: First Conference of the European Nurse Researchers.* Utrecht: National Hospital Institute, 83–94.

Hockey, L. 1987 Issues in the communication of nursing research. In Hockey, L. (ed.), *Current issues.* Recent Advances in Nursing 18. Edinburgh: Churchill Livingstone, 154–67.

Jacox, A. 1974 Theory construction in nursing: an overview. *Nursing Research* **23**, 4–13.

King, I. M. 1981 *A theory for nursing: systems, concepts, process.* New York: Wiley.

Kitson, A. L. (ed.) 1993 *Nursing: art and science.* London: Chapman and Hall.

Kitson, A. L., Hyndman, S., Harvey, G. and Yerrell, P. 1990 *Quality patient care: the dynamic standard setting system.* London: Scutari Press.

Kuhn, T. S. 1970 *The structure of scientific revolutions.* Chicago: University of Chicago Press.

Lang, N. M. and Clinton, J. F. 1984 Quality assurance: the idea and its development in the United States. In Willis, L. and Linwood, M. E. (eds), *Measuring the quality of care.* Recent Advances in Nursing 10. Edinburgh: Churchill Livingstone, 69–88.

Leddy, S. and Pepper, J. M. 1989 *Conceptual bases of professional nursing,* 2nd edn. Philadelphia: Lippincott.

Longman (ed.) 1984 *Dictionary of the English language.* London: Longman.

McFarlane, J. D. 1977 Developing a theory of nursing: the relation of theory to practice, education and research. *Journal of Advanced Nursing* **2**, 261–70.

Marram, G. 1976 The comparative costs of operating a team and primary nursing unit. *Journal of Nursing Administration* **6**, 21–4.

Menzies, I. E. P. 1960 A case study in the functioning of social systems as a defence against anxiety. *Human Relationships* **13**, 95–121.

Miller, A. 1985a The relationship between nursing theory and nursing practice. *Journal of Advanced Nursing* **10**, 417–24.

Miller, A. 1985b Nurse/patient dependency: is it iatrogenic? *Journal of Advanced Nursing* **10**, 63–9.

Morrison, D. P. 1983 The Crichton visual analogue scale for the assessment of behaviour in the elderly. *Acta Psychiatrica Scandinavica* **68**, 408–13.

National Health Service Executive 1993 *A vision for the future: the nursing, midwifery and health visiting contribution to care and health care.* London: Department of Health.

National Health Service Executive 1994 *Research and development in the new NHS: functions and responsibilities.* Leeds: NHS Executive.

Nightingale, F. 1859 *Notes on nursing.* London: Harrison.

Norton, D., McLaren, R. and Exton-Smith, A. N. 1975 *An investigation of geriatric nursing problems in hospital.* Edinburgh: Churchill Livingstone.

Orem, D. E. 1985 *Nursing: concepts of practice,* 3rd edn. New York: McGraw Hill.

Patel, X. S., St. Ledger, A. S. and Schnieden, H. 1985 Process and outcome in the National Health Service. *British Medical Journal* **291**,1365–6.

Pearson, A. (ed.) 1988 *Primary nursing.* London: Croom Helm.

Peplau, H. E. 1952 *Interpersonal relations in nursing.* New York: Putnam.

Polanyi, M. 1958 *Personal knowledge.* London: Routledge and Kegan Paul.

Pursey, A. 1996 Sociological methods: health services and nursing research. In Perry, A. (ed.), *Sociology: insights in health care.* London: Edward Arnold, 83–106.

Rines, A. B. and Montag, M. L. 1976 *Nursing concepts and nursing care.* New York: Wiley.

Rogers, M. E. 1983 *Nursing science: a science of unitary human beings.* Unpublished student handout.

Rogers, M. E. 1989 Nursing: a science of unitary human beings. In Riehl-Sisca, J. (ed.), *Conceptual models for nursing practice,* 3rd edn. Englewood Cliffs: Appleton and Lange, 181–8.

Roper, N., Logan, W. W. and Tierney, A. J. 1980 *The elements of nursing.* Edinburgh: Churchill Livingstone.

Roy, C. 1984 *Introduction to nursing: an adaptation model,* 2nd edn. Englewood Cliffs: Prentice Hall.

Royal College of Nursing 1992 *The value of nursing.* London: Royal College of Nursing.

Sellick, K. J., Russell, S. and Beckmann, J. L. 1983 Primary nursing: an evaluation of its effects on patient perception of care and staff satisfaction. *International Journal of Nursing Studies* **20**, 265–73.

Smith-Marker, C. G. 1988 *Setting standards for professional nursing: the Marker model.* Baltimore, MD: Resource Applications.

Sovie, M. D. 1989 Clinical nursing practices and patient outcomes: evaluation, evolution and revolution. *Nursing Economics* **7**, 79–85.

Statutory Instrument 1983 *The nurses', midwives' and health visitors' rules approval order.* London: HMSO.

Stevens, B. J. 1984 *Nursing theory: analysis, application, evaluation,* 2nd edn. St Louis: Mosby.

Thomas, L. H. and Bond, S. 1995 The effectiveness of nursing: a review. *Journal of Clinical Nursing* **4**, 143–52.

Titchen, A. and Binnie, A. 1993 Changing power relationships between nurses: a case study of early changes towards patient-centred learning. *Journal of Clinical Nursing* **2**, 219–30.

Treece, E. W. and Treece, J. W. 1982 *Elements of research in nursing,* 3rd edn. St Louis: Mosby.

United Kingdom Central Council for Nursing, Midwifery and Health Visiting (UKCC) 1986 *Project 2000: a new preparation for practice.* London: UKCC.

United Kingdom Central Council for Nursing, Midwifery and Health Visiting (UKCC) 1989 *Exercising accountability: a framework to assist nurses, midwives and health visitors to consider ethical aspects of professional practice: a UKCC advisory document.* London: UKCC.

United Kingdom Central Council for Nursing, Midwifery and Health Visiting (UKCC) 1992 *Code of professional conduct for the nurse, midwife and health visitor,* 3rd edn. London: UKCC.

Van Maanen, H. M. 1984 Evaluation of nursing care: quality of nursing evaluated within the context of health care and examined from a multinational perspective. In Willis, L. D. and Linwood, M. E. (eds), *Measuring the quality of care.* Recent Advances in Nursing 10. Edinburgh: Churchill Livingstone, 3–42.

Vaughan, B. and Pillmoor, M. (eds) 1989 *Managing nursing work.* London: Scutari Press.

Wandelt, M. and Stewart, D. 1975 *Slater nursing competencies rating scale.* New York: Appleton-Century-Crofts.

Warnock, M. 1986 Why it is unthinkable to drop philosophy. *Daily Telegraph,* 15 July, p.20 (letters page).

Watkins, M. 1987 In- and day-patient care for elderly people. Unpublished MN thesis, University of Wales, Cardiff.

Watkins, M. 1988 Lifting the burden. *Geriatric Nursing and Home Care* **8**, 18–20.

Watkins, M. 1989 *Operational policy: night hospital elderly care.* Unpublished paper. London: West Lambeth Health Authority (Mental Health Unit).

Wells, J. C. A. 1980 *Nursing: a profession that dislikes innovation: an investigation of the reasons why.* Unpublished MA Thesis, Department of Government, Brunel University, Brunel.

White, T. H. 1939 *The sword in the stone.* London: Collins.

Wright, D. 1984 An introduction to the evaluation of nursing care: a review of the literature. *Journal of Advanced Nursing* **9**, 457–67.

Wright, S. G. 1990 *Building and using a model of nursing.* London: Edward Arnold.

Zarit, S. H., Orr, N. K. and Zarit, S. M. 1985 *The hidden victims of Alzheimer's disease: families under stress.* New York: New York University Press.

Appendix 1.1

Operational Policy – Night Hospital Elderly Care: West Lambeth Health Authority (London), Mental Health Unit (Watkins, 1989)

1. Background

Nurses involved in caring for elderly people are looking towards the future and trying to provide facilities which meet the needs of the community that they serve.

This innovative service aims to offer nursing support for elderly people at night on weekdays, from Monday to Thursday. It is envisaged that the users will be individuals who have difficulty sleeping at night, and who may be noisy and disrupt their carer's sleep. At present, these people are frequently admitted to in-patient care to give carers relief, rather than for the purpose of formal intervention. It is hoped that the Night Hospital will provide sufficient relief to carers without warranting full admission.

Sitting services for elderly confused people have been shown to be effective, in particular for those who are too frail to travel. However, a sitter service does have the dual disadvantages of a stranger going into the home for long periods, denying the carers privacy, and in small homes the noisy confused individual may continue to disrupt carers' sleep. The Night Hospital's service may, therefore, in many instances have advantages over a sitter service.

2. Aims

2.1 To provide, as part of the comprehensive community-orientated mental health services, support for elderly mentally confused people and their families at night.

2.2 To provide relief for relatives who are caring for elderly mentally infirm people at home. The Night Hospital will give relatives the opportunity to have a night free, allowing them to rest or socialise undisturbed.

2.3 To provide individualised programmes of care for each client at night, which are orientated towards facilitating the client's independence and dignity.

2.4 To provide a service which supports informal carers by working in partnership with them to deliver quality care to clients.

3. Philosophy of the service

3.1 That clients should be able to remain in their own homes for as long as possible and be cared for by relatives and friends, who are in turn supported by the statutory health services.

3.2 Where a sitter service would be deemed more appropriate, due to a client's frailty, the Night Hospital staff will arrange appropriate referrals to voluntary and statutory agencies.

3.3 The service will be developed around the individual needs of clients and their families. Each client will have an individualised treatment programme using a nursing intervention approach, the key objective of the service being to meet clients' needs.

Nursing staff will be committed to taking a truly realistic approach to clients' needs, and will be aware of the contribution that both statutory and voluntary services can make to their clients' health.

3.4 Clients will receive care and treatment in the least restrictive setting, with as much freedom as possible.

3.5 Clients will have the right to personal privacy.

3.6 Clients will have the right to be treated with courtesy and respect at all times, and to be addressed as they choose.

4. Referral procedure

4.1 The service will be open to all residents of _ _ _ _ _ _ _ _ _ _ .

4.2 An open referral procedure will be adopted. Referral will be accepted from:

- patients' relatives;
- community nursing staff;
- hospital nursing staff;
- community physicians – general practitioners;
- consultant psychiatrists;
- social services;
- voluntary services.

4.3 A formal system of assessment will be used to find out which professionals or volunteers are also involved, so that liaison can take place.

4.4 Each referred client will be visited at home by a member of the team in order to assess his or her suitability for attendance. Assessment will normally be conducted in conjunction with other members of the community multidisciplinary team.

4.5 In emergency situations, clients may attend the Night Hospital prior to liaison with other members of the health care team involved in their care, although consultation should take place as soon as possible.

4.6 Referrals will only be accepted from the Day Hospital on the basis of attendance at the Night Hospital being an alternative, i.e. not in addition to attendance during the day.

4.7 Referrals should normally be made in writing and addressed to the Charge Nurse.

4.8 The Community Psychiatric Nursing Department Secretary will receive referrals during the day.

5. Attendance periods

5.1 The service will run for four nights a week, from Monday to Thursday inclusive.

5.2 The hospital will cater for a maximum of 15 clients per night, giving a maximum of 60 places per week.

5.3 Clients will be collected by sitting ambulance with a nurse escort between 8.00p.m. and 9.00p.m. They will be returned home the following day between 8.00a.m. and 9.30a.m.

5.4 Clients may be delivered to the Hospital between 8.00p.m. and 9.00p.m. and collected by 9.30a.m. by relatives or friends.

5.5 Clients will attend for a minimum of one night a week and a maximum of four nights a week.

5.6 Each client's progress will be reviewed on a regular basis. Where the prime aim of attendance is respite care, a thorough reassessment after 3 months of attendance will be made in conjunction with the multidisciplinary team and relatives.

6. Programme

6.1 Individual assessments will be completed after four nights of attendance using a stress management/activities of living model of nursing.

6.2 Individual programmes will be drawn up based on clients' assessment. Most programmes will incorporate at least one of the following aims:

- facilitating independence through social activities;
- promoting continence;
- reducing nocturnal restlessness and promoting sleep;
- providing respite care for the carer.

6.3 Individual programmes will be reviewed with the following minimum frequencies:

- at 2-week intervals for programmes aimed at promoting continence;
- at 4-week intervals for programmes aimed at facilitating independence through social activity and/or reducing nocturnal restlessness and promoting sleep;
- at 4-week intervals for programmes aimed at providing respite care. Where the aim is largely orientated towards the carer, attendance will not normally exceed 3 months.

6.4 Light entertainment will be provided for clients, e.g. use of video facilities, television, games and reading material. A hot drink and a light snack will be provided before 11.00p.m.

Hot drinks and snacks will be available throughout the night.

6.5 Between 11.00p.m. and midnight, depending on individual programmes, clients will either be encouraged to prepare for sleep or involved in appropriate activities.

6.6 Most clients will be woken at 7.00a.m. to promote regular sleeping patterns and to ensure that the clients are returned home in time for the hospital to accept day patients. When deemed necessary for an individual, a client will be allowed to sleep on until 8.00a.m. If clients can be collected by a relative or friend, they may be left to sleep until 9.30a.m.

6.7 A light breakfast will be prepared and served by nursing staff for clients in the morning.

7. Managerial organisation

The Community Nursing Manager (Mental Health Unit) will be managerially responsible for the Unit.

8. Staffing

The service will be run by nursing staff consisting of the following:
- one full-time C/N;
- two full-time S/Ns;
- two full-time SENs;
- two part-time qualified nurses;
- one helper.

9. Medical supervision

9.1 Medical supervision will be carried out by the consultant psychogeriatrician.

9.2 Clients will be asked to visit their general practitioner for non-emergency medical care.

9.3 Clients will be referred for psychological medical assessment to the consultant psychiatrist (Elderly Mental Health) from the service when appropriate.

10. Admission and discharge

This will be the responsibility of the clinical nursing team.

11. Evaluation of the Night Hospital

11.1 A part-time project evaluator has been appointed for a 2-year period.

11.2 A comprehensive evaluation of the service will be conducted and a report of the findings presented to the Health Authority in Spring 1991.

11.3 Interim reports will be presented to the project team at 6-monthly intervals.

11.4 The evaluator will receive research supervision from the Department of Nursing, Institute of Psychiatry.

11.5 The evaluator is responsible to the Director of Nursing Services, Mental Health Unit.

Stress management/activities of living model

Although a trained nurse can rapidly assess a patient's nursing requirements using an activities of living model of nursing, to do this without consulting the caregiver would be insensitive and irresponsible.

One method of identifying priority problems for the family unit and planning support for informal caregivers is the dementia stress management model (Zarit *et al.*, 1985).

The dementia stress management model

This is a two-stage model that aims to minimise stress for the caregiver:

- stage 1 – information-giving;
- stage 2 – problem-solving.

In Stage 1 the nurse gives carers information about the patient's disease and the availability of resources to support them.

With regard to Stage 2, the problem-solving cycle can be subdivided into a series of steps and used to help resolve problems caused by a person with Alzheimer's disease in any family unit (see Figure 1.1A).

PATIENT-ORIENTATED NEEDS IDENTIFICATION USING AN ACTIVITIES OF LIVING MODEL

The activities of living model can be used by the nurse and carer to assess each patient's ability to carry out their activities of living, and patients' actual problems are defined in the following categories:

- maintaining a safe environment, including memory and orientation;
- communicating;
- breathing;
- eating and drinking;
- eliminating;
- personal cleansing and dressing;
- controlling body temperature;
- mobilising;
- working and playing;
- expressing sexuality;
- sleeping;
- dying;
- memorising;
- perceiving (Watkins, 1987; after Roper *et al.*, 1980).

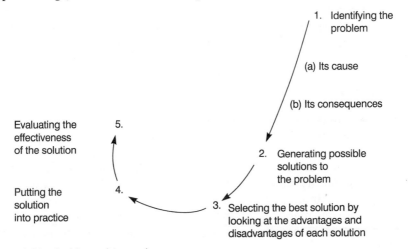

Figure 1.1A   Problem-solving cycle

Carers can be helped to express which patient behaviours cause them most distress. The majority of caregivers report finding certain problems more difficult to cope with than others. For example, most carers can tolerate a patient's inability to dress and to walk unaided, but 60 per cent of carers find it difficult to cope with inappropriate urination and verbal abuse from the sick person.

AIMS OF NURSING/SELECTION OF SOLUTION

Having identified the clients' problems, care can then be organised, with the aim of nursing being:

- to maintain or increase the patient's independence, while ensuring patient comfort; and
- to reduce carers' stress.

It is important that both the nurse and the carer are involved in the selection of a solution, as the carer will frequently be involved in its implementation, e.g. in the case of a continence promotion programme.

IMPLEMENTATION

The selected solution is then implemented by the nurse in the Night Hospital, and in some cases concurrently at home by the carer.

EVALUATION

Finally, the nurse and caregiver evaluate the outcome of the chosen solution. If the strategy is successful, it should be continued; if not, the problem-solving cycle is recommended.

Nursing standards

1. All nurses working in the Night Hospital are aware of the standards of nursing care, have read them, and have been given their own copies of the standards.

ASSESSMENT

2. Each client referred to our service is visited at home, by a member of the nursing team, in order to assess his or her suitability for attendance prior to admission.
3. The assessment is normally conducted in conjunction with all members of the community multidisciplinary team involved in the care of the client. Where immediate admission is deemed to be necessary, and liaison with all members of the multidisciplinary team has not been possible prior to admission, liaison takes place as soon as possible thereafter.

4. Each client is asked during the assessment how he or she wishes to be addressed. If he or she is unable to make his or her wishes known, his or her carer is asked. The name decided upon is recorded and adhered to.

PRIMARY NURSING

5. Each client has a primary nurse who is responsible together with associate nurses, for planning and delivery of his or her care.
6. The primary or associate nurse, who is responsible for the delivery of care to an individual, introduces herself to that client at the beginning of her span of duty, and at intervals throughout.
7. In the absence of the primary and associate nurses for an individual client, any nurse may attend to any client. This applies for a whole span of duty, for part of a span of duty, e.g. during a meal break, or simply when the client's own nurse is occupied with another client.

CARE PLANNING

8. Each client has his or her own individualised care plan which must be in operation by his or her fourth night of attendance at the latest.
9. Individual assessments are completed using a stress management/activities of living model of nursing, in co-operation with the clients' carers.
10. Clear goals are known and recorded on the care plan for each client.
11. Each individualised care plan is evaluated at least once every 4 weeks, or by the eighth night of attendance, whichever occurs sooner. Evaluations are made in consultation with carers.

MANAGEMENT OF INCONTINENCE

12. Incontinence is not regarded as the inevitable consequence of ageing.
13. If the general practitioner has not already investigated the causes of incontinence, such an investigation is requested prior to admission, or as soon as possible after admission.
14. Appropriate medical treatment for problems related to incontinence is given when prescribed, in conjunction with the carer.
15. When medical treatment is not prescribed, or has been completed, and incontinence persists, this is treated by nursing measures.
16. Each client has his or her incontinence needs assessed during care planning, and appropriate nursing measures are prescribed by his or her primary nurse.
17. All clients who are incontinent have clear nursing orders in their care plans for the treatment and/or management of this problem.

PREVENTION OF PRESSURE SORES

18. On admission, every client is assessed on the Norton Scale for susceptibility to pressure sores.

19. Reassessment on the Norton Scale takes place every time the care plan is evaluated, and at the onset of physical illness, and at any time when the client's health is considered to have deteriorated.
20. Every at-risk client has an individualised care plan for the prevention of pressure sores.
21. Pressure-relieving aids are always available, and are used on all at-risk clients who are assessed as being in need of them by their primary nurses.

PERSONAL HYGIENE

22. The personal hygiene needs of each client are discussed with both the client and the carer prior to admission.
23. Whenever possible, the client looks after his or her own personal hygiene needs with minimal help from nursing staff.
24. All clients are bathed at least once a week while in the Night Hospital, unless the client and his or her carer prefer to make their own arrangements.
25. Each client decides when and how he or she is bathed.
26. Each client who is incapable of looking after his or her own personal hygiene needs to be washed thoroughly or bathed every morning unless he or she refuses.
27. Carers are always informed if clients refuse to be washed.

FREEDOM OF MOVEMENT

28. Clients are allowed to decide when they wish to go to bed, and are never awoken before 7.00a.m.
29. When it is impossible to persuade a client to go to bed, he or she is allowed to spend the night reclining in a chair. Blankets and pillows are provided for warmth and comfort.

REALITY ORIENTATION

30. 24-hour reality orientation is practised. All staff understand the full implications of reality orientation and participate in its practice.
31. Formal sessions of reality orientation and reminiscence therapy are available for any patient requiring them, but no one is forced to participate.

GENERAL

32. Every effort is made to maintain the dignity and privacy of each client in our care.
33. The cultural and religious needs of all clients are monitored and planned for.
34. Diversional therapy is available for any patient who requires it, but no one is compelled to participate.

Acknowledgements are due to the Mental Health Team, West Lambeth Health Authority, London.

Research – what it is and what it is not

2

E. Jane Chapman

Introduction

This chapter will introduce the reader to the function and potential of research in nursing. It will address some of the fundamental questions raised by those new to the subject. In a single chapter it is obviously impossible to provide a comprehensive overview of the topic, but it is hoped that many of the major issues will be addressed and discussed and that further investigation of the topic will be stimulated.

The chapter is divided into sections, each of which will address one of the following questions:

- the place of nursing research – why bother with the subject?
- what is nursing research? – definitions and parameters;
- what it is not – limitations of research;
- applications and implementation – how can research findings be used in practice?
- the art and value of critique – is this a skill worth developing?

A short summary reflects on the main themes of the chapter and reviews some of the broad issues facing nurses when considering nursing research.

The place of nursing research (or why bother with the subject?)

Hunt (1981) identified that nurses are becoming increasingly conscious of the need to be able to demonstrate a rational basis for the care that they give. In recent years, increasing pressure on qualified staff to pay more than lip service to the concept of accountability for practice has further fuelled this need.

This chapter will explore the relationship between research and nursing practice and demonstrate that sympathy and understanding for the former can provide the basis for identifying the rationale for, and lead to improvements in, the latter. In common with many others in this book, this chapter will make use of Henderson's (1969) definition of nursing:

> In a broad sense nursing care is derived from what has been called the unique function of the nurse ... to assist the individual, sick or well, in the performance of those activities contributing to health or its recovery (or to a peaceful death) that he would perform unaided if he had the necessary strength, will or knowledge. And to do this in such a way as to help him to gain independence as rapidly as possible. This aspect of her work, this part of her function she initiates and controls; of this she is master.
>
> (Henderson, 1969, p.4)

Assisting patients to achieve goals is accomplished by a variety of nursing care actions – some relatively routine and others requiring specific individualised planning based on information available and the use of professional judgement. How does a nurse determine which are the appropriate nursing actions to undertake for the benefit of the patient?

Tradition and custom dictate much of what nurses do. For we know it to be true that nursing develops by role modelling, being handed down, usually going unchallenged because we have always done it that way (see Chapter 1). In this situation the applicability or usefulness of the action is not generally questioned. The taking of temperatures 4-hourly, or the starving of patients from midnight for operation during the morning session, which may be at any time from seven in the morning to twelve midday, are examples of such practice (see Chapter 6). This source of decision-making is often coupled with authority, either from the Ward Sister, for example 'Sister likes us to use this particular treatment for wounds', 'Sister likes the beds made in this way', or from higher up the management structure through policies and procedures, such as medicine administration policies and catheterisation routines. In these cases, because someone else has made the decision on the course of action to take, there is perhaps no need to understand, or even explore, the rationale for the practice.

Trial and error can also be the source of decision-making for practice. When faced with an unfamiliar situation, the care delivered can often be the result of trial and error, which is generally unsystematic and haphazard, but may be successful in solving individual problems. By working through a random scheme of trying method (a), then (b) and then (c), and so on, the 'right' treatment might eventually be found, or the patient may recover despite the treatment offered. This is analogous to trying to find a way to stop a baby crying in the middle of the night by adopting a succession of different strategies such as rocking, feeding, ignoring, and so on. When success is achieved the situation is not generally analysed and lessons learned for next time; the triumphant person tends just to creep away relieved. The consequence of this route of decision-making is that whilst success may ultimately be achieved, the reason why (the rationale) is obscure, and therefore one is not in a position to be able to predict with confidence whether the same method would work again in the future (see Chapter 1).

It must be said that in certain situations both of these decision-making pathways are acceptable. However, research as an aid for decision-making offers certain features not to be found in these other methods. Research, when properly conducted, can provide unbiased, objective evidence on which to base a decision. It can supply a description of the 'reality' of the current situation, for example, rather than a 'rose-tinted' picture of what is thought to be happening. It can provide predictive information in which an analysis of past events can be used to predict accurately future trends such as recruitment and retention issues, outbreak of certain infectious diseases, or uptake of further education courses. Research can provide objective evaluation of two methods of treatment, or choices of nursing action, and this evidence can be used to make a professional judgement in the clinical situation. Thus tradition, custom, authority and trial and error can be superseded by the delivery of nursing care based on sound scientific evidence of its efficacy.

To illustrate the contribution that research has to make to nursing, three situations will be described.

Research can provide scientifically defensible reasons for nursing actions. Perhaps it is not possible to provide a firm theoretical basis for all nursing actions. However, many clinical practices have now been examined under research conditions and effective, and efficient, courses of action have been scientifically identified. For example, research conducted by Norton et al. (1975), Barton and Barton (1981) and others has determined appropriate action to be taken if pressure sores are to be avoided (regular relief of pressure, the use of pressure-reducing beds and mattresses, and so on). Hayward (1975) and Boore (1978) have conducted widely accepted research which demonstrates that the provision of pre-operative information is a beneficial aid to post-operative recovery.

Research can increase the cost-effectiveness of nursing activities. Nurses, in common with other health care professionals, are being put under ever increasing pressure to provide a value-for-money service, whilst at the same time having to make cuts in the service to constantly strive to keep within target spending levels. With the advent of ward accounting and the responsibility for ward budgets being increasingly invested in the ward sister, research has an important role to play in the provision of sound evidence to help to guide the most prudent use of available funds. Reliance on systematically collected research findings can, where available, save wards and departments considerable amounts of money by reducing poor 'trial and error' spending. In management circles it is often argued that, at times of economic constraints, research is a luxury which cannot be financially supported. The author would argue that it is at these times that research is most valuable. A simple survey of bath additives conducted by Sleep and Grant (1988) clearly demonstrates the savings that can result from the implementation of research findings. Sleep and Grant conducted an experimental study of bath additives used by postnatal mothers for the first 10 days post delivery. Each of the 1800 mothers in the sample was assigned to one of three groups: one group added salt to the bath water, another added Savlon solution, and the third group did not use any bath additive. The results indicated that all three groups found the baths soothing and helpful in reducing discomfort, but the midwives concerned reported no significant differences in the rates of healing or the incidence of any complications such as infection. Based on the results of this study, Health Authorities and individuals can save considerable amounts of money by following a policy of not using any bath additives for this client group. Romney (1982) conducted a similar trial, also focusing on maternity patients. She conducted an experiment to examine the rates of infection amongst groups of women who were shaved pre-delivery and groups who were not. As with Sleep and Grant's (1988) study, no differences were evident between the outcome measure examined, i.e. the rates of infection in the two groups. The study provided a sound scientific basis for not performing pre-delivery shaves. Nursing time and unnecessary expenditure on razors were saved, to say nothing of the increased satisfaction experienced by the future mothers.

Whilst this chapter draws most of its examples from nursing practice research, it is important to outline the potential contribution that research has to make to other areas, e.g. education and management. In the field of nursing education, research studies can provide teachers with research-based evidence on which to select and monitor different teaching strategies and methods. For example, Jacka and Lewin (1987) undertook a study to investigate the nature of the learning that occurred in the classroom and that which occurred in the clinical setting. The study also developed ways of measuring the levels of instruction opportunity and integration within the students' training. Knowledge of nursing practice research can equip the teacher with the ability to teach from a research basis which in turn will provide the student with the 'how' and the 'why' of nursing practice and procedures. Davis (1987) has edited a very useful introductory book which examines a range of research projects and developments currently applicable to nurse education.

Research endeavour is often seen to be in conflict with management endeavour. The main reason for this is a result of the different time perspectives which are commonly adopted by the two groups. The cliche 'management want an answer yesterday' could be coupled with one for researchers – 'researchers can only think in terms of having results in 3–5 years' time'. There is more than a grain of truth in this. Managers, by the very nature of their position, need to resolve current problems immediately. Researchers, on the other hand, by following the scientific rigour of the research process, have to allow themselves time to examine problems in depth. In fact, managers and researchers need to develop an interactive relationship. If managers use researchers to examine certain of their problems, it may be possible for some future problems to be avoided. For example, in the area of recruitment and retention of staff the manager must concern him or herself with ensuring that sufficient nurses are in post to provide a full range of services, but may be faced with different patterns of employment in different areas of the hospital. A researcher could take an objective look at the situation, conduct interviews with staff, follow up people who leave or fail to take up employment when offered it, and investigate any causal relationships which seem to be apparent, thus providing the manager with evidence on which to base further strategies. The researcher needs the manager to generate the research questions worthy of investigation, whilst the manager needs someone to take a look at the overall situation, whilst he or she provides the day-to-day management, and then produces the evidence (or answers) to overcome the problems.

This section has shown that nursing and research should have an interactive relationship. Nursing cannot develop without research to provide scientific knowledge on which to base practice (and education and management), and by the same token research cannot develop without nursing practice to generate the questions which warrant investigation and to implement or utilise the results. The nature of this relationship is summarised in Figure 2.1.

The following section focuses on how research can fulfil this role.

What research is – definitions and parameters

Research means different things to different people. To some it is a way of life – it is an attitude to problem-solving (by being research-minded) which can be applied to almost every area of professional and indeed non-professional problems. In essence, being research-minded means that the individual develops the following attributes:

- an enquiring attitude of mind;
- a logical approach to problems;
- an awareness of the existence of research reports;
- a willingness and ability to read, evaluate, select and make use of research findings.

To others research is an activity pursued by academic nurses in ivory towers remote from reality. No researcher, to my knowledge, has anything approaching an ivory tower; the lucky few may find a quiet corner, possibly a desk and, for the really fortunate ones, possibly a part share in a computer. Practitioners often describe researchers as people who provide complicated pieces of information illustrated by incomprehensible tables and graphs and

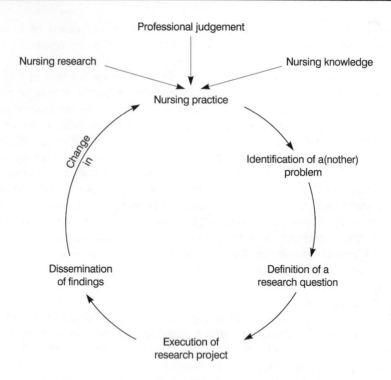

Figure 2.1 Interrelationship between nursing practice and nursing research

littered with unintelligible statistical tests, few of which seem directly trans-latable to practice, but may be used by management or other such groups, and are of no use to themselves.

This section will seek to demonstrate that research is not separate from nursing, but something which must form an integral part of every nurse's professional life. In many situations research is the most appropriate way to solve problems. Research can be defined as:

> an attempt to increase the body of knowledge (i.e. what is currently known about nursing) by discovery of new facts and relationships through a process of systematic scientific enquiry.
>
> (MacLeod Clark and Hockey, 1979, p.3)

This definition specifies a *process* and, in essence, this is what research is; it offers a method (the research process) of problem-solving which has many characteristics to commend it over other problem-solving methods. It is sci-entific, systematic and objective. In the previous section other sources of nursing knowledge were discussed, including tradition, custom, authority, and trial-and-error learning. One way of beginning to understand the value of research is to examine the qualities of research as a basis for problem-solv-ing and decision-making compared to these other sources of knowledge.

Research can provide evidence on which to base selection of appropriate treatment/course of action, whereas tradition and trial and error can, at best, provide experience. Research can provide information to explain why a method, a treatment or a course of action actually works (research-based rationales). Tradition and trial and error are not generally concerned with rationales. If rationales are provided they tend to be subjective and judgemental rather than objective and scientific. Research, through the use of inferential statistics, can provide parameters as to how far the available evidence may be confidently generalised to a wider population. Experiential evidence cannot, with the same reliability, be used in this way.

How does a researcher set out to discover this evidence or nursing knowledge? Research always starts with a question. Of this rather obvious point Lancaster (1975, p.7) said that research 'needs people who ask questions, who have "hunches", who want to find a better way of doing things, who refuse to be put off by platitudinous replies to their questions. Without such people research would never get started.' A topic for research may come from practical experience, from reading, through discussion with colleagues, or just as a 'flash of inspiration'. Whatever the source of the problem, the same series of steps must be systematically followed if reliable and objective scientific evidence concerning the problem is to be revealed. These steps, referred to as the research process, are listed below.

1. The topic of study is identified and the research question posed.
2. A search of relevant literature is undertaken.
3. The research question is refined (and, if appropriate, a hypothesis is formulated).
4. The investigation is planned and data collection methods developed.
5. A pilot study is conducted.
6. The main data set is gathered.
7. The raw data is sorted and analysed.
8. Conclusions and generalisations are drawn from the analysed data.
9. A report containing the findings is prepared.
10. This information is disseminated to the appropriate people.
11. The findings are utilised/implemented as appropriate.

It is not within the scope of this chapter to present more than a brief introduction to the main considerations and components of these steps.

Posing the question

Posing the question follows directly from identification of a particular problem that one wishes to solve, or from an idea or vague hunch one wants to explore. There are three main sources of research questions; they can be generated from experience, from other research or from theory.

Experience may lead to the identification of a specific problem, or perhaps just a 'hunch' as to a way in which care could be improved, or maybe a desire to understand the rationale for the success of a particular course of action. Research questions can be developed from all such suggestions. Investigating the question in a scientific way by following the research process may produce evidence which will help to explain the situation and may indicate a proposed change in practice.

Reading reports of completed research can also be a rich source of research questions. Speculation as to whether the evidence generated by a particular study would apply in the reader's own situation may prompt a desire to repeat the study in a different location to test the validity and the reliability of the original study, and also perhaps to lead to a wider implementation of the recommendation based on the findings.

A third source of research questions is directly from theory. A nursing theory is a set of assumptions put forward to explain events. The explanation is, or should be, the best available summary of the current knowledge on a specific subject. Research questions can be developed by logical deduction from theories. A hypothesis can be generated to test the theory, and if the hypothesis is confirmed then the theory can be supported.

In reality, the nature of the investigation which is undertaken and the actual research question(s) which form the focus of the investigation are determined by a range of external constraining or self-limiting factors. These include:

- time available to be devoted to the problem;
- the levels of knowledge and experience of research within the research team;
- the availability of financial and other resources such as access to expert statistical advice and computing facilities.

In the context of all of these external constraints, the final definition of the research question to be addressed and the methods to be adopted is generally made following the second stage of the research process, i.e. the literature search.

Searching the literature

Searching the literature can be an exciting and illuminating experience or a frustrating and disappointing journey leading nowhere. Keys to successful literature searching include the following:

- a helpful, skilled librarian;
- familiarity with the layout of the libraries to be used, e.g. how far back do the journals on the shelves go to, is there another location for older journals?
- knowledge of the principles of literature searching, familiarity with indexes, bibliographies, methods for computer search (use librarians if needed);
- conscientious indexing of sources investigated – an unrecorded reference source may take many hours to retrace. Index cards or a computerised index of sources examined, including full reference, and comments to remind you of the content should be kept and frequently updated throughout the project.

What should the literature be searched for? In broad terms a literature search is a search for material which provides information on the following aspects of the problem under investigation: the size of the problem; any commentators identifying the problem; whether other research studies have investigated the problem, or whether the problem seems to be unique; if the problem has been previously identified, whether the history of the problem can be traced.

The aim of the literature search is to develop a theoretical framework which encompasses the above factors and provides a justification for the investigation method to be adopted for the project. In practice, the following steps may prove useful.

1. Define the topic in terms of keywords and synonyms which will guide the search through indexes and abstracts.
2. Decide how widely you wish to search. For example, are you going to include just UK research or research from other countries as well? How far is it reasonable to go back to look for material? (The smaller the amount of literature on a topic generally the further back the search needs to go.) Are any foreign language papers to be considered? If so, can translation be arranged?
3. Is it appropriate to search outside recognised nursing literature? For example, should medical, dietetic or physiotherapy literature be included in the search? The topic and the range of reference obtained from the initial investigation of available nursing literature may guide this decision.

A literature search should not be conducted in isolation, but should be coupled with discussion of findings with colleagues, experts, mentors – in fact anyone who is interested in the same problem. A final hint for a student new to the art of literature searching is that time spent discovering the material available from different sources is time well spent. It is useful, for example, to understand what indexes, abstracts, bibliographies, on-line searches, and so on, can offer. Time spent with a librarian or working through a guided study exercise may prove very useful in terms of developing an ability to search the literature efficiently and effectively in the future. Further consideration is given to the art and value of critical reading on pp.47–48.

Refinement of the research question

Following the literature search, the researcher is in a position to decide exactly what the purpose of the study is to be. This involves developing the initial question or idea into a form that is suitable for investigation by the research process. This stage generally consists of defining precisely what one is interested in and narrowing the original question down into a very specific question for which a clear-cut answer is obtainable. For example, a general hunch that some nurses assess wounds in rather different ways can be developed into several widely different research studies. Among many alternatives it could lead to:

- a study of documented records of wounds kept by nurses;
- a descriptive account of the criteria used by nurses when deciding how to manage a wound; or

- an observational study of whether nurses change their practice following a wound-care study day.

In each case the researcher has focused from the initial topic in to a particular, more specific direction. However, in each situation further clear definition of the specific aspects to be studied is required before the research can proceed. The research question should contain a single idea and not several. The final format of the research focus can be in the form of a statement or a hypothesis. A hypothesis is a specific form of research question that states a predicted relationship between variables in such a way that it can be directly tested.

Planning the investigation

At this stage, the research method selected is developed into a reality for the topic of study. In essence this involves choosing the appropriate research method, seeking permission and, where appropriate, ethical approval for carrying out the investigation, the development of the data collection method(s) to be used, the planning and preparation necessary for calculating, identifying and incorporating the sample to be studied, and the training of data collectors where appropriate.

Within the context of this chapter it is not possible to discuss all of the aspects of the range of research methods available. The following brief description of some of the main methods and terms used will, it is hoped, allay some of the confusion often encountered at the early stages of becoming familiar with research, and stimulate further study of a range of these methods.

DESCRIPTIVE METHOD

In a descriptive study the researcher does not change any aspect of the area or subjects being studied. The study aims to describe the current situation. The area to be investigated is generally presented in the form of a research question. Many descriptive studies take the form of surveys. For example, David et al. (1983) surveyed current treatments across England for patients with established pressure sores. A total of 737 wards in 20 health districts were surveyed, and a total of 961 patients with one or more pressure sores were seen by the research team. Descriptive information relating to the (then) current practice of nursing care of patients with pressure sores was collected.

It may be thought that descriptive information of this nature cannot have a direct effect on practice. However, a summary of some of the uses to which the pressure sore data was put may quell such an idea. The findings were used to formulate and focus future research ventures, and have enabled managers and others to rationalise and review resource allocation. The research prompted pharmacists and wound care experts to examine the efficacy of the huge range of products found to be in use for the treatment of sores. A total of 98 products were identified during the survey. In addition, the survey findings provided valuable education material, which in many instances encouraged ward managers and others to review local practices in relation to pressure sore management.

EXPERIMENTAL METHOD

In an experimental study an attempt is made to reveal the existence of a relationship between two or more factors (variables). In its simplest form this might involve establishing whether a particular form of treatment is better than no treatment. The experiment would proceed by giving the treatment to one group of patients and no treatment to another similar group. The effect of the treatment or no treatment would be measured for both groups and the results compared. For example, Romney (1982), in addition to conducting a trial of pre-delivery shaving (see p.36), conducted a similar trial on the value, if any, of pre-delivery enemas. Her hypothesis was that there would be no difference in the rates of faecal contamination, duration of labour, and incidence of infection between mothers who did and did not receive an enema prior to delivery. The research evidence generated supported this hypothesis, and widespread changes in maternity practice resulted.

QUANTITATIVE AND QUALITATIVE RESEARCH

Quantitative research refers to research which involves measurements that can be directly recorded and quantified. In essence, quantitative research is concerned with the measurement of 'facts', e.g. physiological measurements of fluid balance and temperature, tests of knowledge under examination conditions, rates of admission and discharge, rates of recruitment and wastage.

Qualitative research refers to studies which attempt to measure concepts which do not lend themselves to direct measurement, such as pain, anxiety, attitudes and opinions (see Chapter 3). Indicators to represent the concepts need to be developed, and therefore this approach is more subjective than quantitative research. However, it is important to recognise the need for both types of research in nursing, which is concerned with both physiological and psychological dimensions (see Chapters 4, 5 and 6). There is often an inappropriate distinction drawn between these two approaches which supports the belief that quantitative is scientific and reliable in a way that qualitative research can never be. Goodwin and Goodwin (1984) argue that the methods should be seen as opposite ends of the same spectrum, and not mutually exclusive methods. They point out that they are in fact just two different approaches to data collection and analysis, and not two different philosophies of life. In nursing research it is often appropriate to use both quantitative and qualitative data collection methods in order to obtain a realistic picture of the true situation. For example, Boore (1978), when looking at the relationship between the amount of pre-operative information received and the rate of post-operative recovery, collected both physiological (quantitative) and psychological (qualitative) data in order to demonstrate a positive effect between the provision of pre-operative information and the promotion of recovery (see Chapter 4).

ACTION RESEARCH

Action research, a term first used by Kurt Lewin (1948), is a type of applied social research. The main feature of action research is that the researcher and the practitioners collaborate throughout, unlike the majority of other methods where the researcher adopts a 'fly on the wall' role. As evidence becomes available to indicate a possible positive change to practice, practice will be changed during the course of the study. The study continues by investigating the consequences of the change. The advantages of this method for local problem-solving are considerable. However, because of the ongoing developmental nature of the changes in practice, there are limitations to the general application of the findings. Further useful discussions on method can be found in Greenwood (1984), Lathlean and Farnish (1984) and Towell (1979).

DATA COLLECTION METHODS

Data can be collected using a variety of methods, which can be grouped together into four major categories of data collection: by observation; by questioning; by looking things up; and by concurrent recording. A variety of instruments can be used for each of these approaches. For example, observation data can be recorded on video film or directly on to a simple chart, such as that used for recording observed temperature and blood pressure measurements, or on a carefully devised recording sheet which allows a data collector to record a variety of events observed. Data can be obtained by questioning either by the use of a questionnaire which is completed in the absence of the researcher, or by interview when a researcher asks questions face to face. The schedule used needs to be appropriate to the method and to the questions being asked. For example, it is possible to offer clarification in a face-to-face interview, but not in a postal questionnaire, and questions need to be formulated to take account of this. Data can be collected from a wide variety of records which may be patients' care records or management information which is routinely collected. Data may also be collected by asking participants in the study to compile information relating to an aspect of their work/life, e.g. in the form of an activities or food diary.

Pilot study

A pilot study is a small-scale trial of the main data collection methods to be used. During the planning stage many pre-pilot studies may be conducted, but a final 'dry run' should be carried out to ensure that no insoluble problems will be encountered during the main data collection. For example, the pilot study may reveal problems with recruiting suitable subjects, or may reveal that superfluous data is being generated. Steps can be taken to sort out these problems prior to the collection of the main data set. If major modifications are required, then a further pilot study may be necessary. In the event of poor reliability or validity or logistical problems, changes should be made to the data-collecting methods prior to collecting the main data set.

A data collection instrument is said to be reliable *if* it is used on two separate occasions and the same results are obtained, providing that the 'who' or 'what' being measured has not changed. For example, a ruler made of elastic is clearly not reliable, nor is the following question included on a questionnaire: 'Please list qualifications obtained whilst at school'. This may be interpreted as passes obtained in the General Certificate of Education or the General Certificate of Secondary Education examinations, but is open to interpretation to include, for example, all ballet, swimming and piano qualifications obtained between the age of 5 years and leaving school. The reliability of obtaining the required information can be improved if the question states exactly which types of qualifications are being referred to.

A data collection instrument is valid if it actually measures what it is intended to measure. The researcher must ensure that an abstract concept such as pain is validly reflected in the range of information collected, which may include patient report of pain using a numerical indicator (a pain thermometer), timing and nature of analgesia received, reports of previous pain experiences, factors which relate to anxiety status, outcome of definition of the pain (if pain is reported to be low, then is discharge an option? If pain is reported to be high, does the respondent run the risk of further surgery or painful treatment?). Generally a single question or observation can only be a valid data collection method when collecting information relating to a simple construct, e.g. age, sex, height or current weight. In order to be valid, a more complex construct should be operationally defined in such a way as to cover all relevant aspects of the construct.

Problems of reliability and validity must be addressed prior to collecting the main data set.

Collection of the main data set

This is the most tedious part of any project, as it involves the performance of many repetitive tasks. Data must be collected from the subjects in a consistent way, and researchers must not allow themselves to 'drift' into asking new questions, or applying new knowledge gathered as the project evolves.

Analysis of data

Once the data has been collected, it needs to be sorted, analysed and presented in such a way that interpretation of the findings is possible. Plans for analysis should be made throughout all of the preceding stages. The nature of the analysis that can be undertaken depends on the nature of the data collected. Data can be grouped, classified and coded to enable a picture to be built up. Features of the data can be counted and the frequencies of responses calculated. Beyond this, more detailed and sophisticated pictures can be established using statistical methods. Expert statistical advice may be required for this.

Conclusions

Once the data have been analysed and presented in an easily assimilated form, e.g. by the use of tables, graphs and histograms, conclusions can be drawn. Conclusions should summarise all that has been learned from the data set and all the inferences and generalisations that can be drawn.

Report

A report should summarise all of the stages of the research project. Readers of the report should be able to follow the research process through and to understand how the conclusions were reached. The findings then need to be disseminated by publication, presentation of the report to appropriate groups, and through education channels via seminars, study days and conferences.

Implementation

The final stage of the research process, namely implementation, is discussed on pp.49–52.

What it is not – limitations of nursing research

Broadly speaking, the limitations of nursing research can be divided into three main groups:

- those limitations which are a consequence of the problem being unsuitable for investigation by the research methods;
- those limitations which result from attempting to 'measure the unmeasurable';
- those limitations which result from the failure, for whatever reason, to adhere to the research process.

One of the first hurdles faced by a student of research method is that of learning to pose a 'researchable question'. Not all nursing problems are directly, or indeed indirectly, researchable. Scientific research cannot be used to answer questions of a moral or ethical nature, many of which are faced by nurses throughout their professional lives. Such problems include the following. How do you determine which patient should be offered a kidney transplant when only a limited number of transplants are possible? Is it appropriate to carry out HIV testing in certain circumstances without the patient's consent? Should nurses be allowed to withdraw from certain medical procedures, such as termination of pregnancy, on moral or religious grounds?

Secondly, there are limitations which result from the problems of conducting qualitative research, e.g. research which seeks to investigate phenomena which cannot be directly measured, such as pain, anxiety or aggression. If you adopt the maxim that pain is what the patient says it is, then it is impossible, at present, to measure pain in a purely quantitative way. It is therefore necessary to ask the patient to attempt to interpret his or her feeling of pain in a measurable form. Hayward (1975) developed a pain thermometer which the patient could use to indicate the intensity of the pain being experienced. This is a qualitative measurement of pain and, as people are not consistent either in the way they feel pain or in the way they describe pain, it is not possible to use this measurement to determine accurately how much analgesia is required in all cases.

Thirdly, research has limitations in that the value of evidence produced will be influenced by the way in which the problem was investigated. Polit and Hungler (1985) point out that 'virtually every research study contains some flaw' (p.18). All studies are bound by certain constraints of time, financial resources, personnel to conduct the research, and the skills and knowledge of such personnel, with regard to both the topic under investigation and the research methodology. From the outset the problem under investigation can be approached in a variety of ways, and at each stage of the research process decisions and compromises must be made. For example, which variables can be controlled? Which can be left to random variation? How should the sample be selected? How large a sample should be taken? What is the most appropriate and most feasible method(s) for data collection? How many revisions of the data collection can be allowed for, and when must the main data collection be started? How much time is there for the training of data collectors? What support from a competent statistician is available, at both the design and the data-handling and analysis stage? What material is to be included in the final report? How widely is the report to be circulated? At each stage, decisions have to be made and the limitations of the methods are faced. Flaws of design, or the introduction of certain biases either knowingly or unknowingly, can completely change the value of the research, and may lead to inappropriate conclusions being drawn.

It must be remembered by any reader of research that, whilst the researcher may have tried his or her hardest to conduct an objective and unbiased study, certain compromises will have been made and the resultant product must be examined with care in order to weigh up the value of the evidence produced to support the claims made in the report. The following discussion on critical reading examines these ideas in more depth.

Art and value of critique

Critique is a judgement of merit of works of literature, and expression (statement) and exposition (interpretation) of such judgement. By no means does the word only refer to negative criticism – it is the overall judgement of the good, the bad, the value and not least the applicability of the work being reviewed.

The art of critique

The art of critique is not as mystical and intangible as it sounds. It is an acquired skill which will develop with practice and, it has been argued, should be part of the basic mental equipment of every practising nurse (Committee on Nursing, 1972) and not just a skill confined to nurse researchers and graduate nurses. A research report cannot benefit nursing care unless its contents are carefully examined, its conclusions considered, lessons learned and nursing practice changed where appropriate.

The development of the art of critique lies in the maxim of practice makes perfect, and the following are a few guiding principles. The adoption of a questioning approach to one's reading may or may not come easily; to many it does not. The presentation, in print, of a plausible set of conclusions, coupled with some incomprehensible statistics and an author with several letters after his or her name may lead to an unquestioning acceptance of the correctness of the claims made. In research, as has been previously stated, all that is produced is evidence and this evidence *must* be carefully scrutinised before changes in practice can confidently be made. A basic understanding of the research process provides the key to the development of a questioning approach. In the early stages of developing this skill a check-list, such as that produced by Hawthorn (1983), can be very helpful. A further principle to aid success is the adoption of a rigorous note-taking habit, either on index cards, in a notebook, or using a word processor. A note of the author, title, full reference and brief summary of content of all useful articles read (and a note of location of the volume if using several libraries) will do much to enhance the review of the material covered, and may avoid hours of frustration.

In essence, a research report should provide sufficient information to enable the reader to weigh up in his or her own mind the nature of the problem/hypothesis under investigation, the background to the problem, the why and wherefore of the methodology adopted, the reliability and validity of the data obtained, the appropriateness of the analysis performed and the conclusions drawn. The reader should guard against making allowances for information not included in the report. The author is in control of the evidence which he or she chooses to provide in order that the reader may assess the conclusions reached, and if the information is incomplete it is undesirable to infer too much. For example, in a study of the effectiveness of pressure sore treatment, McClemont et al. (1979) report a marked difference in time taken to de-slough sores for groups of patients receiving different treatments. The clear implication is that the difference is due to the treatment. However, it is possible that the difference is due to some other factor which differs between the patient groups, e.g. that one group is more seriously ill. The authors provide no information on the basis of which it can be decided whether or not this is a possibility. The authors' conclusions lead the reader to believe that the results are not affected by other factors – this is a dangerous assumption.

The critical reader should develop the skills of a detective, backing judgements with other reading and sound professional knowledge and experience. It is an art that develops with practice.

The value of critique

Many of the values of critique have already been referred to. Research should not be allowed to sit on shelves of libraries and offices, never to be used. It should be published and disseminated to as wide an audience as possible so that it may directly or indirectly improve the quality of patient care. A reader of research should have a specific goal in mind, for example:

- reading for general interest;
- the development of a theoretical framework for a proposed project or investigation;
- completion of an academic exercise;
- looking for answers to specific problems.

All of these may be achieved by critically reading research. The value of critical reading is that it may provide the reader with the answers that he or she is searching for.

Implementation

Nursing research cannot implement itself. Implementation requires that nurses identify the research relevant to their area of work or responsibilities, weigh up the evidence presented and then formulate a plan to best utilise the findings (if appropriate). What is required is truly research-minded practitioner nurses who seek out, evaluate, interpret and then utilise the research which is available.

An examination of these four stages of implementation reveals the reality of problems which will be encountered. Finding time to seek out relevant research is not always seen as a priority by many practitioners. Studies such as those conducted by Myco (1980) and Barnett (1981) have shown that nurses tend to read very little in the way of professional material of any kind. In the author's experience, when questioning groups of nurses at the beginning of a research course/lecture as to the professional reading they have undertaken in the preceding week, many will admit to having looked at the weekly journals only. On further questioning the respondents tend to identify that, within these journals, the news pages and the job advertisements have received attention, and few are able to recount the content or even the subject matter of any research reports contained in the journal. A possible solution to this problem is the establishment of a 'journal club' in which a group of nurses agrees to review a range of professional journals relevant to their sphere of work. Each member is responsible for examining just one or two journals to identify any papers which may be relevant to the group. As many professional journals are issued only monthly or bi-monthly, the journal club should meet about six times a year. At the meeting each member should report the content of any relevant findings to the group, whose members can together reflect on the possible implications of the study. For example, is it just interesting or does it warrant further consideration, or possible implementation? This can be a very successful venture and many other research-related activities may be able to be carried out by and through the group, e.g. arranging seminars and developing proposals for small-scale studies.

Where should nurses be looking for material? In the UK there are two refereed general journals in which researchers may choose to publish their report – the *Journal of Advanced Nursing* and *The International Journal of Nursing Studies*, both of which cover research on all aspects of nursing practice, education and management from the UK and abroad. Several nursing research journals are produced in the USA, including *Nursing Research, Research in Nursing and Health* and the *Western Journal of Nursing Research*.

In addition, most nursing specialities are served by specialist journals, and it is appropriate for many nurses to seek information from journals that are not specifically on nursing but are from related disciplines. These journals are not generally found at railway stations or in the newsagents alongside the weekly publications, and their price is too prohibitive to recommend the purchase of individual copies. Hence the visiting of professional libraries will be required in order that the available material can be reviewed. Knowing about relevant research demands an interest and a willingness to seek out the information. The feeling that 'somebody else' will keep one up to date does not bode well for progress. Teaching from a research-based curriculum which encourages questioning and examination of available evidence for the theories and practices being taught may go some way to alleviate the apathy and encourage individuals to see that keeping up to date with relevant research is the responsibility of all practitioner nurses.

The second step towards successful implementation is an ability to weigh up the evidence in an informed way. Hunt (1981) argues that one of the inhibitory factors to successful implementation is that nurses do not believe research findings. It could be argued that, in order not to believe research findings, such findings need to have been critically read and understood, and the evidence weighed up in such a way that one is in a position not to believe the findings. In reality this is not often the case. Unwillingness to accept research findings which directly challenge traditionally held beliefs and practices is not uncommon. The disbelief of the findings is a defence for the accepted practice. For example, a traditional approach to wound care was to keep the wound clean and dry, and therefore nurses may be unwilling to accept research findings which support the idea that a moist wound environment will encourage more rapid healing than a dry wound environment.

One way of overcoming this scepticism is to encourage nurses to accept research for what it is, namely evidence, and to ask them to be prepared to weigh up objectively the strengths and weaknesses of the evidence, as they would if they were in the position of jury member in a court of law. Nurses need to decide if the results and conclusions appear to be reasonable, formulated from an appropriate sample, and of sufficient statistical significance. At the same time, they need to learn to re-examine practices for which they are unable to provide a sound rationale or research basis, and be prepared to examine new evidence as it becomes available, which may indicate a possible change in practice.

A further component in the process of implementing research findings is the need to understand them. The ability to understand research findings arises from a sound understanding of the subject under study, a basic knowledge of research theory and methods, a modicum of statistical appreciation and a willingness to read carefully and thoroughly and exercise a professional judgement whilst reading. Understanding does not come easily at first but, with wide reading, more and more research methods are encountered and basic knowledge and skills will develop over time. The novice may well be advised to seek more experienced help, e.g. from a nurse researcher or a statistician.

Only when these stages have been successfully negotiated can action plans for implementation be drawn up. It is perhaps pertinent to be reminded that not all research can be directly implemented, for a variety of reasons previously discussed. Lelean (1982, p.228), when writing about the implementation of research, suggests that there would be fewer problems if the word 'implementation' was replaced with 'utilisation'. Lelean illustrates this point with a quotation from MacLeod Clark and Hockey (1979) – a quotation which still holds true:

> To make use of research does not necessarily mean to implement findings – the use of research implies the reading of research reports with insight and comprehension in the first place – sometimes it will encourage the reader to pursue some of the references – sometimes, the reader will be motivated to replicate the research in his or her own area of practice – on occasions, the reader may simply be directed to situations which warrant special attention.
>
> (MacLeod Clark and Hockey, cited in Lelean, 1982, p.228)

Thus using research rather than thinking that research is only useful if it can be directly implemented can stimulate the reader to:

- deepen his or her knowledge of the subject by further reading;
- examine his or her practice with a view to possible modification;
- consider whether replication of the study is warranted/necessary/desirable, and if so by whom;
- be made aware of an aspect of care which may warrant a closer look;
- consider implementation.

If implementation is contemplated, the following steps should be observed:

1. The weight of the evidence for the conclusions of the study should be carefully considered.
2. The feasibility and resource implications of the proposed implementation should be identified.

3. The desirability and cost-effectiveness of the proposed change should be considered, and the reassurance of quality of care as a result of the proposed change – does the proposed implementation have a direct positive effect on the quality of patient care or is it something that just makes for an easier life for the nurses?
4. A strategy for implementation needs to be developed which pays particular attention to the education and training needs of the staff who will be involved.
5. Finally, a review programme should be established to formally evaluate the effectiveness of the change.

Summary

This chapter has provided an overview of research in nursing, and has outlined the methods by which researchers explore problems to generate evidence which will increase the body of nursing knowledge. In summary, it is appropriate to reiterate some of the major points raised and to reflect on the overall potential contribution that research can make to nursing.

Nurses need research to enable them to identify and demonstrate a rational basis for the care that they give. There must be a move away from tradition and custom as the basis for what nurses do and a striving to develop scientific knowledge for practice. This will serve to improve the care delivered to patients and clients and strengthen the knowledge base on which the profession of nursing is based.

With the increasing pressures on nurses, in common with other health care professionals, to establish quality assurance programmes, research has a vital role to play. Inherent in quality assurance is the concept of the delivery of care at predetermined levels. This presupposes that levels can be set, and that it is possible to measure care delivered in the work-place to determine whether the level is attained. It is not appropriate to dwell on the complex issues surrounding quality assurance. However, it is relevant to spell out what should by now be obvious. Research-based knowledge and its application provide a vital key to the success of quality assurance, and hold the route to the scientific and objective basis for the selection of appropriate courses of action, and also provide the methods for objective measurement, e.g. by audit, questionnaire, structured observation or systematic integration of written records.

In order that nurses can make the best use of research, there is a need to develop research-mindedness. It is not appropriate or indeed desirable for all nurses to be able to carry out research, but it is important that they can use the research findings generated by others. To achieve this state of affairs, a serious examination of nurse education at both basic and post-basic levels needs to occur. The advent of Project 2000 provides a clear opportunity (see Chapter 9). However, nursing will not become a research-minded profession overnight. Many of the skills will only develop with practice; for example, developing the art of critique (see p.48). Thus it must be the responsibility of each individual, both nurse teacher and nurse practitioner, to develop his or her own research skills and to share this developing expertise with others.

Research needs to be read and used. It has already been stated that not all research is suitable for instant implementation in a clinical setting, but if research is to fulfil its potential for nursing it must be tried, tested, challenged, developed and, when appropriate, rejected. This will only come about if nurse practitioners, nurse researchers and nurse managers each have sympathy for the role that the others have to play, and each realises that together they can interact to the benefit of patients and clients. Nurse practitioners can identify problems which are appropriate for study, nurse researchers can systematically study the problem and generate scientifically based recommendations and nurse managers have the potential to act on the recommendations. These three branches of the profession can work together to the benefit of patients and clients.

References

Barnett, D. E. 1981 Do nurses read? *Nursing Times* **77**, 2131–3.

Barton, A. and Barton, N. 1981 *The management and prevention of pressure sores.* London: Faber and Faber.

Boore, J. 1978 *Prescription for recovery.* London: Royal College of Nursing.

Committee on Nursing 1972 *Report.* London: HMSO.

David, J. A., Chapman, R. G., Chapman, E. J. and Lockett, B. 1983 *An investigation of the current methods used in nursing for the care of patients with established pressure sores.* Harrow: Nursing Practice Research Unit, Northwick Park Hospital and Clinical Research Centre.

Davis, B. (ed.) 1987 *Nursing education: research and development.* London: Croom Helm.

Goodwin, L. D. and Goodwin, W. L. 1984 Qualitative vs. quantitative research or qualitative and quantitative research. *Nursing Research* **33**, 378–80.

Greenwood, J. 1984 Nursing research: a position paper. *Journal of Advanced Nursing* **9**, 77–82.

Hawthorn, P. J. 1983 Occasional paper. Principles of research: a checklist. *Nursing Times* **79**, 41–3.

Hayward, J. 1975 *Information: a prescription against pain.* London: Royal College of Nursing.

Henderson, F. 1969 *Basic principles of nursing care,* revised ed. Basel: Karger.

Hunt, J. 1981 Indicators for nursing practice: the use of research findings. *Journal of Advanced Nursing* **6**, 189–94.

Jacka, K. and Lewin, D. 1987 *The clinical learning of student nurses.* Nursing Education Research Unit Report No. 6. London: Nursing Education Research Unit, University of London.

Lancaster, A. 1975 *Guidelines to research in nursing. No. 1. Nursing, nurses and research,* 2nd edn. London: King Edward's Hospital Fund.

Lathlean, J. and Farnish, S. 1984 *The ward sister training project: an evaluation of a training scheme for ward sisters.* London: Nursing Education Research Unit, Department of Nursing Studies, King's College, University of London.

Lelean, S. R. 1982 The implementation of research findings into nursing practice. *International Journal of Nursing Studies* **19**, 223–30.

Lewin, K. 1948 *Resolving social conflict*. New York: Harper and Row.

McClemont, E. J. W., Shand, I. G. and Ramsay, B. 1979 Pressure sores: a new method of treatment. *British Journal of Clinical Practice* **33**, 21–5.

MacLeod Clark, J. and Hockey, L. 1979 *Research for the enquiring nurse*. Aylesbury: HM + M Publishers.

Myco, F. 1980 Nursing research information: are nurse educators and practitioners seeking it out? *Journal of Advanced Nursing* **5**, 637–46.

Norton, D., McLaren, R. and Exton-Smith, A. N. 1975 *An investigation of geriatric nursing problems in hospital*. Edinburgh: Churchill Livingstone.

Polit, D. F. and Hungler, B. P. 1985 *Essentials of nursing research: methods and applications*, 3rd edn. Philadelphia: Lippincott.

Romney, M. L. 1982 Nursing research in obstetrics and gynaecology. *International Journal of Nursing Studies* **19**, 193–203.

Sleep, J. and Grant, A. 1988 Occasional paper. Effects of salt and savlon bath concentrate post-partum. *Nursing Times and Nursing Mirror* **84**, 55–7.

Towell, D. 1979 A 'social systems' approach to research and change in nursing care. *International Journal of Nursing Studies* **16**, 111–21.

Health and health promotion – consensus and conflict

3

Sue McBean

We use the words 'normal' and 'healthy' when we talk about people, and we probably know what we mean. From time to time we may profit from trying to state what we mean, at risk of saying what is obvious and at risk of finding out we do not know the answer.

(Winnicott, 1986, p.21)

Health is one of the most frequently used words in our vocabulary – yet it is something prone to assumption, preconception and misconception. Explicitly or implicitly, health is one of the four major assumptions of all nursing models (Keck, 1989), and it should thus be of significant interest to all nurses. From the late 1980s onwards the previously limited research on health as a belief has become richer, although only 10 years ago the body of knowledge was still described as 'scarce' and in need of 'further systematic research' (Calnan, 1987, p.40). In addition, the literature on health often consists of only a few pages or at best a short chapter in any one text, for example Naidoo and Wills (1994). Students commonly turn to Seedhouse (1986), which is one of the largest and best written accounts available, but the work is mainly a philosophical debate, and much of it is not overtly applied to health care. This chapter, which is the result of over a decade of reading and development, will expose the reader to a broad range of ideas and analysis about health which might otherwise take many months of study.

Until the early 1990s, health promotion was an over-used and abused term about which there was much confusion. Since then several excellent texts have been published, but it is still timely to clarify the meaning and implications of a term which represents one of the most rapidly expanding and important areas of health care. The literature on health promotion over the last 15 years suggests that criticism is more in order than congratulation (Rodmell and Watt, 1986). Commitment to the principles of health promotion espoused by the World Health Organisation from government department level downwards has to be more than rhetorical, but some would question this commitment (McBean, 1992a; Stone, 1989; Young, 1996). With regard to health promotion this chapter should be viewed more as a signpost for the major areas of consensus and contention than as a route map. Table 3.1 summarises some of the issues, most of which will be discussed in the text.

What is truth?

> Put yourself on the margins but don't be endlessly naming them ... choose ... but be prepared to be flexible here.
>
> (Riley, 1985, p.53)

History is often thought of as fact. Writing in *What is History?*, E. H. Carr (1964) informed a discussion of truth: 'It used to be said that facts speak for themselves. This is, of course, untrue' (p.11). He reasoned that the historian selects which facts will speak and decides the order and context of presentation. Facts then speak only through the interpretation of the author. Along a slightly different but related line, Beattie (1986) wrote of a modern, sophisticated phenomenon which allows 'selective presentation of scientific evidence to support an official position' (p.8). His concern was that the government had publicly asserted that it is acceptable to be 'economical with the truth' (p.8). Anxious that people should be allowed to make 'reasoned choices', Seedhouse (1986) argued that this comes only from possession of the 'fullest relevant information' 'about factors which affect their lives' (pp.84–85). He argued that health education without a complete explanation becomes indoctrination and propaganda.

Table. 3.1   Health promotion and nursing – some areas of consensus and conflict

Consensus	Conflict
Nurse role in patient education: past – poor track record; current – expanding; future – great potential	Among professionals, *and* between the public and professionals – views on the measurement and maintenance of health
The roles of nurses in health promotion should expand	Definitions of health: lay vs. professional
A disease-centred approach is limited: health promotion is more than simply the prevention of ill-health	The relative importance of policy vs. individual action and self-care vs. social care
Health promotion roles are for all nurses, not just those in the community	Concern about the value and effectiveness of various health promotion approaches – glossy, individualistic, shocking, authoritarian
Individual behaviour changes may be impossible or ineffective without politico-economic and socio-cultural changes	The importance of positive and negative role modelling: parents, professionals and the media
The value of certain methods: facilitation, discussion, above all participation and consultation, healthy alliances (multisectoral work)	The use of a risk/epidemiological approach The significance of the health belief model

Farrant and Russell (1986) gave a lengthy exposition of their deep concerns about the basis of truth in health information offered to the public on heart disease. Evidence has accumulated that the conventional individual risk factors, such as diet and smoking, cannot *alone* explain the incidence of heart disease. What is needed is an hypothesis that includes:

- a large emphasis on chronic psychosocial stress (especially in relation to poverty);
- the role played by the food retail, agricultural and tobacco industries.

If the 'do-it-yourself lifestyle' stance is the only one taken with regard to the prevention of heart disease, then these two additional factors have not been reflected honestly. Farrant and Russell (1986) described health information as being a politically defined compromise rather than being based on scientific evidence. One should question the usefulness of giving only clear, simple, perhaps simplistic guidelines which avoid conflict while there are still areas of inconclusiveness, uncertainty and contention which exist within the scientific literature on heart disease.

Most people in the UK believe that stress is the major cause of heart disease. This has been used by 'experts' as evidence of an inadequate understanding. However, Manicom suggested that, 'The public may have a more sophisticated understanding of the causes of disease than the medical profession' (Manicom, cited in Farrant and Russell, 1986, p.45). The World Health Organisation believe that health professionals have a role in making information about healthy lifestyles better known to the public who 'have the right to be informed' (World Health Organisation, 1985, p.150), as they 'may not have the necessary knowledge to make an informed choice of lifestyle' (World Health Organisation, 1985, p.54). However, one must proceed with caution if Williams (1984) is correct: 'there are relatively few cases where there is unequivocal evidence that certain courses of action will lead to health' (p.193).

Seedhouse quoted Professor Oliver (then President of the British Cardiac Society) as saying, in 1985, that he rejected the 'currently favoured idea that low fat diets can save people from heart attacks' (Seedhouse, 1986, p.84). In 1982 Oliver wrote: 'Much as we might like to think otherwise, it is not yet possible to prevent coronary heart disease in the community – let alone in an individual' (p.1066). Compare this with advice from the Health Education Council in 1984: 'Another way to beat heart disease is to watch what you eat .... The best thing to do is to cut down on the total amount of fat you eat by up to a quarter'. Oliver (1982) suggests that lifestyle changes with regard to smoking, fat consumption, obesity and sloth are at best *prudent*, but that 'the falling mortality from coronary heart disease in the United States remains largely unexplained and cannot be wholly ascribed to preventive measures' (Oliver, 1982, p.1066).

A review of the medical literature shows that this distinguished cardiologist has maintained a position of concern regarding low fat diets. He is particularly worried about women, adolescents and the elderly following the kind of dietary advice in standard health education material such as *Beating Heart Disease* (Health Education Council, 1984). From someone working as a Professor in the Cardiovascular Research Unit of the University of Edinburgh and, later, the Wynn Institute for Metabolic Research in London, the article titles alone should confirm that health educators must refrain from dogmatism: 'Dietary fat and coronary heart disease: there is much to learn' (Oliver, 1987); 'Reducing cholesterol does not reduce mortality' (Oliver, 1988); 'Might treatment of hypercholesterolaemia increase non-cardiac mortality?' (Oliver, 1991); 'Cholesterol and coronary disease – outstanding questions' (Oliver, 1992); and 'Lowering cholesterol for prevention of coronary heart disease – problems and perspectives' (Oliver, 1993).

What is health? The importance of health beliefs

To be admitted to the UK register of nurses requires competence both in 'advising on the promotion of health and the prevention of illness' and the recognition of 'situations that may be detrimental to the health and well-being of the individual' (Statutory Instrument, 1983; see Chapters 1 and 2). Although the nine competencies are not necessarily prioritised, interestingly these points are the first two on the list.

Promotion, prevention, health, illness and well-being are concepts which need detailed examination, thought and discussion. Familiarity with these terms is not enough – intimacy and commitment through reflection, analysis and thorough understanding are required. The components of the word 'competent' derive from Latin and mean *comm* 'to come', and *petere* 'to seek' (Chambers Dictionary, 1993). How much of the curriculum for diploma and pre-registration/professional development degree courses should be set aside for *seeking* to understand these concepts? Actually, it is not simply a case of time allocation or degree of emphasis. What is required is a radical reform (see Figure 3.1) to match the paradigm shift currently occurring in health care (Seedhouse, 1988). As Bradshaw (1986) put it, for nurses 'to be convinced that the determinants of better health lie outside the NHS ... the pathogenic orientation of nurse training' must become a 'healthy orientation to nurse education'(Bradshaw, 1986, p.9).

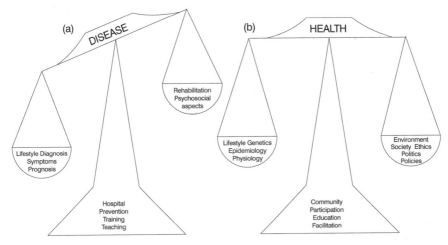

Figure 3.1   Imbalance and balance in nursing education: (a) pathogenic orientation; (b) health orientation

It is important to be aware of different views on health before giving health advice, for the same reason that the nursing model chosen will inform and underpin planning and the giving of care. This is demonstrated by the following example. The nurse who believes it is healthy to be slim, physically fit and *normotensive* might expect to do health teaching about stress and salt reduction, diet and exercise. The client or patient being approached about these subjects may, on the other hand, believe that health is concerned with coping, adapting and having a strong network of support. Health teaching about therapy or counselling, self-esteem and self-help groups would therefore be more appropriate than an overture on lifestyle (see Chapter 5). In any nurse–patient interaction which is centred on promoting health, an assessment of health beliefs is vital. The writer believes that an amazing paradox frequently exists. In giving health advice from a medical, disease-oriented paradigm the nurse is taking a professional stance that is in direct conflict with her own internal lay belief system. Preliminary work on *folk health beliefs* of health professionals supports this view (McBean, 1992b; Roberson, 1987).

Objective vs. subjective health

It is arguably enough to feel better now rather than to concentrate on ... disease prevention.

(Tannahill 1984, p.197)

Despite the fact that the UK has had a National Health Service (NHS) for over 40 years, and Health Visitors for even longer, relatively little is known about the health beliefs held by the public. Even less information is available about the health beliefs of professionals. The most researched area of health is the absence of it. For many professionals, particularly epidemiologists, health is defined in terms of morbidity and mortality statistics (see Chapter 7). This is epitomised in the following quotes from Blaxter (1987): 'the first British health survey, the Survey of Sickness' and 'Traditionally, the measure of health used is mortality' (p.5). Most documentation of professional views is about an objective, measurable state – the absence of clinical abnormality, ailment and disease. Research on lay views clearly reveals an anomaly. Unlike the 'experts', the public usually rely on subjective estimates of health.

Blaxter's (1987) separation of terms related to ill health may help here:

- disease – biological or clinical abnormality;
- illness – the subjective experience of symptoms of ill health;
- sickness – the functional consequences of disease or illness (causing a change in lifestyle);
- disability – a permanent change in lifestyle.

Blaxter (1987) wrote that 'it is obviously possible to have disease without illness, and to have illness without disease' (p.5). An example of disease without illness would be a woman with early cervical cancer. Illness without disease could be observed in a person with gross physical symptoms due to AIDS-paranoia. The former would be objectively unhealthy but could subjectively feel well, while the reverse would be true for the person with symptoms of AIDS.

It is critical that one distinguishes between these views when talking about promoting health. Is the role of the nurse to pursue measurable health (i.e. the absence of disease) or subjective health? Obviously the answer has to be that *both* goals are important. However, the second area has been much neglected in the past, yet it is the goal which can have most impact on the quality of people's lives. The aims of *Health for All by the Year 2000* (World Health Organisation, 1988) (commonly abbreviated to 'Health For All 2000' or 'HFA 2000') are only partly about measurably reducing preventable ill health, i.e. adding years to life. These aims also include improving the lived experience or subjective health of people – 'adding life to years' and 'health to life'. The essence of this relatively recent approach to quality rather than just quantity is embodied in the book title *To Live Until We Say Goodbye* (Kübler-Ross, 1978) and in the phrase 'living with AIDS' rather than 'dying with AIDS'.

Defining health?

It has been suggested that if health cannot be defined, then health professionals cannot evaluate their work (Noack, 1987). It also becomes difficult even to use the term professionals of *health* care. What does the 'health' in health care worker and *Health For All 2000* mean? The former stems from the setting up of the National Health Service. The theory was that by detecting, curing and preventing disease people would be made healthy, so health and disease were placed at opposite ends of a continuum (see Figure 3.2). Being disease-free equated with health in the minds of planners and politicians. Although there has been a reduction in some diseases prevalent in 1948, new problems have arisen, e.g. auto-immunity, diseases of affluence, and AIDS, while menstruation and the menopause have been medicalised. 'Health' in *Health For All 2000* relates to a very different philosophy to the one involved in setting up the NHS. It is actually about a 'positive sense of health' (World Health Organisation, 1985, p.5). It is also about people not the nation and about communities not populations. It is more about access, equity, participation and opportunity than about medical treatment *per se*.

To define health would be to deny its breadth as an issue. Robinson (1983) suggested an analysis would be more appropriate than definitions. Analysis means discovering the general principles (Chambers Dictionary, 1993). Moreover, what is needed is a resolution of the many and varied dissertations on health into a framework which can be used to improve the planning and evaluation of health care (Noack, 1987).

Analysing beliefs about health

It is important to realise just how high health is on the agenda of most people in this country. Health is one of the most talked about subjects, apart from the weather. 'How are you?' is a common greeting, and on departing we often say 'Keep well' or 'Take care' (Richman, 1987). It is uncommon to talk of 'hailing' someone now. However, the greeting 'Hail' comes from the Old English *hal* meaning 'whole'. 'Your health' is a welcome toast for all occasions, and health is also derived from *hal*.

Newman (1986) wrote that 'we have become idolatrous of health' (p.7). This worship goes on in health farms, health gyms and health food stores. Beauticians wear white coats symbolising their 'medical' power to heal. A beauty salon sighted in Wales was called 'Panacea', meaning 'a potion for all ills'. Chemist shops (also with white-coated assistants) commonly have signs inside and outside declaring 'health and beauty'. We talk of having a healthy

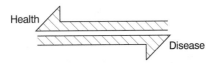

Figure 3.2   A health–disease continuum

bank account, a healthy atmosphere, a healthy outlook and healthy attitudes. The word 'sick' is applied to the acts of some criminals. Envious of the dangerous but seductive skin tan, it is hard to refrain from the comment, 'You look healthy'.

Four models of health beliefs

'What does being healthy mean to you?' is the question most studies of beliefs about health seek to answer. Woods *et al.* (1988) refer to the *lived experience of health*. This concept, which was developed and researched by Parse *et al.* (1985), is about describing the way in which people perceive, conceive and 'experience health in everyday life' (p.27). The answers given are the subjective thoughts and feelings of individuals. Woods *et al.* (1988) used the four models of health developed by an American nurse academic, Judith Smith, to analyse their data. Smith (1981) proposed that these four models of health consistently emerge from theorists. Since using her framework in the first edition of this book, I have become even more convinced of its utility after reading her 1983 text, in which she developed these ideas considerably (Smith, 1983). These four models will be used to give clarity and structure to the following review of what might otherwise appear to be a mêlée of dissimilar lay and professional beliefs.

Clinical model of health

> Health and disease are not symmetrical concepts .... And, while there are many diseases, there is in a sense only one health.
>
> (Engelhardt, cited in Noack, 1987, p.6)

Health as the absence of ailments and disease is reflected in the *clinical model*. Smith (1983) wrote that this is the narrowest model as it 'views individuals within the boundary of their skin' (p.89). This rather negative view of health is subscribed to by at least two important nursing theorists. Although Orlando does not define health, her work implicitly assumes health to be partially about 'freedom from mental or physical discomfort' (Orlando, cited in Marriner-Tomey *et al.*, 1989, p.231). Dycus *et al.* (1989) cite the beliefs of Adellah about health as: 'a state mutually exclusive of illness (with) no unmet needs and no anticipated or actual impairments' (p.97). For Helman (1994) the clinical model is similar to a numerical definition in which health is described 'by reference to certain physical and biochemical parameters, such as weight, height, circumference, blood count, haemoglobin level, levels of electrolytes or hormones, blood pressure, heart rate, respiratory rate, heart size' (Helman, 1994, p.103). Health, then, is conformity to a range of normal values.

Margaret Newman (1986) abhorred the portrayal of dichotomised health and illness, where the former is a positive state to be desired and the latter is a negative state. She believed it is a view which 'has pervaded most of our thinking from very early in life' (p.7). In being brought up to believe that not only is health a personal responsibility but also within individual control, those who do not have it tend to be viewed as inferior, irresponsible or even repulsive. In a recent rewrite of the classic text, *Teaching for Health*, Kiger (1995, p.7) provides a perfect, if surprisingly rather uncritical, example of a polarised health continuum. At one end of the continuum, Kiger claims, is optimal health and at the other end are ill health and disability. Newman (1986) proposed a synthesised view of health and disease rather than a polarised one. Thus, for her, disease is a 'meaningful aspect of health' (p.9). Newman (1986) placed great emphasis on the view of Martha Rogers that 'health and illness are "simply" expressions of the life process – one no more important than the other' (p.4).

Syred (1981, p.27) took the polarisation of health and illness one step further by saying that the continuum starts 'with "good" health at one end of the scale and death at the other' (see Figure 3.3). In this case, nursing intervention would be more about changing the course of disease processes than about promoting health. The idea that death is the opposite to health seems shockingly negative. However, before this clinical model of health is deemed worthless by professionals, it is important to consider research which suggests that it is a view held by many lay people. Noack (1987) wrote that 'Worldwide, health is defined in negative terms as the absence of disease' (p.5). Although Seedhouse (1986) described the health–disease continuum as the most limited model available, research into lay definitions of health finds positive health to be an elusive concept.

Health as the absence of disease was a view held by the socially disadvantaged families studied by Blaxter and Paterson (1982). In their sample of nearly 50 mothers and grown-up daughters, they found that 'both generations tended to think of health *only* in the ... sense of not (being) ill' (p.27). Indeed, there was 'little evidence, in either generation, of health as a positive concept' (p.29). Both Herzlich (1973), studying in France in the 1960s, and Williams (1990), surveying the views of the elderly in Aberdeen in the 1980s, found beliefs about health as the absence of illness or disease: 'Health is strictly speaking not something positive, it's simply not being ill' (Herzlich, 1973, p.56); 'From one angle they thought of it (health) as being free from illness or disease' (Williams, 1990, p.31). Woods *et al.* (1988), while emphasising the positive views of health held by their large sample of American women (*n*=528), admitted that clinical health was the most frequently cited model, used by more than 50 per cent of respondents.

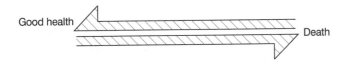

Figure 3.3   Syred's (1981) health–death continuum

Role performance model of health

In this model the emphasis is on health being the *ability to perform socially defined roles*. Thoughts on this model fall into three categories.

The most negative approach and the one which has received most criticism is the functionalist or sociological view of health (see Chapter 7). In 1951 Parsons wrote that health is the 'state of optimum capacity for an individual for the effective performance of the roles and tasks for which he has been socialised' (Parsons, cited in Morgan *et al.*, 1985, p.33). The central belief here is that people should be well not for their own sakes, but because they have role obligations to others and the cost to society is high when they are ill (Richman, 1987). Seedhouse (1986) was heavily critical of this opinion, partly because it infers that people with incapacitating disability cannot be healthy. He also felt that the roles and tasks which people perform may cause them to become unhealthy, as with exposure to coal dust or noise. A worrying implication of this concept is that those who are no longer fit or able to work due to disability or age may receive a health service in proportion to their reduced value to society (Morgan *et al.*, 1985).

A second approach to this model reflects opinions expressed by the lay population. In 1979 Dubos first published *Mirage of Health* (Dubos, 1995). He summarised this view of health as 'the ability of the individual to function in a manner acceptable to himself and to the group of which he is part' (p.9). This suggests that people want to function for what it brings themselves and those close to them, rather than as a duty and for the good of society in general. Blaxter and Paterson (1982) found that women considered themselves to be healthy, despite reporting high levels of morbidity, as long as they could carry out their normal roles and their children could continue to attend school. The women were of working-class background and it may be that denial of symptoms and continuing to function is a survival strategy (Richman, 1987). It is one thing for people to feel unhealthy while fulfilling their role as mother or employee. However, it is less satisfactory that people should, while continuing to function, have to deny illness in order to avoid poverty and hunger. The ability to perform roles was low on the list of views about health generated by the research of Woods *et al.* (1988). It may be that the value of role performance is only realised when it is threatened by ill health. Most people, in taking it for granted, may not spontaneously mention it. However, 17 per cent of the 528 respondents mentioned the following points:

- able to be as active as you want;
- able to perform usual functions;
- able to get through it;
- predictably being able to do things.

The third approach to the role performance model is about people having a right to sufficient health to be able to carry out roles. The philosophy of *Health For All 2000* is based on this approach. Health enables people to make full use of their abilities (World Health Organisation, 1985). Smith and

Jacobson (1988) wrote that people would be healthy if they were capable both of meeting their obligations and of 'enjoying the rewards of living in their community' (p.3). This is a complete reversal of Parsons' view. Instead of people having a duty to society, society has a duty to people.

Adaptive model of health

Several nurse theorists believe health to be about the *ability to adapt or cope*. Ackermann *et al.* (1989) refer to the views of King as follows: 'Health implies continuous adaptation to stress' (p.350); as such, illness interferes with the dynamic state of health. Levine wrote that, 'Change is characteristic of life, and adaption is the method of change' (Levine, cited in Foli *et al.*, 1989, p.395). According to Creekmur *et al.* (1989), Adam took the work of Virginia Henderson and developed her concept of nursing into a conceptual model. Although health is not defined within this model, it is referred to implicitly in the following statement: 'The goal of nursing is to maintain or to restore the client's independence in the satisfaction of his fundamental needs' (Adam, cited in Creekmur *et al.*, 1989, p.140). Ashworth (1997) wrote of Virginia Henderson as an outstanding nurse whose influence will continue despite her death. Henderson made several statements about health, one of which was that it 'requires independence and interdependence ... strength, will, or knowledge' (Henderson, cited in DeMeester *et al.*, 1989, p.84). Sister Callista Roy, the author of one of the models most well known to UK nurses, was a firm supporter of the view of health as adaptation: illness results from ineffective coping which consumes energy; when adaptation occurs, coping is effective and energy is released for healing (cf. Blue *et al.*, 1989).

One of the most widely read critics of modern medicine, Ivan Illich (1976), believed health to be the process of adaptation, rather than a state. Health for him was about healing when damaged, growing up, ageing, and coping with change and autonomy. This is similar to the view of Dubos (1995), that life and health are about independence, free will, the struggle with danger, finding new solutions and responding positively to life's challenges. Seedhouse (1986) described all of these views of health as an ability to adapt as vague, with a 'sugar-coating of ambiguity' (p.42). He condemned the writers for not describing exactly what the ability to adapt is, or how it might be created or enhanced by health workers.

As there is little support for health as adaptive ability in the literature on lay beliefs, it is possibly a professional conception with unclear relevance to clients. In the study by Woods *et al.* (1988), as few as 14 per cent of the women reported using an adaptive image for health. They used words such as flexibility, putting things in perspective, acceptance of life's situation, ability to accept anything mentally, and being in control.

At first sight the health *ease/dis-ease* continuum of Antonovsky (1987) (see Figure 3.4) appears to be similar to those described for the clinical model of health (see Figures 3.2 and 3.3 above). Believing that well-being (ease) is reduced to a level of being pain free and able to function fully, Noack (1987) was critical of the concept. However, Sullivan (1989) evaluated the model from a nursing perspective, and in contrast found it to be *health-oriented* rather than from the *pathogenic paradigm*. The focus is not on why someone develops a disease, but on a new question: Why do some people remain well 'despite omnipresent stressors'? (Sullivan, 1989, p.336). The answer to this question seems to be related to the possession of a strong sense of coherence. Sullivan described this *health-promoting coherence* as feeling that events are under some kind of control (not necessarily one's own), so that they are 'comprehensible rather than bewildering' (p.338). Thus the stimuli that one experiences are predictable, explicable and are to be seen as challenges worth facing, in the knowledge that one has the resources available to meet the demands being made.

The focus of this model is not the position at either end of the continuum, but the process of creating health (*salutogenesis*). If the movement towards health ceases, one does not have a state of disease. There is instead a potential for health breakdown. In aiming to promote health in a client, the nurse using this model would assess and reinforce their sense of coherence. The extent of coherence may be explored using certain issues for discussion, such as the following questions taken from Helman (1981), who was writing about folk models of illness.

- What has happened?
- Why has it happened?
- Why has it happened to me?
- Why now?
- What would happen if nothing was done about it?
- What should I do about it?

Littlewood (1989) wrote that: 'To date nursing models have not incorporated the importance of the patient's own model of illness causation' (p.228). She believed that psychological models root problems in an individual's personality, whereas in using an anthropological model one is looking more at an individual's understanding and the meanings that they ascribe to events. Sullivan (1989, p.341) described the sense of coherence, the individual's understanding, as 'the link between personality and health' (see Chapter 5). As the empirical testing of this *salutogenic model* progresses (see, for example, Lundberg and Nyström Peck, 1994) it is set to

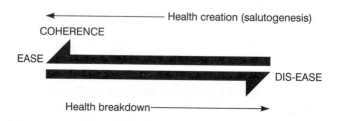

Figure 3.4 Antonovsky's (1987) salutogenic model

become increasingly popular in the UK, and is already being favoured in Nordic countries and in the USA.

Closely associated with the ideas of health as an ability to adapt are those which surround the concept of health as a strength or internal reserve. Dubos (1995) defined this in Darwinian terms as a fixity of the internal environment which controls and maintains an individual despite a need to adapt to changes in the external environment. Research suggests that views about a reserve of health or inner strength are an important tenet in lay beliefs. Some people believe a lack of internal strength makes one susceptible to AIDS (Aggleton *et al.*, 1989). Thus it is not a virus *per se* which causes AIDS, but an inherent weakness with which one is born, or which develops as a result of adopting certain lifestyles.

Nurses are frequently heard to say that they tend not to deal adequately with patients' spiritual needs (see Chapter 6). Reporting on the work of Oliver Sacks with regard to the Viennese sleeping sickness epidemic of 1916, Seedhouse (1986) wrote that, 'He was frequently overwhelmed by the impression of a tremendous inner strength in his patients'. He makes the case that 'this spirit is ... a quality ... which drives people to continue to develop in the face of apparently insurmountable odds' (p.38). It may be that spiritual strength could be tapped by nurses in developing a salutogenic sense of coherence.

Physical strength is commonly encountered as a lay belief about health. Williams (1990) found, in his research on elderly Aberdonians, that weakness was perceived as the opposite of health but that this was not in itself disease, more a proneness to be ill. Similarly, of the three dimensions of lay beliefs identified by Herzlich (1973), one was a combination of physical strength and a potential for resistance to illness. Many of the people who are learning to live with AIDS are working from a similar belief about health. Improvements in health status and quality of living are being produced by an immuno-supportive lifestyle, in other words getting plenty of sleep, eating well, cutting down on caffeine, nicotine and alcohol, encouraging plenty of social contact and maintaining a positive self-image.

Eudaemonistic model of health

Woods *et al.* (1988) wrote that this model has connotations of exuberant well-being. Although the term *eudaemonism* is not one familiar to most nurses, the model has proved useful in nursing research. The meaning of this word is happiness – it is of Greek origin, derived from the words for *well* and *spirit* (Chambers Dictionary, 1993). The results of the research on women's health beliefs by Woods *et al.* (1988) showed an overwhelming identification with this model. The women in their study used nine subdivisions of the model, and 88 per cent of all health images given were eudaemonistic. Some examples of phrases given within each category of the model are shown in Table 3.2. Positive affect was reported by 49 per cent of respondents, fitness by 44 per cent, healthy lifestyle by 24 per cent and harmony by 24 per cent.

Table. 3.2   Some examples of phrases used for each of the categories within the eudaemonistic model of health (after Woods *et al.*, 1988)

Positive affect	**Fitness**
Happy	Stamina
Exhilarating	Strength
Affectionate	Energetic
Feel good	Rested
Positive mental attitude	In good shape
Sense of well-being	Able to be active
Healthy lifestyle	**Harmony**
Taking care of self	Spiritually whole
Good eating habits	Sense of purpose
Not smoking	Relaxed
Moderate intake of alcohol	Peace of mind
Exercising	Satisfied
Eating balanced diet	Balance
Social involvement	**Cognitive function**
Liked by others	Think rationally
Involved in the community	Creative
Able to love and care	Alert
Feel good about relationships	Having many interests
Able to enjoy family	Inquisitive
Body image	**Positive self-concept**
Ideal weight	Self-confident
Look good	High self-esteem
Good feelings about one's body	Sense of self-worth
Self-fulfilled	
Able to achieve goals	
Reaching optimum	
Productive	
Self-aware	

The positive concepts of health embodied in the *eudaemonistic model* are extremely attractive, but it must be remembered that there are still relatively few studies of lay beliefs, and in these there is only limited evidence for a positive view of health. The lack of a positive view of health in the findings of Blaxter and Paterson (1982) was characterised by (and perhaps therefore attributed to) 'apathy, a feeling of powerlessness, and low norms of health' (p.195).

Writing in 1989, Clarke and Lowe reviewed the literature and found no accepted methods for researching beliefs about positive health. They followed a suggestion by Blaxter and asked:

- Who is the healthiest person you know?
- How do you know that they are healthy?
- What do people do to keep healthy?

The responses that they received, mainly from young people, closely agreed with some of the categories of Woods *et al.* (1988). Comments were mostly about appearance (body image), particularly of the eyes and face, physical activity (fitness) and diet (healthy lifestyle). However, areas of dissimilarity were the use of local folklore escape clauses about alcohol intake and smoking, and infrequent comments on obesity.

Common themes in the eudaemonistic model are independence, interdependence (family, friends and community) and control. Responses may depend on whether or not those being interviewed feel healthy, and thus 'in control', at the time of the research. Too few studies mention current *health status*. Van Maanen (1988) compared the views of healthy American elderly subjects with a group of elderly British subjects whom she defined as unhealthy because of their temporary residence in a community hospital. The American group had a positive eudaemonistic opinion about health as a state of mind (positive affect), healthy lifestyle and social involvement. The British elderly held a eudaemonistic outlook in relation to the past when talking of a state of well-being and independence (positive affect), hard work and accomplishments (positive self-concept). However, their social involvement was currently reduced to giving the staff sweets, and health was regarded primarily as the absence of disease.

From the same study of a group of middle-aged working-class women cited earlier, Blaxter wrote in 1984 about control being striking in its absence. The women talked of how they believed disease is caused (and from this, beliefs about health may be inferred). They believed ill health to be caused by such factors as infections, poisons in the environment, poverty and childbirth. Individual behaviour and responsibility for oneself were rarely mentioned, which denotes an almost total absence of belief about power and control to enhance health. The research findings of Calnan (1987) reinforce those of Blaxter. Women in social classes I and II held eudaemonistic views of health, but the views of women in social classes IV and V were overwhelmingly about not being ill and 'getting through the day' (Blaxter, 1984, p.32).

Cognitive function was cited as a health image by only 10 per cent of the women in the study by Woods *et al.* (1988). Dubos (1995) wrote of the Greek goddess, Hygeia, that: 'She was the guardian of health and symbolized the belief that men could remain well if they lived according to reason' (p.7). Thus health depends on wisdom and reason – having a healthy mind would give one a healthy body. Indeed, a state of eudaemonia is defined as 'a full and active life governed by reason' (Chambers Dictionary, 1993). Dubos also described how the sister of Hygeia, Panakeia (from whom the word 'panacea' is derived), became more powerful, representing healing through drugs. A change in the status and power of Panakeia is taking place now at the start of a new millennium across all Western health services, with the reorientation from acute to primary health care (Department of Health, 1994; National Health Service Executive, 1996; World Health Organisation, 1985).

Beliefs about health as harmony, balance or equilibrium are mentioned by many authors, such as Dubos (1995), Calnan (1987) and Herzlich (1973). This is also a common theme with nurse theorists. The work of Parse draws heavily on that of Martha Rogers. Parse (1981) wrote of health as an interchange of energy which can enable or limit 'becoming', growing and choosing who one will be; health is the 'unique perspective of each human being experiencing self in the man–environment energy interchange' (p. 30). Of Martha Rogers, Daily *et al.* (1989) wrote that, although she used the word health in many of her earlier writings, she never really defined the term. However, Rogers describes the role of the nurse as promoting the *symphonic* interaction between man and the environment. Betty Neuman used a word to describe health (or wellness) with the same root as symphony, namely *harmony* (Neuman, cited in Harris *et al.*, 1989, p.366). Conner *et al.* (1989) wrote of beliefs about health underpinning the systems model of Dorothy Johnson as 'an elusive, dynamic state' involving 'the organisation, interaction, interdependence and integration' of subsystems (p.313). A lack of balance in the system causes poor health; this balance can be described as existing when 'a minimal amount of energy' is required for maintenance.

Health as self-fulfilment is frequently cited in the literature. Axline (1966), in *Dibs – In Search Of Self*, gives the following description of what it means to be a complete person: 'I guess Dibs only wanted what we all want on a world-wide scale. A chance to feel worthwhile. A chance to be a person wanted, respected, accepted as a human being worthy of dignity' (p.195). It seems that this category of the eudaemonistic model is one of the areas of health beliefs most favoured by nurse theorists. The following are all taken from chapters in the book edited by Marriner-Tomey (1989).

Nurse theorist	Health definition
Parse[3.1]	Growth, increasing complexity
Peplau[3.2]	Creation, construction, production, maturation
Wiedenbach[3.3]	Self-direction
Fitzpatrick[3.4]	Heightened awareness of the meaningfulness of life
Newman[3.5]	Expanded consciousness

Exogenous health beliefs – a fifth dimension

There are several other rather disparate conceptions of health which merit attention. They do not fit Smith's (1983) four models but have the unifying link of being very much external to the individual, or *exogenous*. The clinical, role performance, adaptive and eudaemonistic models are all *endogenous* beliefs. There are four main exogenous beliefs: health as an ideal; health as a commodity; health as a moral condition; and health as luck. The first two views are held mainly by professionals and the media, while the second two are mainly lay beliefs.

Health as an ideal

This is reflected in a description of health by Abdellah as a state with no unmet needs (Abdellah, cited in Dycus *et al.*, 1989). The often quoted, often criticised, World Health Organisation definition of health incorporated into the Declaration of Alma Ata in 1978, and now 50 years old, is usually categorised as an idealistic view of health (Seedhouse, 1986): 'a state of complete physical, mental and social well-being and not merely the absence of disease or infirmity' (World Health Organisation, 1988, p.7). However, the supposedly idealistic nature of this non-dynamic 'complete' state is mistaken. Laughlin and Black (1995) infer that the quote is almost always taken out of context causing its real meaning to be 'overlooked' (p.39). The World Health Organisation actually declared health to be 'not merely the absence of disease or infirmity', but *'a fundamental human right and that the attainment of the highest possible level of health is a most important world-wide social goal whose realization requires the action of many other social and economic sectors in addition to the health sector'* (World Health Organisation, 1988, p.7; author's italics). This statement could be the subject of a whole chapter in itself. Taking the entire quote, it is clear that the World Health Organisation definition fits more closely the third section of 'Role performance models of health' described earlier – society has a duty to provide people with the health which is their right.

Dubos (1995) likened the state of perfect health to a mirage or an illusion. He condemned contemporary dreamers who try to draw people to a Utopia which, by definition, is imaginary, so that the health we supposedly once held in some past 'golden age' could be reclaimed. Those who set up perfect health as the objective are usually trying to sell something. Dubos believed that the health service was 'selling' magic bullets of medicine or miracle cures that do not really exist. The fashion trade, cosmetic and food industries also set up, through advertising, an ideal that few can attain even if they buy the products. One of the hallmarks of the current era is the philosophy of 'wanna be' (I want to be) – a dissatisfaction with what one has because the media make it seem that most people have more. If self-esteem is one of the more important elements of health (Dickson, 1982), nurses must be cautious in promoting a view of *health for tomorrow* that by definition devalues what someone has today. Consider the following statement, written by Sally Brampton of *The Observer*, and found on the dust cover of a book by Walker and Cannon (1984): 'We have lost touch with what is naturally good for us to such an extent that few of us remember what the boundless energy and optimism engendered by good health actually feels like'.

Health as a commodity

Phrases such as 'clean bill of health' and 'healthy, wealthy and wise' epitomise this view of health as a commodity which is very closely linked by advertisers to health as an ideal. There is a very broad range of purchases which will supposedly help individuals to achieve perfect health. These include vitamins, membership of a gym, ionisers, water filters, track suits, books about diet, beds, bracelets, eye lotions, herbal products and anything which is organic or preservative free. The aim of the manufacturers is profit, not health. Thus arguments to buy are very persuasive, and often omit the drawbacks, such as the high fat and sugar content in some high fibre cereal bars, and the risks of food poisoning when preservatives are omitted. Snack manufacturers, hoping that sales can be increased if products are perceived as healthy, advertise on their packets with phrases such as 'jacket potatoes', 'baked potatoes', 'higher in fibre than traditional crisps', 'free from artificial colours, flavours and preservatives', 'natural vinegar flavour', 'nutritious snack' and 'cooked in the finest vegetable oil'.

The average low fat yoghurt is likely to contain ten times less fat than a packet of crisps. 'Low fat' crisps now have to be described as 'lower fat', as they still contain 60 per cent of the usual fat level of crisps. An interesting approach to this marketing dilemma has been taken by some firms, who have incorporated the supposed low fat nature of their product into the title of the organisation. Containing hardly any fat, and no salt, a medium-sized banana has twice as much fibre as high fibre crisps.

Patients are now clients and consumers of health care. Talk is of purchasing, buying in expertise, tenders and the right to private health care for those who can afford it. Seedhouse (1986), in his critique of this model, said that health as a commodity means that it is outside the responsibility of the individual. Thus health can be bought, sold, given, taken and lost, but the only personal investment required is money. Losing health might be just bad luck, like losing a wallet.

Health as luck

Richman (1987) wrote of the lay belief that ill health might be caused by bad luck or fate. Helman (1994) mentions the emphasis that some people place on the supposed health influence of the moon, sun and other planets in the form of astrology. Blaxter (1984) found that working-class women believed that tuberculosis or cancer could occur at random. Comments were made reflecting this fatalistic view: 'It could happen to anyone' and 'I'm just the type'. When studying beliefs about health and illness among working-class Londoners, Cornwell (1984) heard frequent comments about fate, destiny and health being a matter of luck or a lottery. Beliefs about chance and bad luck being a cause of AIDS have been found among young people (Aggleton et al., 1989). The obvious dangers of all of these views are that people will be less likely to feel empowered to promote health or to avoid illness than they would if a more rational belief existed.

Health as a moral condition

Lay belief that one is morally responsible for one's own health is common. Health, or the lack of it, is caused not by a healthy lifestyle but by being a good or bad person. The terms 'good health' and 'bad health' reinforce the notion that one may be rewarded according to the kind of person one is. Cornwell (1984) found that 'being good' was about hard work, moderation, virtue, cleanliness and decency. If people were 'good', she found that reports of their ill health were described as unjust and undeserved. Cornwell also reported that people wished to hide illness as if they were ashamed of it, and were prone to making excuses about symptoms. One man with eczema was at pains to explain the cleanliness of the house he lived in and that his eating habits were good. The morality of health hinges on beliefs about ascribing guilt. A current example of this is seen in ideas about some people with HIV being 'innocent' (haemophiliacs and babies) and others being 'guilty' (gay men and drug users) (Aggleton *et al.*, 1989). Guilt inducement is used in some health education campaigns to manipulate people's behaviour. Examples of this include the television advertisement aimed at men who, in risking heart disease, risk the livelihood and comfort of their family, and also the poster showing a smoking pregnant woman with the slogan 'Do you want this cigarette more than you want this baby?' Charles and Kerr (1986) describe how 'good' and 'bad' food are used as issues with women who are caught between salads and quiches or feeding their husbands with 'proper' food because they 'deserve' it.

Implications of this discussion of health beliefs

It should be apparent from reading the first half of this chapter that beliefs about health are very varied and are frequently defended with passion. Preparing people to be health care professionals for the future has to be as complex as these beliefs are diverse. Indeed, writing about what it means to be healthy, the subtitle of the book by Stainton Rogers (1991) is *An Exploration of Diversity*. Those who are developing a health-oriented curriculum for the education of nurses will find in these pages much to digest about the need for the inclusion of a very different knowledge base. This will include, for example, ethics, politics, sociology, ethnography, media studies, history, economics, epidemiology, philosophy, self-reflection, values clarification and, above all, the ability to view health as a multifaceted issue. Meleis (1991) believed that the way forward has to be with health as a central concept in nursing. She argued that, to make progress with this approach, 'the unity and diversity among these models need to be addressed, compared, and contrasted' and above all *integrated* (Meleis, 1991, p.112).

Health and well-being into the next millennium?

With the simple addition of a question mark, this section draws its title from the *Regional Strategy for Northern Ireland* (Department of Health and Social Services, 1996). This publication is the updated equivalent of *The Health of the Nation* White Paper (Department of Health, 1992). It seems appropriate to ask two central questions, although it is not the remit of this chapter to provide comprehensive answers. These are, 'Have the words and actions of the people (from politician to field worker) with the power to change and improve the lot of the disadvantaged been more than rhetoric?' and 'What have we learned about the art and science of creating, maintaining and promoting health which would be of value to take into the future?'

With regard to the first question, the sincerity of the values underpinning initiatives or the pragmatism of the planners and implementers is not in question, but where adequate finance does not follow proposed change there is, realistically, little which can be done. Should we do a little for many people or a lot for a few people? We have mainly been doing the former and have thus, many would argue, increased the health divide between the 'haves' and the 'have nots' (Townsend *et al.*, 1988; Whitehead, 1991).

The main problem with the second question is that practice appears to be lagging about 20 years behind the visionaries. We are only now in the last couple of years comfortable using phrases such as community participation, targeting, profiling community need, healthy alliances, disadvantage, empowerment and equity. Meanwhile, global problems continue to escalate and concerns have moved rapidly on to the environmental issue of *sustainability*. The basis of *Health For All 2000* is *equity*. Inequity has been defined as unfair, avoidable differences between people (Whitehead, 1990). Crombie (1995) asserted that equity is a more practical goal than equality – the idealistic term with which it has often been confused. Having barely encroached on the problems of equity for individuals, groups, communities and countries we must urgently take up the challenges of *intergenerational* equity. Crombie (1995) wrote:

> While health professionals have been concerned with the health of people in the here and now, for obvious reasons, equity and sustainability now require a longer term view of human health.
>
> (Crombie, 1995, p.7)

Some of the areas of conflict outlined in the first edition of this text have been long resolved, for example the debate over definitions of *health promotion* and *health education*. Even so, practice has lagged behind research and theory development. It is still not uncommon to see health care professionals and even planners, purchasers and authors using the two terms as if they are synonymous. Thus a brief discussion of an old kernel starts this section.

What is health promotion?

It is obviously vital to decide what the term health promotion covers, as it is something all registered nurses must be competent to advise on (Statutory Instrument, 1983). It most definitely should not be used synonymously with health education (Tones, 1996). Clarification of the meanings of both these terms should enable nurses to become more aware of the extent of our role.

Strehlow (1983) was an early writer on the role of the nurse in the achievement of health. She was ahead of her time in her knowledge of the importance of the *Health For All 2000* movement. However, in her text this was mixed up with an individualistic approach based on government beliefs about where the responsibility for health should be focused (Department of Health and Social Security, 1976). While she wrote of 'the promotion of health' (Strehlow, 1983, p.4), other authors had very different concepts in mind when using the phrase 'health promotion' (Walt and Constantinides, 1983, paragraph 24). Strehlow was in fact talking only of health education, and even this she seemed reluctant to define, stating that, 'There is no consensus regarding health education' (Strehlow, 1983, p.7). She argued that health education is a pervasive, flexible activity which is not bounded by custom or tradition. The limitless unpopular scope of health education was the daily life of the recipients. Strehlow saw health education as health professionals teaching about health to individuals and groups of all ages and at all stages of life. Compare this with a state of the art definition from authors currently involved in health promotion from national, strategic, managerial and moral philosophical approaches:

> Health education is communication activity aimed at enhancing positive health and preventing or diminishing ill-health in individuals and groups through influencing the beliefs, attitudes, and behaviour of those with power and of the community at large.
>
> (Downie *et al.*, 1996, p.28)

The beliefs that Walt and Constantinides (1983) held about health promotion are summarised in Figure 3.5. They described it as being at one end of a continuum, with health education near the opposite end. Health education places the responsibility for health on individuals who, once informed of unhealthy behaviour, are then at fault if they do not act to improve their health. The basis of health promotion is a belief that people do not always have the power to change their behaviour. The prerequisite enabling people to change is a transformation of the environment in which they live and work. One of the problems inherent in health promotion is its all-pervasiveness. A decade on, using words reminiscent of those Strehlow used to critique health education, Jones (1994) took a similar line when writing about this 'healthy public policy approach': 'The territory of health, it seems, has been redefined as bound up with the whole of life' (p.544). Furthermore, '"caring for health" has expanded into a potential surveillance of all aspects of daily life' (Jones, 1994, p.545).

Are health education and health promotion poles apart as a continuum might suggest? Noack (1987) polarised the activities in a very similar way to Walt and Constantinides (1983). He wrote of two major types of health promotion. The individual health approach is about personal behaviour change in response to health education. A community (i.e. population) health approach is described as being very different to the personal one in terms of its goals and strategies. It involves different sectors of society such as housing, pollution control, traffic safety and the production, taxation and sale of products which affect health. Promotion of health by this approach is achieved by seeking changes in policy, legislation and administration to

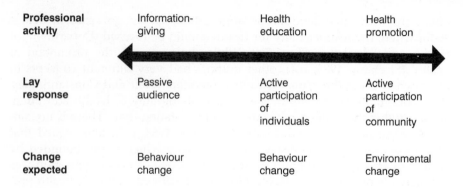

Professional activity	Information-giving	Health education	Health promotion
Lay response	Passive audience	Active participation of individuals	Active participation of community
Change expected	Behaviour change	Behaviour change	Environmental change

Figure 3.5 Walt and Constantinides' (1983) view of health education and health promotion

improve working conditions and to reduce the negative consequences of industrialisation, urbanisation and the distribution of wealth.

A preliminary analysis of the *health promotion model* (HPM) developed by an influential American nurse (Pender, 1996) indicates that it, too, is a polarised model. The HPM has been extensively tested and refined over the last 10 years. In the model, Pender describes health protection as action related to illness – avoiding illness, detecting it at an early stage, or learning to live with it. Health promotion for Pender is about increasing well-being.

Tannahill (1985) proposed a concept of health promotion which *included* health education, rather than polarising it. Health education as part of health promotion means the latter becomes a broader umbrella expression that includes other activities apart from the communication of health information to the public. This model 'is widely accepted by health care workers' and is essentially 'descriptive of what goes on in practice' (Naidoo and Wills, 1994, p.97). In this model, health promotion is defined as:

> efforts to enhance positive health and reduce the risk of ill-health, through the overlapping spheres of health education, prevention and health protection.
>
> (Downie *et al.*, 1996, p.60)

The three overlapping spheres of activity of which health promotion is composed are discussed extensively by Downie *et al.* (1996). A practical example of its application to family planning is given by McBean (1992c), as it can be difficult to tease all seven elements of this model apart.

The priorities

It has been suggested that the appropriate emphasis of health promotion in developing countries would be the *population approach,* whereas in developed countries it should be the *individual approach* (Noack, 1987; World Health Organisation, 1986). However, population-oriented activity is directed at ensuring that the prerequisites for health exist as a context within which individual choices about behaviour can be made. After examining a list of health prerequisites, it is abundantly clear that the deficits in the UK also require a population approach (see Table 3.3).

In 1986, the World Health Organisation adopted a resolution defining *intersectoral cooperation* in national strategies for *Health For All 2000* as the recognition 'that factors which influence health are found in all major sectors of development' (World Health Organisation, 1986, p.9). The World Health Organisation (1986) submitted that changing to a healthy lifestyle in a non-conducive environment is like trying to roll an impossibly heavy ball up a steep incline (see Figure 3.6). Changes in behaviour can only realistically occur if the slope of the incline is reduced by improvements in sectors of society such as agriculture, housing, education and employment.

Nursing education – imperatives

The word 'imperative' is very powerful, and has been used here to signify the critical nature of the response of nurse educators and nursing as a whole to the issues raised in this chapter. The Chambers Dictionary (1993) gives several meanings for the word, all of which reinforce this point, namely 'command', 'urgently necessary', 'calling out for action', 'authoritative' and 'obligatory'. The 1986 World Health Assembly met to discuss 'the role of intersectoral cooperation in national strategies for health for all' (World Health Organisation, 1986, p.7). The UK was called upon, along with other Member States of the World Health Organisation, to:

> ensure that the training of health professionals at all levels encompasses an adequate awareness of the relationships between environment, living conditions, life-styles and local health problems in order to enable them to establish a meaningful collaboration with professionals in other health-related sectors.
>
> (World Health Organisation, 1986, p.10)

The term 'intersectoral cooperation' can be taken broadly to mean multiagency or interagency collaboration, and indeed can be taken to mean healthy alliances in the current terminology of the government. Examples of sectors include housing, education, retailers, health and transport. Sectors of society often have a government department guiding and controlling affairs.

Table. 3.3   Health prerequisites (after World Health Organisation, 1985, pp. 14–21)

Decent food at prices within people's means
Basic education to increase levels of literacy
A continuous supply of safe drinking water
Proper sanitation
Decent housing at a reasonable price
Secure work and a useful role in society providing an adequate income
Freedom from the fear of war (particularly nuclear war)

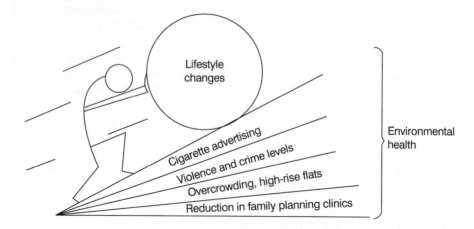

Figure 3.6   Changing to a healthy lifestyle in a non-conducive environment (adapted from World Health Organisation, 1986)

Agencies tend to be more local to a community. Examples of agencies include social work, probation, police, ministers of religion, community nurses, public health doctors, environmental health, youth workers and teachers. Change requires everyone involved to analyse the costs and benefits to themselves. Not involving local representatives can mean that initiatives may be blocked. Collaborative working can potentially harness much power for change. The need for an holistic approach to the care of individuals is widely accepted because individuals are more than the sum of their parts. Similarly, the social context in which people make decisions is more than the sum of *its parts* – it is a multidimensional and multifaceted existence. The World Health Organisation edict above means that nurse education must help future practitioners not only to understand the need for, but to be skilled at, working together with the many stakeholders who each hold a different key to unlocking the potential for change.

In 1989, an English National Board document sought to guide the development of the (then) new Project 2000 curricula along the above lines. The Common Foundation Programme should include an exploration of power and social change and an examination of local, national and international policies (English National Board for Nursing, Midwifery and Health Visiting, 1989). However, social, political and environmental influences were said to be only *in addition* to other subjects. Frost and Nunkoosing (1989), in setting out a framework of possible areas to be included in a Common Foundation Programme, mentioned the word 'health' only three times – as a goal of nursing, in relation to recreation and as various health care policies. These seem to be extras rather than core issues. In addition, nursing suffers from the problem of attempting too much. We require our completing students to have some of the skills of technician, manager, teacher, counsellor, family therapist and researcher. Little time is left for an understanding of social policy, politics, ethics, history, epidemiology and, in particular, the collaborative skills in question.

When the first edition of this book was written, the UK government, unlike Australia, Canada and the USA, had failed to respond with written guidelines on how to meet the targets we had signed up to some 5 years previously (World Health Organisation, 1985). However, with the publication of the White Paper, *The Health of the Nation* (Department of Health, 1992), and similar regional papers in Scotland, Northern Ireland and Wales, national priorities for health have now been explored. In common with the other nations listed above (Epp, 1987; Gott, 1988; Robbins, 1987), there is now some clarity about the health-promoting responsibilities of health care workers. There are three documents in particular which contribute to an understanding of the health promotion roles and responsibilities of nurses, midwives and health visitors. These are *Targeting Practice: the Contribution of Nurses, Midwives and Health Visitors* (Department of Health, 1993), *Making it Happen: Public Health – the Contribution of Nurses, Midwives and Health Visitors* (Department of Health, 1995) and *Primary Care – The Future* (National Health Service Executive, 1996).

Over two decades ago a then popular nursing text (Pearce, 1971) highlighted the significance of *public health measures*. Until recently, public health as part of the curriculum has been in decline. Educationalists should note the arguments that a 'New Public Health' is needed – a restoration of the UK's public health heritage (Public Health Alliance, 1988). It is only in this way that it will be possible to face new and old challenges, such as food poisoning and homelessness, poverty and sustainability. Discussion about the New Public Health can be found in journals such as *Health Promotion International* and *Critical Public Health*, and via membership of the Public Health Alliance (information can be obtained from Public Health Alliance, 138 Digbeth, Birmingham, B5 6DR). The text, *The Nation's Health: a Strategy for the 1990s*, is also excellent (Jacobson *et al.*, 1991).

Encouragingly, literature to support curriculum developments in promoting health is much more evident than at the time of writing for the first edition of this book, although the best materials are still unlikely to be widely available. There are now a few American health promotion texts specifically for nurses (Edelman and Mandle, 1994; Pender, 1996) but they tend to take a personal approach to promoting health, and thus the emphasis is more on assessment and teaching of individuals than on community approaches. However, a number of health promotion texts aimed at a multidisciplinary readership complement the ones for nurses, and these take a broader intersectoral and community participation approach (Katz and Peberdy, 1997; Naidoo and Wills, 1994; Pike and Forster, 1995; Scriven and Orme, 1996; Wass, 1994). *Health Visitor, Health Education Journal* and *Primary Health Care* increasingly carry articles of interest to nurses with a health promotion remit. Nursing students at pre- and post-registration stages need ready access to the kind of books and journals listed above on the New Public Health and community approaches to promoting health.

High profile, high gloss

Williams (1984) was aware of the possibility of health promotion evolving in an unsatisfactory direction when she wrote of slick salesmanship. Similarly, Tannahill (1987) warned of the dangers of dashing off on the latest bandwagon. The practice of health promotion by specialists is perhaps only now emerging from a decade of difficulty brought about by changes in NHS culture superimposed on global edicts for new emphases in methods and priorities.

In the late 1980s and early 1990s, most local departments and staff with specialist training changed their title from Health Education to Health Promotion. Health Education Units, until the early 1980s, were like Aladdin's Caves. A visit could produce a wealth of free, high quality material for use with groups of any age, on any subject – from poisonous toadstools to safety on the beach. Now one might have to pay to borrow loan materials, or to obtain disposable items such as posters and leaflets. Furthermore, it is likely that help will be confined to a limited number of key areas identified as priorities for policy, namely heart disease, smoking, substance misuse, immunisation, stress, exercise, cancer, dental health, HIV/AIDS and sexual health. Most staff were acutely aware of the need for the time consuming, slower, community and population approaches to take priority over individual, purely educational strategies. While the underpinning philosophy may have been that health cannot be improved by education alone, with limited staff numbers and funds a glossy, media 'educative' approach was often necessary for survival. As the NHS grappled with the internal market, health promotion specialists struggled to work out whether they should be purchasers or providers, and groaned under the burden of specialist work wherein each member of staff had to attend to giving their particular lifestyle message to all major groups of society.

What's in a name?

When the Health Education Council (England) demised in 1987, why did we see the creation of a Health *Education* Authority (HEA), not a Health *Promotion* Authority? What do the words mean? 'Council' means deliberation, discussion and advice (Chambers Dictionary, 1993). Is the HEA *in* authority or *an* authority, that is in control or a knowledgeable expert? Prior to the NHS reforms, it was probably the former, and subsequently only the latter. A major difference between the HEA when it first took over and the old HEC was a much higher level of expensive mass media advertising to attempt to get health messages across to the public. However, Aggleton and Homans (1987) argued that mass media campaigns generally produce only short-term increases in knowledge, and only a slight shift in attitudes. Anomalies exist in the other countries of the UK. In 1987, freed from central London administration with the loss of the HEC, Wales set up a new regional body, interestingly called the Health Promotion Authority for

Wales. In 1991, Scotland chose to retain the 'education' title when it set up a Health Education Board to replace a Health Education Group. Northern Ireland, however, chose newer terms and opted for Health Promotion Agency.

If Health Promotion Units work around a group of disease topics, and focus on the behaviour and responsibility of the individual, their use of the word 'promotion' does not fit the broad community-oriented concepts outlined above. Williams (1984) made a strong case for *promotion* in the Health Promotion Unit sense to mean hard sell and salesmanship. This technique, she believed, may trade on our fears and insecurities as well as our eternal optimism about health. Williams advised caution in continuing to sell ideas for health. When people purchase goods there is usually a tangible product for the outlay. However, if we 'buy' healthy lifestyles the immediate effects may be only pain and effort. Caution is also advisable with regard to manipulating lives to improve statistics. Dental health may improve if sweets are cut out but, if children eat more nuts and crisps instead, cholesterol levels will increase. Williams advocated a more appropriate style of health promotion in activities such as lobbying to have sugar and salt removed from canned foods.

Tannahill (1987) claimed that having diseases or behaviours as priority topics does not make sense. Recently, in a short discussion paper about how Scotland made the transition, *From Priorities to Programmes*, he criticised the topic-based approach as 'seriously flawed' (Tannahill, 1994, p.3). A topic basis results in staff titles such as Health Promotion Officer (HPO) for Coronary Heart Disease, HPO for HIV/AIDS, HPO for Smoking and HPO for Substance Misuse. Two staff would be working on disease prevention and two on behaviours. All four staff would be targeting health promotion programmes in schools and workplaces! A far more holistic, positive and, more importantly, efficient and effective programme would use key community settings such as schools, workplaces and large public institutions, such as hospitals and universities. Staff titles thus become, for example, HPO for Youth Settings and HPO for Workplaces. This move to a settings approach is probably the biggest change to affect health promotion specialists during the last decade. It is important for nurses to adopt for their own work the strengths of this more holistic model as opposed to a medical model or behaviourist approach.

Issues requiring action or clarification

Redman (1993, p.725), when reviewing 25 years of research into patient education, argued that it was far from being a 'mature technology'. Health promotion as a broader discipline with a longer history and deeper roots *is* maturing now. Some of the issues and problems which remain are outlined below. One of the greatest of these (see also Figure 3.7) is that 'Official support for different approaches to health promotion is given in inverse relation to their effectiveness' (Stone, 1989, p.890).

Other issues and problems include the following:

First, in the previous edition of this book it was suggested that whenever the term 'health promotion' is used the underlying assumptions and interpretations should be clarified (Tannahill, 1987). There has been much progress over the past few years, some of it documented in this chapter. When the term health promotion is used now it should be possible to assume that it has the broad meaning discussed earlier (Downie *et al.*, 1996) and is not being used *instead of* health education. The worst situation, to be avoided, is the not uncommon tendency to use the two terms together. For example, to speak of 'the role of the nurse in health promotion and health education' suggests a misunderstanding of the fact that the former *includes* the latter!

Secondly, clarification is also required concerning the goals of pre-registration courses. Butterworth (1989) described the Project 2000 diploma programme as a 'child' of *Health For All 2000*. The World Health Organisation (1985) stated that pre-registration education should particularly emphasise primary health care and community needs. In the 'Heathrow Debate' it was argued that 'Project 2000 is in its early days. It will need to be fully bedded in and ... carefully reviewed' (Department of Health, 1994, p.18). This infers that Project 2000 may need some further changes if it is really to take nursing practice into the next millennium. Orr (1995) expressed concern that first, there may be too much health promotion in pre-registration courses, to the detriment of input on high dependency skills, and secondly, student nurses should be prepared for patient teaching and health education, but a pre-registration course could not be expected to deliver health promotion skills. However, Luker and Caress (1989) argued that it is beyond the scope of nurse training to acquire a high level of ability in teaching patients when such skills take up to 4 years to acquire. They wrote that:

> the wisdom of involving all nurses ... in patient education is challenged as an unrealistic and undesirable goal ... a course of anything up to 4 years in length is presently considered the minimum necessary to acquire the skills in the teaching of schoolchildren ... . Adult educationalists have argued that the teaching of adults involves concepts which make it yet more complex than the teaching of children ... it seems unreasonable to suggest that nurse training ... as detailed in the proposals for ... *Project 2000* ... can encompass the breadth and depth of knowledge necessary to teach patients.
>
> (Luker and Caress, 1989, pp.711–712)

The World Health Organisation (1985) also suggested that teachers would have training needs for designing and implementing the new curricula. This would be very reasonable because, in the 1970s, when many of our current nurse teachers began nursing, only around one third of them had any community experience. Orr (1995) suggested that problems in pre-registration courses may exist because of scarce community qualifications among teachers. Even in the mid-1980s, pre-registration community experience was counted in hours, not weeks. Perhaps the lack of extra training for nurse teachers contributes to the problematic situation in which we still appear to expect most nurses from the adult branch to work in acute services on qualifying. Student nurses seem to be too worried about their physiology and pharmacology examinations to have the time to take a copy of *The Black Report and The Health Divide* (Townsend *et al.,* 1988) off the shelves.

Thirdly, Robbins argued that 'The National Health Service ... has little control or influence over the determinants of health ... . Health is gained, maintained or lost in the worlds of work, leisure, home and city life' (Robbins, 1987, p.17). Debate has taken place over the advisability of using NHS staff to promote health, when clearly most of those staff work mainly with individuals rather than with groups, communities and populations. In addition, contact with people is mainly as patients, 90 per cent of them in acute care areas, leading to the tendency for a medical model approach. Despite this, in *The Health of the Nation* (Department of Health, 1992) the government placed great emphasis on the importance of the NHS:

> The success of this strategy will depend to a great extent on the commitment and skills of the health professionals within the NHS.
> (Department of Health, 1992, p.5)

Despite the emphasis on a primary care led NHS (National Health Service Executive, 1996), it seems that the main developments envisaged for community nurses concern issues such as nurse prescribing, clinical developments such as minor injuries clinics and secondary prevention such as screening and the management of chronic diseases. However, public health nursing is listed as one of three broad areas for practice in the future. This would include working at the level of communities for needs assessment and for meeting those needs.

Tannahill (1984) suggested that free rational choice is illusory. The Conservative government from 1979 onwards showed that they believed individuals *do* have freedom, control, power and choice. The previous Labour government had similar beliefs about people's health (Department of Health and Social Security, 1976). In contrast, Rodmell and Watt (1986) wrote that choice had been *reified*, that is described as a real and almost concrete object instead of as an abstract potential.

One of the important roles for nurses is helping people to *make sense* of their choices (see Antonovsky's model in Figure 3.4). Other roles for nurses have been described by various authors. Edelman and Milio (1994) suggested the roles of advocate, facilitator, coordinator, consultant, educator, researcher and collaborator. Skills in leadership, creativity, health assessment and mediation will also be required (Edelman and Milio, 1994; Gott, 1988; Morton, 1989). Above all, nurses must first become whole themselves (Chinn, 1988), so that they can release the power they have to promote healing in others (see Chapter 6). Milio (cf. Draper, 1986) suggested that nurses move along a continuum which has love and caring at one end and power and coercion at the other. She wrote that this love 'provides that minimal level of social trust that allows individuals to work together sufficiently to turn decisions into a lasting, sustained reality' (Milio, cited in Draper, 1986, p.105). Nurse theorists make much of the special therapeutic relationships which nurses can engender. Presumably health messages should spring from this philosophy of therapy and care, mutual support and social trust. Nurses must have the time that is required to build and nurture these special relationships – time which can so easily be lost in the current drive for efficiency. Otherwise 'we are tattering the social fabric that sustains us, and in the process the most disadvantaged among us are the first to topple into uncertainty, want and illness' (Milio, cited in Draper, 1986, p.105).

Fourthly, it is necessary to be 'more explicit about where responsibilities for health rest as well as about what those responsibilities are' (Smith and Jacobson, 1988, p.1). Since the publication of *Prevention and Health: Everybody's Business* (Department of Health and Social Security, 1976), the conclusion has been that this responsibility lies with the individual. However, the most important health determinants have been shown to relate to socio-environmental engineering of public health issues by legislation and taxation (McKeown, 1979). Stone (1987) asserted that, while attempts to change individual behaviour receive high levels of support from professionals, these methods are relatively ineffective (see Figure 3.7). He also argued that immunisation and monophasic screening, such as cervical smears, have proven value, but multiphasic screening, for example work done in a well man clinic, has not been shown to have significant effects, despite trials lasting for many years. Care needs to be taken in case so much time is spent pulling drowning individuals out of the river that no one remembers to look upstream to see who is pushing them in or why they fall in (McKinley, cited in Tones, 1981).

A universal model of health promotion?

The framework presented in Figure 3.8 is a combination of Tannahill's (1985) model of three overlapping spheres of activity and a model proposed by the World Health Organisation (1984). Tannahill (1987) sees health education as the key sphere, while Stone (1989) argues that health protection is the most effective area for effort (see also Figure 3.7). These three lines of approach give a subtle, useful and dynamic view of health promotion which is a long way from the idea that it is something different to, or simply the same as, health education.

Some key issues in health education

The risk approach

Because most people are concerned more with the threat of illness than with health, the notion of risk has become part of our thinking about

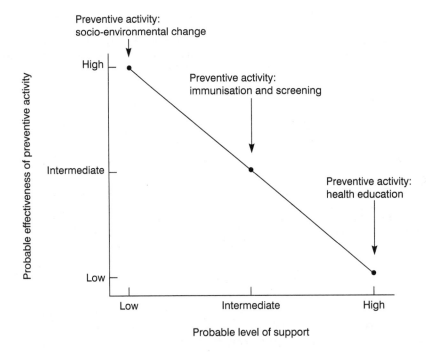

Figure 3.7 The inverse relationship between different approaches to health promotion and their effectiveness (after Stone, 1989)

the prevention of disease – the *chances* of health being thought of as a low risk of illness. We do not speak of our 'vulnerability to health'.

(Backett *et al.*, 1984, p.1)

Dwore and Matarazzo (1981) asserted that practice in health promotion had preceded theory development. There is some evidence that this is still the case more than 15 years later, for example the difficulty in predicting outcomes related to behaviour (Williams, 1984) and in particular concerns regarding diet and heart disease (Oliver, 1982, 1987, 1988, 1991, 1992, 1993).

The type of advice about which such concerns have been raised can still be seen in health education materials today, but was epitomised by a leaflet circulated by the Health Education Council, *Beating Heart Disease* (Health Education Council, 1984). The message to the public in this leaflet included accusing people of *gambling* with life because of their behaviour, suggesting that risky behaviour means every day holds a life-or-death question, and assuring the reader that the risk of developing heart disease and dying can be reduced. In fact, the language of *reducing* is lost on the reader. The gambling/life-or-death phrases are likely to make the reader think that it is all or nothing, and therefore a potentially false hope that change will bring certain health (and perhaps longevity). Several authors cited in this chapter have questioned these suppositions, for example Farrant and Russell (1986) and Williams (1984).

Insurance companies and the military have been using the concept of *susceptibility to risk* since the turn of the century (Alexander, 1988). Although the

Tannahill (1985)	World Health Organisation (1984)
(1) *Health education* Educational activity aimed at positively enhancing well-being and the use of preventive and non-preventive health services	*Promotion of self-help and self-care* What people *do* themselves to promote their own health
(2) *Prevention* Preventive procedures such as immunisation and screening	*Extended opportunities, more accessible services* Actions which make it *easier* for people to promote their health, by providing cycle tracks, family planning facilities, immunisation, safe play areas, etc.
(3) *Health protection* Decisions by local, national and international government or other influential bodies in industry and commerce which promote health	*Creation of a healthier environment* Improving the environment without necessarily requiring individual effort, by reducing lead levels, imposing speed limits, improving housing, etc.

Figure 3.8　A universal model of health promotion

concept of risk is not new, it should be remembered that its application in the health service is recent (Backett *et al.*, 1984). Use of the *risk approach* in health education has only been subjected to research processes in the last two decades, and is not yet thoroughly underpinned by theory. In 1976, the Department of Health and Social Security wrote of risk factors for coronary heart disease, saying that 'we have little real evidence as yet to show that getting rid of these attributes reduces the statistical risk' (p.62). Reducing risk factors may be a plausible means of decreasing morbidity but it is not yet proven, except perhaps in the case of smoking. In extensive studies, Peto *et al.* (1994) have shown that stopping smoking, even in middle age after half a lifetime of smoking, means that most of the risk of death from tobacco is removed.

Backett *et al.* (1984) described the situation thus: 'The hypothesis on which the risk approach rests, therefore, is that the more accurate these measures of risk are the more readily will the need for help be understood and the better or more effective will be the response' (p.2). The assumptions in this hypothesis and the use of the high-risk strategy have been questioned by many authors. Rose (1981) disputed the value of using the risk approach with individuals. He advocated a mass approach to dealing with risk, such as reducing salt intake. Rose suggested that the individual approach may be much more limited than was initially realised. Large benefits are conferred on only a few people with high-risk factors, while in fact a major part of the morbidity and mortality figures is comprised of large numbers of people exposed to only a low-risk. This he called a *prevention paradox*. Rose wrote that, 'The mass approach is inherently the only ultimate answer to the problem of a mass disease' (p.1850). He argued that the downward shifting of diastolic blood pressure by a mere 2–3 mmHg might equal all the life-saving benefits of current antihypertensive treatment. A decade later, Rose (1992) was still just as convinced of the 'irony' (p.12) of the fact that many people must change their behaviour in order to bring a benefit to a few. He was not only concerned about flaws underpinning the concept of risk applied to individuals but also in the application to populations.

Alexander (1988) also questioned the ascendancy of the risk factors notion which ignores the issue of the link between disease causation and socio-economic status. On this point, Farrant and Russell (1986) argued for the reduction of the effects of chronic psychosocial stress to be considered in reducing coronary heart disease (see Chapters 4 and 5). Seedhouse (1986) suggested a need to assess the degree of *risk of the intervention*. Drug treatment for hyperlipidaemia is apparently relatively safe, but Rose (1981) estimated one death per 1000 patients treated.

Rose posited difficulties for health education message framing: 'a risk which has not materialized within the individual's own experience is unlikely to be regarded seriously' (Rose, 1992, p.22). McLeroy (1989) argued for the importance of framing health messages correctly, otherwise the public might develop an aversion to the concept of risk. Conflicting information with regard to recommendations for behaviour would thus cause confusion or irritation. Wilson *et al.* (1988) discussed three ways of framing messages of health:

- *Gain* – if you change to this new behaviour there will be a positive consequence;
- *Loss*– if you fail to change to this new behaviour you will not experience a positive consequence;
- *Fear* – if you continue to engage in the old behaviour you will experience a negative consequence.

However, there are no indications from research as to which approach might prove most effective with different client health beliefs. Mikhail (1981) and Hill and Shugg (1989) believed that nurses should provide clients with information on the *benefits of change*. Research by Sennott-Miller and Miller (1987) suggested that the opposite is the case. What health workers have failed to do in the past is to frame messages in a fourth way: to help clients to focus on, and overcome, the difficulties of new lifestyles. They often know what the consequences of behaviours are, but need help with the *means of change*.

Another problem with the concept of medical and educative intervention after screening for high-risk factors is that the largest recent trial to demonstrate the effectiveness of this measure for coronary heart disease was inconclusive (Oliver, 1982). This American trial lasted for 7 years and involved nearly 13 000 participants. It may be that social pressure to *conform* could be more effective in reducing levels of risk factors such as obesity and smoking than advice to change behaviour for medical reasons (Rose, 1981). Morgan *et al.* (1985) wrote that campaigns which aim to reduce the likelihood of developing disease use an epidemiological model. This explanation of disease causation used by experts was not found in the constructs (see Chapter 5) of any lay beliefs examined by Calnan and Johnson (1983). People either had general fears of diseases to which they did not feel personally vulnerable, or they believed that they were vulnerable because a disease was present in the family. This theory of inheritance presumably indicated a fatalistic view, with little likelihood of being able to alter the risk by changing behaviour.

The Oxford Prevention of Heart Attack and Stroke Project used nurse facilitators to encourage a systematic case finding approach to hypertension, smoking and obesity (Fullard, 1989). So far this has only shown an increase in recording of these indices in patients' notes. Tudor-Hart (1985) argued that 50 per cent of the people who are known to have hypertension are not being treated, and of those being treated 50 per cent are not well controlled. The persistent problem of payments to general practitioners being based on the *recording* of risk factors rather than on effective interventions was criticised by Toon (1995). Referring to 'massive indiscriminate collection of data of no proven value', Toon (1995, p.1084) argued that this strategy is flawed, not least because effective interventions for these noted risk factors have not yet been identified.

On the smoking front, the work of Macleod Clark *et al.* (1987) suggested that health care workers would need additional training to assist a move away from a prescriptive form of health education, if their interventions are to be successful. However, heightened susceptibility to disease will not necessarily be associated with intentions to act (Hill and Shugg, 1989). In addition, it may be the perceived or real difficulty of changing which has more impact on behaviour than potential benefits (Sennot-Miller and Miller, 1987). Thus simply identifying people with risk factors does not mean that they will necessarily receive the treatment they need or an effective form of health education, and they may focus more on the real problems of new behaviour than on the more abstract advantages of reducing risk. Reducing difficulty and increasing social pressure may facilitate change more effectively than an individual risk approach. The targets of *Heartbeat Wales* were those of a mass strategy, and included 'restricting smoking in public places, better food labelling, price incentives, increasing availability of "healthy" foods in shops, workplace canteens and restaurants' (Catford and Parish, 1989, p.129).

With question marks hanging over the risk reduction approach, it may be useful to differentiate between *health-protecting behaviours* which are risk and disease prevention oriented and the more positive concept of a *health-promoting lifestyle*. This is discussed by Cohen and Jaffe (1994), McKeown (1979) and Walker *et al.* (1988). They describe seven habits for good health:

- sleeping for 7 to 8 hours per night ;
- eating breakfast;
- avoiding snacks between meals;
- maintaining near optimal weight;
- exercising daily;
- consuming alcohol moderately;
- avoiding smoking.

Research in America showed that adopting six or seven of these habits halved mortality rates compared with people who followed zero to three habits. The health of elderly people who followed most of the habits was said to be as good as the health of people 30 to 40 years younger who followed only a few of them. However, uptake of all seven habits was thought to be as low as 10 to 20 per cent of the population. It has not yet been clarified why health promoting lifestyles should be more successful than health protecting behaviours. It may be that risk reduction is attempted too late, after much damage has already been done, while health promoting lifestyles may have been ongoing for many years, thus preventing damage. There are, however, many unanswered questions. What is the role of sleep? Why is a general approach to health effective in reducing the incidence of many diseases, while a specific approach to one disease, such as cardiovascular disease, shows mixed results? While awaiting answers to these questions it is important that we note the implications of being over-prescriptive, and that we avoid dogmatism about risk factors in the absence of more assurance.

Individualism

Naidoo (1986) wrote that individualism is 'the dominant ideology underlying modern health education practice' (p.17). She argued that there are three main criticisms of this approach:

- the denial of social effects on health;
- the assumption that people have free choice; and
- its general ineffectiveness.

Rodmell and Watt (1986) suggested that, as 'lifestylism', individual approaches involve the pathologisation of typical conduct. In causing a sense of moral failure and inadequacy, lifestylism is unhealthy and unhelpful.

Arguing for a new focus for strategies to improve health, Chapman (1987) compared health education to a *host-directed approach* such as the administering of antimalarial drugs. He advocated vector and environment directed strategies, such as draining the swamps in which mosquitoes live. With smoking, for example, vector and environment directed strategies would be aimed at the tobacco industry and the socio-cultural and political climate. In the case of malaria, this would mean the reduction or eradication of mosquitoes. If ill health is directly attributed to individual behaviour alone, then it becomes easy to blame people as they have supposedly inflicted damage on themselves (Naidoo, 1986). Examples of this kind of guilt inducing victim blaming are common, for example smoking during pregnancy, obesity, HIV and AIDS, and almost all conditions that are directly or indirectly related to stress, from gastric ulcers to arthritis. Even hypothermia in the elderly has been suggested as being caused by them leaving windows open at night and not wearing enough clothes (*Guardian*, 1988). However, this last point may be an example of victimising an unpopular health minister by misrepresentation, rather than victim blaming the elderly, if Edwina Currie is to be believed (Currie 1989, pp. 203–207).

Ewles and Simnett (1995) offer further criticisms of the individualistic or behaviour change approach to health education:

- it assumes that experts know best and that lay people believe this;
- it often means imposing middle-class values on working-class people;
- rebelliousness may occur, causing behaviour opposite to that intended;
- it assumes that ill health is caused by behaviour, not by socio-economic conditions.

A powerful argument was offered by French and Adams (1986). They wrote that so far there is no convincing evidence that changes in behaviour facilitated by health education have improved levels of health. Robbins (1987) believed that individualism or *healthism*, as he called it, is a narrow approach which treats health as a goal and not as a resource (see Chapter 7). The focus of education, then, is to search and strive for something ideal which one does not have rather than enhancing what one already has.

Tones and Tilford (1994) offered a note of caution and concern about the vehement dismissal of the individual focus of conventional preventive health education. They argued that the most radical views on individualism go too far and are 'often intolerant and doctrinaire' (p.18). They suggested that individually focused preventive health education should be reassessed objectively, rather than simply dismissed as being part of the dominant ideology of capitalism.

The health belief model

The *health belief model* (HBM) was first described in the 1950s (Mikhail, 1981). Attributed to Becker and Rosenstock (cf. Becker and Maiman, 1975), it is an attempt to predict health behaviour in response to prevention services such as immunisation and screening (Harris and Middleton, 1995). Given the common situation whereby clients do not do what health professionals expect them to, Shillitoe and Christie (1989) argue that the HBM explains these discrepancies. The model implies that knowledge of a client's health beliefs may help a health worker to influence health-related behaviour in the 'right' direction. However, Mikhail (1981) advises caution in applying any theory uncritically to nursing, especially as in this case the HBM is only partially developed and in need of some refinement. Although individual elements of the model have much empirical support, most studies have been conducted retrospectively and depend on self-reported information. Hence what people say at one point in time caused their behaviour change may not be what *actually* caused it some time before. In addition, Mikhail (1981) warned that research had still not determined the conditions under which health beliefs are acquired and altered, or how stable such beliefs are. Shillitoe and Christie (1989) summarised the model as describing a relationship between an action, the expected outcome(s) of that action and the value of that outcome to the individual.

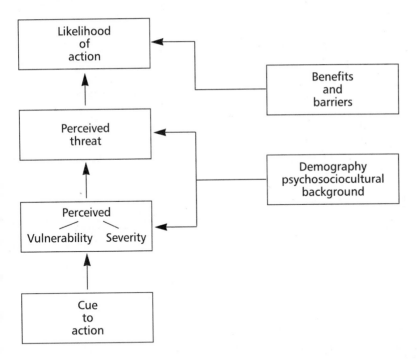

Figure 3.9   The health belief model (after Becker and Maiman, 1975)

In Figure 3.9 it can be seen that the model combines subjective beliefs about illness, in terms of vulnerability to, and severity of, disease, with a weighing up of the advantages and disadvantages of changing behaviour.

The points on the model where a health worker might expect to have most effect are:

- on the initial stimulus or cue to action;
- in changing beliefs about the perceived threat;
- in exploring the cost implications of both benefits and difficulties.

An example of the model in action is shown in Figure 3.10.

The HBM is a more detailed version of the knowledge–attitude–practice (KAP) model which was popular in the 1950s and 1960s (Walt and Constantinides, 1983), and may still be found underlying modern health education. The assumption was that once someone had a certain knowledge, attitudes would change and the outcome would be a new healthier behaviour. This is a form of individualism and can lead to victim blaming. The KAP model suggests that people smoke cigarettes because they do not know the damage this can cause. The model indicates that if they were to be informed of the danger, they would stop smoking. This approach is obviously simplistic and naive. There can be immense problems with its application, as has been shown by Obeid (1996). It ignores the

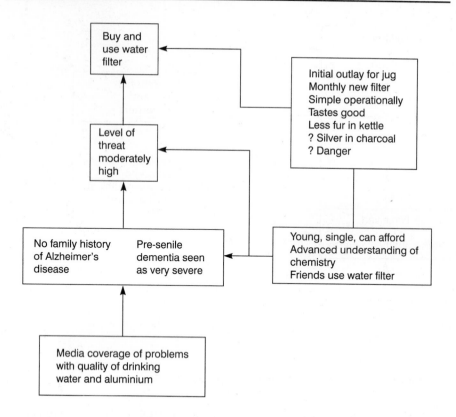

Figure 3.10   The health belief model in action – to drink or not to drink?

probability that the links between knowledge, attitudes and behaviour are neither consistent nor unidirectional (Coutts and Hardy, 1985).

Shillitoe and Christie (1989) provide four major criticisms of the HBM. First, it assumes that the relationship between threat and action is linear, whereas it is likely to be curvilinear – at maximum levels of threat, action is likely to be inhibited, not enhanced. Secondly, health behaviour is seen only as an avoidance of negative or unpleasant experiences, while it seems probable that society's perceptions of healthy behaviour are changing, and may now also be about reinforcing positive feelings. Thirdly, past behaviour may be more powerful than beliefs in predicting behaviour. Finally, despite the fact that over 40 years have elapsed since the construction of the HBM, there is very little research-based information on how health care workers can use the model to help clients' behaviour to change.

Harris and Middleton (1995) described the HBM as a dominant and influential framework not just for understanding health behaviour but also for predicting it. In contrast to Shillitoe and Christie (1989), Harris and Middleton (1995) report that empirical support for the HBM is widespread. However, they highlight many problems with HBM research, including a lack of agreement between different researchers as to how the key components of the model should be measured. Moreover, there is no consensus about the processes or principles that link the stages. For example, if numerical values for the factors included in the HBM could be obtained, it is not even clear if prediction would best be estimated by addition or multiplication (Brannon and Feist, 1992).

Hunt and Macleod (1987) added to the controversy surrounding the HBM. They referred to the idea that people change to health-related behaviour directly after a cue to action for reasons of health. It seems much more likely that other factors, such as financial worries, a new job or a new relationship, may trigger the change, sometimes a long time after the initial cue (Hunt and Macleod, 1987). They proposed a useful model of stages of behaviour change based on work by Prochaska *et al.* (1992) (see Figure 3.11). Nursing interventions may prove valuable at any stage of the model, but again, as with the HBM, there are no conclusive research studies to assist the development of nursing theory here. Interestingly, this stages of change model takes into account the possibility that people may relapse. With regard to the HBM example shown in Figure 3.10, the water filter jug has become a prized bath toy for a toddler and so presumably *perceived threats* may not be constant over time!

The stages of change model

While Naidoo and Wills (1994) depict the *stages of change model* as cyclical, Prochaska *et al.* (1992) show it to be a spiral. This model has been developed over 15 years of research into addictive behaviours, but it is likely to have a much wider application. It seems most applicable to nursing. Success should not be measured simplistically *only* as the number of patients who change their behaviour, for example the number who give up smoking or lose weight after patient education interventions. The key to success, as with all nursing, is the subtlety, richness and depth of *assessment*. In using the stages of change model, it is important to find out where, in the process of change, the patient is currently located. The communication shared between nurse and patient is likely to be very different in the case of a patient who is precontemplative, compared to someone who is ready to make a change in lifestyle. Rather than explaining why people do not change their behaviour, the model explores *how* people change (Naidoo and Wills, 1994).

The different stages of the model shown in Figure 3.11 are described by Prochaska *et al.* (1992) as follows.

Precontemplation

The patient is unaware or under-aware of his or her problems. Other people may be very aware of the behaviour causing problems to the patient and/or others, and may exert undue pressure for change. When the pressure is reduced, the patient reverts to their old ways. Thus change from this point

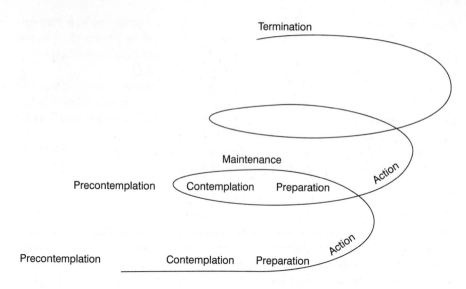

Figure 3.11   The stages of change model (after Prochaska *et al.*, 1992, p.1104)

on the model is unlikely to occur at all if the person is unaware, and unlikely to be maintained if it is caused by pressure from others rather than as a result of working through issues personally. Prochaska *et al.* (1992) regarded as pre-contemplative anyone who was not seriously thinking of making a change within the next 6 months.

Contemplation

In this stage, commitment to changing behaviour has not taken place, but awareness of the problem exists, and the person is seriously considering making a change. A major problem with this stage, identified by Prochaska *et al.* (1992, p.1103), is that people often seem to remain 'not quite ready yet' for years. They describe the person's struggle with a cost-benefit analysis of change as characterising this stage.

Preparation

In this stage, the person intends to make a change in behaviour during the next month, and may already have unsuccessfully attempted to change within the last year.

Action

This is the stage when behaviour is overtly different. This requires significant effort by the person. Prochaska *et al.* (1992) advise caution at this point because the person and the professionals mistakenly equate action with change. Change is something which is happening throughout the model, except during precontemplation. Belief that action *is* the change may lead to underemphasis at the next vital stage.

Maintenance

It is most important that this stage is viewed not as the absence of a behaviour, but as a continuation of change. The prevention of relapse may require effort for the rest of the person's life.

Relapse

With addictive behaviours, relapse is the rule rather than the exception. This may be true of many health-related behaviours. Prochaska *et al.* (1992) cite smoking as an example where it is common for three to four cycles to occur through the stages of action and relapse before long-term maintenance is achieved.

Into the next millennium?

It has been argued that the most practical model of health promotion is that of Tannahill (Downie *et al.*, 1996), and that the model of behaviour change most suited to nursing is that of Prochaska *et al.* (1992). This chapter would not be complete without brief reference to the useful conceptual framework that is usually known as 'Beattie's boxes' (Beattie, 1991). This representation of ideas about health promotion on opposing axes forms a map to guide theory and practice (Beattie, 1991; see Figure 3.12).

In 1985, Dr Mahler, then Director General of the World Health Organisation, argued that *Health For All 2000* would only be possible with the collaboration of nurses at all levels. He believed that nurses were more ready for change than any other professional group, and that they could lead the way through a better understanding of the use of primary health care (Mussallem, 1985). At any given time, about 10 per cent of the population is in acute care, with about 90 per cent of nurses caring for them. During preparation for practice, most of these nurses are likely to have had limited experience of community care, little emphasis on health education, and almost no input on health promotion. In Project 2000 there is a rich opportunity to redress this imbalance.

It is appropriate to acknowledge one further model of health, namely the *ecological model*. This will be crucial for the next millennium. De Leeuw (1989) made interesting comparisons between the principles of ecology and a term with which nurses are more familiar – *holism*. Indeed, he argued that the terms may be used interchangeably. The Ottawa Charter on Health

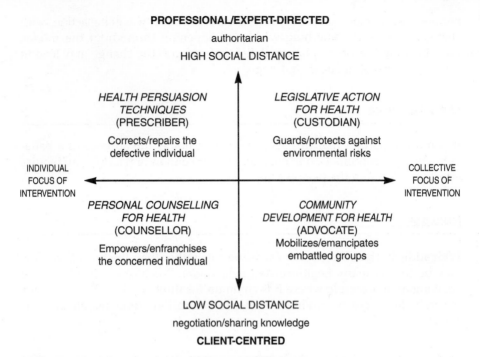

Figure 3.12   A theoretical framework for health promotion (after Beattie, 1991, pp. 184–185)

Promotion (de Leeuw, 1989; Dines and Cribb, 1993) made inextricable links between caring, holism and ecology:

> The overall guiding principle for the world, nations, regions and communities alike, is the need to encourage reciprocal maintenance – to take care of each other, our communities and our natural environment.
>
> (Ottawa Charter, cited in Dines and Cribb, 1993, pp.207–208)

In a similar vein, Milio (cited in Draper, 1986) linked caring (love), ecology and sustainability:

> Love and power relations set the pace and course for modern life and thereby control 'time' in human experience. Without taking account of this resource of time, no individual or community can create health; no people can maintain the many interconnected relations with environments, groups, and individuals that ultimately sustain them.
>
> (Milio, cited in Draper, 1986, p.105)

This relates to comments made at the start of this chapter about sustainability. For many, sustainable development is a precontemplative issue. Others who have contemplated the meaning have been misled into believing that one can buy a way into it using 'green' products (Labonté, 1991). Labonté argued that the cure will not be pain free as with the medical model. He raised concerns about a common fallacy that we can find ways to continue economic growth without environmental damage. Ecosystems, Labonté argued, do not grow indefinitely. The idea of *sustainable growth* is an excuse to carry on as before, and does not fit an ecological model. McCormack (1995) announced with some justifiable bitterness that the only thing which seems to be sustainable is poverty.

Endnotes

3.1 Parse (cf. Lee and Schumacher, 1989).
3.2 Peplau (cf. Carey *et al.*, 1989).
3.3 Wiedenbach (cf. Danko *et al.*, 1989).
3.4 Fitzpatrick (cf. Beckman *et al.*, 1989).
3.5 Newman (cf. Hensley *et al.*, 1989).

References

Ackermann, M. L., Brink, S. A., Clanton, J. A. *et al.* 1989 Imogene King: theory of goal attainment. In Marriner-Tomey, A. (ed.), *Nursing theorists and their work*, 2nd edn. St Louis: Mosby, 345–60.

Aggleton, P. and Homans, H. 1987 *Educating about AIDS*. Bristol: NHS Training Authority.

Aggleton, P., Homans, H., Mojsa, J., Watson, S. and Watney, S. 1989 *AIDS: scientific and social issues*. Edinburgh: Churchill Livingstone.

Alexander, J. 1988 The ideological construction of risk: an analysis of corporate health programs in the 1980s. *Social Science and Medicine* **26**, 559–67.

Antonovsky, A. 1987 *Unraveling the mystery of health – how people manage stress and stay well*. San Francisco: Jossey-Bass.

Ashworth, P. 1997 Virginia Henderson. *Edlines* (Royal College of Nursing Newsletter of the Education Consortium) **14**, 6.

Axline, V. M. 1966 *Dibs – in search of self*. Harmondsworth: Penguin.

Backett, E. M., Davies, A. M. and Petros-Barvazian, A. 1984 *The risk approach in health care*. Geneva: World Health Organisation.

Beattie, A. 1986 Foreword. In Farrant, W. and Russell, J. (eds), *The politics of health information*. London: Institute of Education, 7–8.

Beattie, A. 1991 Knowledge and control in health promotion: a test case for social policy and social theory. In Gabe, J., Calnan, M. and Bury, M. (eds), *The sociology of the health service*. London: Routledge, 162–202.

Becker, M. H. and Maiman, B. A. 1975 Sociobehavioural determinants of compliance with health and medical care recommendations. *Medical Care* **13**, 10–24.

Beckman, S. J., Chapman-Boyce, P., Coleman-Ehmke, S. *et al.* 1989 Joyce J. Fitzpatrick: life perspective model. In Marriner-Tomey, A. (ed.), *Nursing theorists and their work*, 2nd edn. St Louis: Mosby, 420–31.

Blaxter, M. 1984 The causes of disease: women talking. In Black, N., Boswell, D., Gray, A., Murphy, S. and Popay, J. (eds), *Health and Disease*. Milton Keynes: Open University Press, 34–43.

Blaxter, M. 1987 Self-reported health. In Cox, B. D., Blaxter, M., Buckle, A. L. J. *et al.* (eds), *The health and lifestyle survey*. London: Health Promotion Research Trust, 5–16.

Blaxter, M. and Paterson, E. 1982 *Mothers and daughters: a three-generational study of health attitudes and behaviour*. London: Heinemann.

Blue, C. L., Brubaker, K. M., Fine, J. M., Kirsch, M. J., Papazian, K. R. and Riester, C. M. 1989 Sister Callista Roy: adaptation model. In Marriner-Tomey, A. (ed.), *Nursing theorists and their work*, 2nd edn. St Louis: Mosby, 325–44.

Bradshaw, P. 1986 Agents of positive health. *Senior Nurse* 4, 8–9.

Brannon, L. and Feist, J. 1992 *Health psychology: an introduction to behavior and health*, 2nd edn. Pacific Grove, CA: Brooks/Cole.

Butterworth, T. 1989 Of public concern. *Nursing Times and Nursing Mirror* 85, 19.

Calnan, M. 1987 *Health and illness: the lay perspective*. London: Tavistock.

Calnan, M. and Johnson, B. 1983 Influencing health behaviour: how significant is the general practitioner? *Health Education Journal* 42, 34–45.

Carey, E. T., Noll, J., Rasmussen, L., Searcy, B. and Stark, N. L. 1989 Hildegard E. Peplau: psychodynamic nursing. In Marriner-Tomey, A. (ed.), *Nursing theorists and their work*, 2nd edn. St Louis: Mosby, 203–18.

Carr, E. H. 1964 *What is history?* Harmondsworth: Penguin.

Catford, J. and Parish, R. 1989 'Heartbeat Wales': new horizons for health promotion in the community – the philosophy and practice of Heartbeat Wales. In Seedhouse, D. and Cribb, A. (eds), *Changing ideas in health care*. Chichester: Wiley, 127–42.

Chambers (ed.) 1993 *The Chambers Dictionary*. Edinburgh: Harrap.

Chapman, S. 1987 Small fish in big ponds. In Campbell, G. (ed.), *Health education, youth and community: a review of research and developments*. London: Palmer, 24–8.

Charles, N. and Kerr, M. 1986 Issues of responsibility and control in the feeding of families. In Rodmell, S. and Watt, A. (eds), *The politics of health education*. London: Routledge and Kegan Paul, 57–75.

Chinn, P. L. 1988 Promoting health. *Advances in Nursing Science* 11, vi.

Clarke, R. and Lowe, F. 1989 Positive health – some lay perspectives. *Health Promotion* 3, 401–6.

Cohen, J. and Jaffe, D. T. 1994 Holistic health strategies. In Edelman, C. L. and Mandle, C. L. (eds), *Health promotion throughout the lifespan*, 3rd edn. St Louis: Mosby, 324–49.

Conner, S. S., Magers, J. A. and Watt, J. K. 1989 Dorothy E. Johnson: behavioral system model. In Marriner-Tomey, A. (ed.), *Nursing theorists and their work*, 2nd edn. St Louis: Mosby, 309–24.

Cornwell, J. 1984 *Hard-earned lives*. London: Tavistock.

Coutts, L. C. and Hardy, L. K. 1985 *Teaching for health*. Edinburgh: Churchill Livingstone.

Creekmur, T., DeFelice, J., Doub, M. S., Hodel, A. and Petty, C. Y. 1989 Evelyn Adam: conceptual model for nursing. In Marriner-Tomey, A. (ed.), *Nursing theorists and their work*, 2nd edn. St Louis: Mosby, 133–45.

Crombie, H. 1995 *Sustainable development and health*. Birmingham: Public Health Alliance.

Currie, E. 1989 *Lifelines: politics and health 1986–1988*. London: Sidgwick and Jackson.

Daily, J. S., Maupin, J. S., Satterly, M. C., Schnell, D. L. and Wallace, T. L. 1989 Martha E. Rogers: unitary human beings. In Marriner-Tomey, A. (ed.), *Nursing theorists and their work*, 2nd edn. St Louis: Mosby, 402–19.

Danko, M., Hunt, N. E., Marich, J. E., Marriner-Tomey, A., McCreary, C. A. and Stuart, M. 1989 Ernestine Wiedenbach: the helping art of clinical nursing. In Marriner-Tomey, A. (ed.), *Nursing theorists and their work*, 2nd edn. St Louis: Mosby, 240–52.

de Leeuw, E. J. J. 1989 *The sane revolution. Health promotion: backgrounds, scope and prospect*. Maastricht: Van Gorcum.

DeMeester, D. W., Lauer, T., Neal, S. E. and Williams, S. 1989 Virginia Henderson: definition of nursing. In Marriner-Tomey, A. (ed.), *Nursing theorists and their work*, 2nd edn. St Louis: Mosby, 80–92.

Department of Health 1992 *The health of the nation: a strategy for health in England.* London: HMSO.

Department of Health 1993 *Targeting practice: the contribution of nurses, midwives and health visitors: the health of the nation.* London: Department of Health.

Department of Health 1994 *The challenges for nursing and midwifery in the 21st century: the Heathrow Debate.* London: Department of Health.

Department of Health 1995 *Making it happen: public health. The contribution, role and development of nurses, midwives and health visitors. Report on the Standing Nursing and Midwifery Advisory Committee.* London: Department of Health.

Department of Health and Social Security (DHSS) 1976 *Prevention and health: everybody's business.* London: HMSO.

Department of Health and Social Services (DHSS) 1996 *Health and wellbeing into the next millennium: regional strategy for health and social wellbeing 1997–2002: Northern Ireland.* Belfast: Department of Health and Social Services.

Dickson, A. 1982 *A woman in your own right.* London: Quartet.

Dines, A. and Cribb, A. (eds) 1993 *Health promotion: concepts and practice.* Oxford: Blackwell Scientific Publications.

Downie, R. S., Tannahill, C. and Tannahill, A. 1996 *Health promotion: models and values*, 2nd edn. Oxford: Oxford University Press.

Draper, P. 1986 Nancy Milio's work and its importance for the development of health promotion. *Health Promotion* **1**, 101–6.

Dubos, R. 1995 Mirage of health. In Davey, B., Gray, A. and Seale, C. (eds), *Health and disease – a reader.* Buckingham: Open University Press, 4–10.

Dwore, R. and Matarazzo, J. 1981 The behavioural sciences and health education. *Health Education* May/June, 4–7.

Dycus, D. K., Schmeiser, D. N., Taggart, F. M. and Yancey, R. 1989 Faye Glenn Abdellah: twenty-one nursing problems. In Marriner-Tomey, A. (ed.), *Nursing theorists and their work*, 2nd edn. St Louis: Mosby, 93–108.

Edelman, C. L. and Mandle, C. L. (eds) 1994 *Health promotion throughout the lifespan*, 3rd edn. St Louis: Mosby.

Edelman, C. L. and Milio, N. 1994 Health defined: objectives for promotion and prevention. In Edelman, C. L. and Mandle, C. L. (eds), *Health promotion throughout the lifespan,* 3rd edn. St Louis: Mosby, 4–24.

English National Board for Nursing, Midwifery and Health Visiting 1989 *Project 2000 – a new preparation for practice; guidelines and criteria for course development and the formulation of collaborative links between approved training institutions within the National Health Service and centres of higher education.* London: English National Board for Nursing, Midwifery and Health Visiting.

Epp, J. 1987 Achieving health for all: a framework for health promotion. *Canadian Nurse* **83** (Supplement), 1–13.

Ewles, L. and Simnett, I. 1995 *Promoting health: a practical guide.* London: Scutari Press.

Farrant, W. and Russell, J. 1986 *The politics of health information.* London: Institute of Education.

Foli, K. J., Johnson, T., Marriner-Tomey, A. et al. 1989 Myra Estrin Levine: four conservation principles. In Marriner-Tomey, A. (ed.), *Nursing theorists and their work*, 2nd edn. St Louis: Mosby, 391-401.

French, J. and Adams, L. 1986 From analysis to synthesis: theories of health education. *Health Education Journal* **45**, 71–4.

Frost, S. and Nunkoosing, K. 1989 Quest. Building a strong foundation. *Nursing Times and Nursing Mirror* **85**, 59–60.

Fullard, E. 1989 The facilitator of prevention in primary care: the birth of a new professional. In Seedhouse, D. and Cribb, A. (eds), *Changing ideas in health care.* Chichester: Wiley, 195–210.

Gott, M. 1988 *Nursing, distance learning, and health promotion in Western Canada.* Unpublished report. London: Winston Churchill Trust.

Guardian (ed.) 1988 Currie reaffirms responsibility of individual in preventive medicine. *Guardian* 29th October, p.4.

Harris, P. and Middleton, W. 1995 Social cognition and health behaviour. In Messer, D. and Meldrum, C. (eds), *Psychology for nurses and health care professionals.* Hemel Hempstead: Prentice Hall, 107–30.

Harris, S. M., Hermiz, M. E., Meininger, M. and Steinkeler, S. E. 1989 Betty Neuman: systems model. In Marriner-Tomey, A. (ed.), *Nursing theorists and their work,* 2nd edn. St Louis: Mosby, 361–88.

Health Education Council 1984 *Beating heart disease.* London: Health Education Council.

Helman, C. G. 1981 Disease versus illness in general practice. *Journal of the Royal College of General Practitioners* **31**, 548–52.

Helman, C. G. 1994 *Culture, health and illness: an introduction for health professionals,* 3rd edn. Oxford: Butterworth-Heinemann.

Hensley, D., Keffer, M. J., Kilgore-Keever, K. A., Langfitt, J. V. and Peterson, L. 1989 Margaret A. Newman: model of health. In Marriner-Tomey, A. (ed.), *Nursing theorists and their work,* 2nd edn. St Louis: Mosby, 432–47.

Herzlich, C. 1973 *Health and illness: a social psychological analysis.* London: Academic Press.

Hill, D. J. and Shugg, D. 1989 Breast self-examination practices and attitudes among breast cancer, benign breast disease and general practice patients. *Health Education Research* **4**, 193–203.

Hunt, S. M. and Macleod, M. 1987 Health and behavioural change: some lay perspectives. *Community Medicine* **9**, 68–76.

Illich, I. 1976 *Limits to medicine. Medical nemesis: the expropriation of health.* London: Marion Boyars.

Jacobson, B., Smith, A. and Whitehead, M. (eds) 1991 *The nation's health: a strategy for the 1990s,* 2nd edn. London: King Edward's Hospital Fund.

Jones, L. J. 1994 *The social context of health and health work.* Basingstoke: Macmillan.

Katz, J. and Peberdy, A. (eds) 1997 *Promoting health: knowledge and practice.* Basingstoke: Macmillan and Open University Press.

Keck, J. F. 1989 Terminology of theory development. In Marriner-Tomey, A. (ed.), *Nursing theorists and their work,* 2nd edn. St Louis: Mosby, 15–23.

Kiger, A. M. 1995 *Teaching for health,* 2nd edn. Edinburgh: Churchill Livingstone.

Kübler-Ross, E. 1978 *To live until we say goodbye.* London: Prentice-Hall.

Labonté, R. 1991 Econology: integrating health and sustainable development. Part one: theory and background. *Health Promotion International* **6**, 49–65.

Laughlin, S. and Black, D. 1995 *Poverty and health: tools for change.* Birmingham: Public Health Alliance.

Lee, R. E. and Schumacher, L. P. 1989 Rosemarie Rizzo Parse: man-living-health. In Marriner-Tomey, A. (ed.), *Nursing theorists and their work,* 2nd edn. St Louis: Mosby, 174-86.

Littlewood, J. 1989 A model for nursing using anthropological literature. *International Journal of Nursing Studies* **26**, 221–9.

Luker, K. and Caress, A. 1989 Rethinking patient education. *Journal of Advanced Nursing* **14**, 711–18.

Lundberg, O. and Nyström Peck, M. 1994 Sense of coherence, social structure and health; evidence from a population survey in Sweden. *European Journal of Public Health* **4**, 252–7.

McBean, S. F. 1992a A team approach to health promotion. *Primary Health Care* **2**, 18–21.

McBean S. F. 1992b *Health beliefs of learner nurses – an ethnographic approach.* Unpublished MSc Thesis, King's College, University of London.

McBean, S. F. 1992c Promoting positive health. *Primary Health Care* **2**, 10, 12, 14.

McCormack, C. 1995 *War without bullets ...: the opposition of a global community activist to the injustices of the exploitation of the planet and its inhabitants.* Videocassette tape. Glasgow: The Popular Democracy Education and Resource Centre.

McKeown, T. 1979 *The role of medicine: dream, mirage or nemesis?* Oxford: Basil Blackwell.

Macleod Clark, J., Haverty, S. and Kendall, S. 1987 *Helping patients and clients to stop smoking. Phase 2. Assessing the effectiveness of the nurse's role: final report.* London: Department of Nursing Studies, University of London.

McLeroy, K. R. 1989 Issues in risk communication. *Health Education Research* **4**, 169–70.

Marriner-Tomey, A. (ed.) 1989 *Nursing theorists and their work*, 2nd edn. St Louis: Mosby.

Marriner-Tomey, A., Mills, D. I. and Sauter, M. K. 1989 Ida Jean Orlando (Pelletier): nursing process theory. In Marriner-Tomey, A. (ed.), *Nursing theorists and their work*, 2nd edn. St Louis: Mosby, 228–39.

Meleis, A. I. 1991 *Theoretical nursing – development and progress*, 2nd edn. Philadelphia: Lippincott.

Mikhail, B. 1981 The health belief model: a review and critical evaluation of the model, research, and practice. *Advances in Nursing Science* **4**, 65–82.

Morgan, M., Calnan, M. and Manning, N. 1985 *Sociological approaches to health and medicine.* London: Croom Helm.

Morton, P. G. 1989 *Health assessment in nursing.* Springhouse, PA: Springhouse Publishers.

Mussallem, H. K. 1985 Prevention and patterns of disease: prospects and research directions in nursing for the future. In Willis, L. E. and Linwood, M. E. (eds), *Prevention and nursing.* Edinburgh: Churchill Livingstone, 147–62.

Naidoo, J. 1986 Limits to individualism. In Rodmell, S. and Watt, A. (eds), *The politics of health education.* London: Routledge and Kegan Paul, 17–37.

Naidoo, J. and Wills, J. 1994 *Health promotion: foundations for practice.* London: Baillière Tindall.

National Health Service Executive 1996 *Primary care: the future.* Leeds: National Health Service Executive.

Newman, M. A. 1986 *Health as expanding consciousness.* St Louis: Mosby

Noack, H. 1987 Concepts of health promotion. In Abelin, T., Brzezinski, Z. J. and Carstairs, V. D. (eds), *Measurement in health promotion and protection.* Copenhagen: World Health Organisation, 5–28.

Obeid, A. 1996 Critique of the health beliefs model. *Primary Health Care* **6**, 20–23.

Oliver, M. F. 1982 Does control of risk factors prevent coronary heart disease? *British Medical Journal* **285**, 1065–6.

Oliver, M. F. 1987 Dietary fat and coronary heart disease: there is much to learn. *Cardiology* **74**, 22–7.

Oliver, M. F. 1988 Reducing cholesterol does not reduce mortality. *Journal of the American College of Cardiology* **12**, 814–17.

Oliver, M. F. 1991 Might treatment of hypercholesterolaemia increase non-cardiac mortality? *Lancet* **337**, 1529–31.

Oliver, M. F. 1992 Cholesterol and coronary disease – outstanding questions. *Cardiovascular Drugs and Therapy* **6**, 131–6.

Oliver, M. F. 1993 Lowering cholesterol for prevention of coronary heart disease: problems and perspectives. *Cardiovascular Drugs and Therapy* **7**, 785–8.

Orr, J. 1995 Ill-prepared for health promotion. *Health Visitor* **68**, 398.

Parse, R. R. 1981 *Man–living–health: a theory of nursing.* New York: John Wiley.

Parse, R. R., Coyne, A. B. and Smith, M. J. 1985 *Nursing research – qualitative methods.* Bowie, MD: Brady Communications Company.

Pearce, E. 1971 *A general textbook of nursing.* London: Faber and Faber.

Pender, N. J. 1996 *Health promotion in nursing practice,* 3rd edn. Stamford: Appleton and Lange.

Peto, R., Lopez, A. D., Boreham, J., Thun, M. and Heath, C. 1994 *Mortality from smoking in developed countries (1950–2000): indirect estimates from national vital statistics.* Oxford: Oxford University Press.

Pike, S. and Forster, D. (eds) 1995 *Health promotion for all.* Edinburgh: Churchill Livingstone.

Prochaska, J. O., DiClemente, C. and Norcross, J. C. 1992 In search of how people change: applications to addictive behaviours. *American Psychologist* **47**, 1102–14.

Public Health Alliance 1988 *Beyond Acheson: an agenda for the New Public Health.* Birmingham: Public Health Alliance.

Redman, B. K. 1993 Patient education at 25 years; where we have been and where we are going. *Journal of Advanced Nursing* **18**, 725–30.

Richman, J. 1987 *Medicine and health.* London: Longman.

Riley, D. 1985 *Dry air.* London: Virago.

Robbins, C. 1987 *Health promotion in North America: implications for the UK.* London: Health Education Council and King Edward's Hospital Fund.

Roberson, M. H. B. 1987 Folk health beliefs of health professionals. *Western Journal of Nursing Research* **9**, 257–63.

Robinson, K. 1983 What is health? In Clark, J. and Henderson, J. (eds), *Community health.* Edinburgh: Churchill Livingstone, 11–18.

Rodmell, S. and Watt, A. 1986 Conventional health education: problems and possibilities. In Rodmell, S. and Watt, A. (eds), *The politics of health education.* London: Routledge and Kegan Paul, 1–16.

Rose, G. 1981 Strategy of prevention: lessons from cardiovascular disease. *British Medical Journal* **282**, 1847–51.

Rose, G. 1992 *The strategy of preventive medicine.* Oxford: Oxford University Press.

Scriven, A. and Orme, J. (eds) 1996 *Health promotion: professional perspectives.* Basingstoke: Macmillan.

Seedhouse, D. 1986 *Health: the foundations of achievement.* Chichester: Wiley.

Seedhouse, D. 1988 *Ethics: the heart of health care.* Chichester: Wiley.

Sennott-Miller, L. and Miller, J. L. L. 1987 Difficulty: a neglected factor in health promotion. *Nursing Research* **36**, 268–72.

Shillitoe, R. W. and Christie, M. J. 1989 Determinants of self-care: the health belief model. *Holistic Medicine* **4**, 3-17.

Smith, A. and Jacobson, B. 1988 *The nation's health: a strategy for the 1990s: a report from an Independent Multidisciplinary Committee.* London: King Edward's Hospital Fund.

Smith, J. A. 1981 The idea of health: a philosophical inquiry. *Advances in Nursing Science* **3**, 43–50.

Smith, J. A. 1983 *The idea of health: implications for the nursing professional.* New York: Teachers College Press.

Stainton Rogers, W. 1991 *Explaining health and illness: an exploration of diversity.* Hemel Hempstead: Harvester Wheatsheaf.

Statutory Instrument 1983 *Nurses', midwives' and health visitors' rules approval order.* London: HMSO.

Stone, D. 1987 Screen fantasy. *New Society* **82**, 12–13.

Stone, D. 1989 Upside-down prevention. *Health Service Journal* **99**, 890–91.

Strehlow, M. S. 1983 *Education for health.* London: Harper and Row.

Sullivan, G. C. 1989 Evaluating Antonovsky's salutogenic model for its adaptability to nursing. *Journal of Advanced Nursing* **14**, 336–42.

Syred, M. E. J. 1981 The abdication of the role of health education by hospital nurses. *Journal of Advanced Nursing* **6**, 27–33.

Tannahill, A. 1984 Health promotion – caring concern. *Journal of Medical Ethics* **10**, 196–8.

Tannahill, A. 1985 What is health promotion? *Health Education Journal*, **44**, 167–8.

Tannahill, A. 1987 Regional health promotion planning and monitoring. *Health Education Journal* **46**, 125–7.

Tannahill, A. 1994 *From priorities to programmes: the experience of the Health Education Board for Scotland.* Edinburgh: Health Education Board for Scotland.

Tones, B. K. 1981 Health education: prevention or subversion? *Journal of the Royal Society of Health* **101**, 413–16.

Tones, K. 1996 The anatomy and ideology of health promotion: empowerment in context. In Scriven, A. and Orme, J. (eds), *Health promotion: professional perspectives.* Basingstoke: Macmillan, 9–21.

Tones, K. and Tilford, S. 1994 *Health education: effectiveness, efficiency and equity,* 2nd edn. London: Chapman and Hall.

Toon, P. D. 1995 Health checks in general practice: time to review their role. *British Medical Journal* **310**, 1083–84.

Townsend, P., Davidson, N. and Whitehead, M. 1988 *Inequalities in health: the Black Report 1980 and the Health Divide.* Harmondsworth: Penguin.

Tudor-Hart, J. 1985 When practice is not perfect. *Nursing Times* **81**, 28–9.

Van Maanen, H. M. T. 1988 Being old does not always mean being sick: perspectives on conditions of health as perceived by British and American elderly. *Journal of Advanced Nursing* **13**, 701–9.

Walker, C. and Cannon, G. 1984 *The food scandal.* London: Century.

Walker, S. N., Volkan, K., Sechrist, K. R. and Pender, N. J. 1988 Health-promoting life styles of older adults: comparisons with young and middle-aged adults, correlates and patterns. *Advances in Nursing Science* **11**, 701–90.

Walt, G. and Constantinides, P. 1983 *Community health education in Commonwealth countries.* London: Commonwealth Secretariat.

Wass, A. 1994 *Promoting health: the primary health care approach.* London: W.B. Saunders/Baillière Tindall.

Whitehead, M. 1990 *The concepts and principles of equity and health.* Copenhagen: World Health Organisation.

Whitehead, M. 1991 The concepts and principles of equity and health. *Health Promotion International* **6**, 217–28.

Williams, G. 1984 Health promotion – caring concern or slick salesmanship? *Journal of Medical Ethics* **10**, 191–5.

Williams, R. 1990 *A protestant legacy – attitudes to death and illness among older Aberdonians.* Oxford: Clarendon Press.

Wilson, E. K., Purdon, S. E. and Wallston, K. A. 1988 Compliance to health recommendations: a theoretical overview of message framing. *Health Education Research* **3**, 161–71.

Winnicott, D. 1986 *Home is where we start from – essays by a psychoanalyst.* Harmondsworth: Penguin.

Woods, N. F., Laffrey, S., Duffy, M. *et al.* 1988 Being healthy: women's images. *Advances in Nursing Science* **11**, 36–46.

World Health Organisation 1984 *Health promotion: a discussion document on the concept and principles.* Copenhagen: World Health Organisation.

World Health Organisation 1985 *Targets for Health For All 2000.* Copenhagen: World Health Organisation.

World Health Organisation 1986 *Intersectoral action for health.* Geneva: World Health Organisation.

World Health Organisation 1988 *From Alma Ata to the year 2000:   reflections at the midpoint.* Geneva: World Health Organisation.

Young, L. 1996 Healthy alliances. *Primary Health Care* **6**, 11.

Biological sciences in nursing

4

Jennifer Boore

The place of the biological sciences in nursing

Nursing has been described as an art and a science (Rogers, 1989) drawing on a range of underlying disciplines from both the biological and behavioural sciences. It has been stated that, while some other professions also draw on the same theoretical disciplines, nursing is a 'unique mix of other sciences with the uniqueness lying in the mix' (Hockey, 1973). Having said that, the range of the fundamental disciplines applied in different branches of nursing also varies. For example, those working in the mental health field require an in-depth understanding of psychology, while those working in intensive-care units need a detailed comprehension of physiology in order to provide high-quality care.

The different disciplines that inform nursing practice are widespread, ranging from physics to philosophy (Smith, 1981), but with the greatest dependence on the biological and behavioural sciences. The broad range of the nature of knowledge relevant to nursing makes it impossible for any one nurse to acquire the full range of understanding involved. However, as a profession we should have such knowledge available within our members, to be drawn upon as necessary. Each student practitioner needs to be provided with a foundation of the relevant sciences which can be developed and extended as is appropriate for the area of practice into which that individual practitioner moves. The knowledge of different disciplines is needed in order to understand the patient and to provide care to maintain or promote health. This requires the ability to integrate an understanding of pathophysiological changes and treatment with knowledge of normal structure and function and age-related change (Carnevali and Thomas, 1993).

The biological sciences within the nursing curriculum

CURRENT POSITION

In recent times, the profession of nursing in the UK has increased in autonomy and has acquired the self-confidence to permit greater decentralisation in determining the range and depth of the underpinning disciplines in preparation for professional practice. This is demonstrated in the move away from a single state examination for registration and greater variability in the content of programmes of nurse education seen in the Project 2000 programmes offered. In a swing away from the previous situation, the social sciences and psychology have, rightly, increased in importance within the nursing curriculum, but this has been at the expense of the biological sciences (Trnobranski, 1993). Yet many of the ways in which nursing practice is developing towards specialist practice rely on a depth of knowledge of the biological sciences (Clarke, 1995).

The teaching of the biological sciences in nursing programmes has been identified as an area of difficulty by both staff and students in Colleges of Nursing (Courtney, 1991) and on degree programmes (Wharrad et al., 1994). This is partly because few nurse teachers have academic backgrounds within the biological sciences (Akinsanya, 1987a) and much of the teaching in this area of the curriculum is taught either by nurses without the most appropriate biological science knowledge base, or by non-nurse biologists. There is difficulty in achieving an appropriate balance between teaching complexity and detail with a resulting lack of understanding, and imparting material that has been simplified to the point of inaccuracy which can then be clearly understood.

The biological sciences are identified as one of the scientific areas underpinning nursing practice. However, this is far too simplistic a description. Table 4.1 indicates the range of biological sciences relevant to nursing, and several of these disciplines can be subdivided still further. The problem is that each of these different biological sciences can be studied as a degree programme in its own right, so that the breadth and depth of knowledge from each of these subjects for nursing education has to be selected. Furthermore, while these can be, and usually are, defined as separate disciplines, so far as nursing is concerned it is a unified amalgam of selected knowledge from these different biological sciences that is needed for practice. In addition, there is a tendency for each of the different sciences (within both biological and behavioural realms) to be taught separately, particularly where the education of nurses is taking place within the higher education sector (Chandler, 1991), and this raises potential problems for nursing education. It is important to recognise that biological and behavioural sciences are not totally separate (see Chapter 5), and that there is considerable interaction between them, as there is between the different biological sciences.

Traditionally, physiology is taught using a systems approach and, while this may be suitable for medical education where the focus is on diagnosing disorders of particular organs or systems, it is less appropriate for nursing. Nursing is more concerned with the functions of the body and the effect of various disorders on these activities and on the individual as a whole; relatively few essential bodily functions depend on only one organ or system. The fact that this is recognised is demonstrated by the general organisation of some of the physiology books primarily focused for nurses, which have functional headings (e.g. Hinchliff and Montague, 1988; Tortora and Grabowski, 1993). The difficulty of the task is clearly illustrated by the fact that there is still a tendency to adopt the usual systems approach within those sections. However, it is also a fact that nurses care for patients with disorders of particular organs or systems of the body. Nursing education needs an approach to teaching of the biological sciences that enables the developing professional to integrate an understanding of the different functions of the body with knowledge of the effects of disorders on specific organs or systems.

At present, there is a tendency for the biological sciences to be perceived as 'medical property'. However, in order to use this knowledge base to provide high-quality nursing care, nursing needs to incorporate the biological

Table. 4.1   Biological science disciplines in nursing

Subject title	Content of discipline
Anatomy	Structure of human body
Physiology	Function of human body
Biochemistry	Chemical make-up and function of body cells and organs
Genetics	Determination of individual characteristics and transmission of characteristics to succeeding generations
Pathology/ pathophysiology	Causes and effects of disease
Microbiology	Microscopic organisms and their contribution to disease
Pharmacology	Drug actions and interactions
Nutrition	Dietary requirements and provision
Ergonomics	Suiting the individual to the environment and the environment to the individual
Epidemiology	Disease in relation to populations

sciences fully into the *gestalt* of nursing, including the theoretical frameworks used to guide practice (Jordan, 1994). Akinsanya (1987b) has proposed a model for linking the biological sciences into nursing under the title *bionursing*, which identifies the levels of decision-making for which biological science knowledge is required. While this is a useful model, it does not relate clearly to other nursing models and it does not identify the specific areas of knowledge required from the biological sciences.

Concepts in the biological sciences in nursing

In this chapter, the task of identifying concepts applicable to nursing from the different biological science disciplines is set out and it becomes necessary to find a structure for ordering these concepts. The aim is to begin to incorporate a framework for the biological sciences within a nursing theoretical paradigm. A natural structure for ordering these biological concepts is within conceptual areas that are comparable to the four key concepts of *Person, Environment, Health* and *Nursing* identified by Fawcett (1984) within the metaparadigm of nursing (see Chapter 10). Table 4.2 shows the relationship between these key concepts and the conceptual areas within this paper. As in theories of nursing, there is considerable interaction within the broad area of the biological sciences between the conceptual areas and between individual concepts.

In order to incorporate knowledge from the biological sciences into nursing, the relevant concepts drawn from the biological sciences must first be identified and synthesised in some way that makes the wealth of information manageable and applicable to nursing. Secondly, the detail needed for

Table. 4.2   Relationship between key conceptual areas in biological sciences in nursing and key concepts in nursing

Key concepts in nursing metaparadigm	Conceptual areas within biological sciences in nursing

Person	Individual
	    Homeostasis
	    Age-related change
	    Individual within the population

Environment	Environment–individual interaction
	    Stress and adaptation
	    The microbiological environment

Health	Health–illness
	    Themes in pathophysiology
	    Disordered body function
	    Risk factors

Nursing	Treatment and care
	    Drug therapy
	    Surgical intervention

the appropriate level of practice at practitioner, specialist practitioner and advanced practitioner levels (United Kingdom Central Council for Nursing, Midwifery and Health Visiting, 1994) must be identified. It is this detailed work on curriculum development that, so far as can be ascertained, has been undertaken only by individual teachers in preparation for teaching their own students. This chapter cannot possibly undertake the whole task which is needed, but will begin the first stage by identifying and discussing briefly some of the relevant concepts within the proposed grouping.

Person (individual)

Nursing is essentially an interpersonal activity (Peplau, 1988) which aims to enhance the health status of individuals. To achieve this, it is necessary to understand how the human body normally functions. It is also important to have a fundamental grasp of the way in which social and psychological factors also influence health and illness (Davey et al., 1995), although these issues are not discussed here (see relevant chapters in this volume).

Homeostasis

The major biological concept in relation to the individual is that of *homeostasis* (Cannon, 1939), a state first described by Claude Bernard, the father of modern physiology, in 1857 (Vander *et al.*, 1994). He stated that:

> it is the fixity of the internal environment which is the condition of free and independent life ... all the vital mechanisms, however varied they may be, have only one object, that of preserving constant the conditions of life in the internal environment.
>
> (Vander *et al.*, 1994, p.5)

The 'internal environment' identified by Bernard is the fluid surrounding each cell, i.e. the extracellular fluid.

PHYSIOLOGY AS MAINTENANCE OF HOMEOSTASIS

Essentially, the maintenance of homeostasis is what physiology is all about. The importance of this lies in the requirements for normal cell functioning to continue (see Figure 4.1). Although human beings are multi-celled organisms, the body is still composed of millions of individual cells, each of which must continue to carry out the basic activities of life of a free-living single-celled organism. In addition, each individual cell co-operates with others of its specialised type in order to carry out the activities necessary to maintain the organ and system functions needed to maintain the requirements for life within a multi-celled organism.

At the cellular level and also at organ, system and organismic levels, both structure and function are dynamic in nature. There is a continual turnover

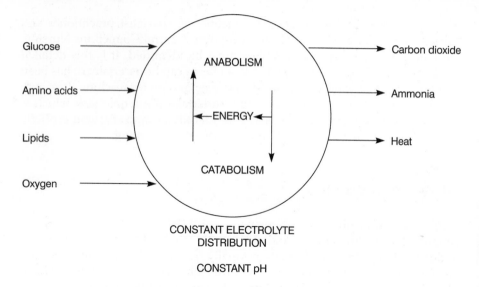

Figure 4.1　Requirements for normal cell function

of bodily components, with structures being broken down (*catabolism*) and (some of) their components being reused, together with additional material being provided, to build up new structures (*anabolism*). This continual turnover allows adaptation in response to change. For example, an increased physical workload results in the building up of muscle structure to enable the activity to be carried out adequately. These anabolic activities require energy, which is mainly produced by the catabolism of glucose in the presence of oxygen. The myriad of both catabolic and anabolic activities are maintained in equilibrium through the activity of enzymes whose level of activity is closely regulated.

The term homeostasis seems to imply that all of the different characteristics (such as levels of electrolytes, temperature and pH) necessary for the continued health of each cell and of the whole body are maintained in a fixed condition. However, this view is misleading. In health they are maintained within limits and display some variation above and below a stable point. The amount of variation about that point is related to the critical nature of the level of that particular characteristic. For example, the pH (the measure of acidity or alkalinity) of the fluid surrounding the cell is tightly regulated between 7.35 and 7.45 because the cell enzymes function normally only within very narrow pH limits. On the other hand, the level of sodium in the extracellular fluid varies to a considerably greater extent (135–150 mmol/L) because, although it is important, the precise level of this electrolyte is less critical.

REGULATION OF HOMEOSTASIS

All of the systems of the body contribute to the maintenance of homeostasis through a range of different activities, as indicated in Figure 4.2. The systems of the body that are mainly involved in these different activities are listed in Table 4.3.

Control and co-ordination of the different bodily functions represent the most important issue in relation to regulation of homeostasis. The two major systems involved are the nervous and endocrine systems which, although they function in very different ways, interact in the regulation of body activities. The central nervous system (i.e. the brain and spinal cord) is the integrating or controlling centre of the nervous system, and it controls muscle activity and secretion from some glands through impulses that are rapidly transmitted along the nerve fibres of the motor side of the peripheral nervous system and of the autonomic nervous system. The peripheral motor nerve fibres initiate conscious activity, while the autonomic nervous system regulates activities that maintain bodily functions of which we are generally unaware.

The endocrine system acts less rapidly in regulating metabolism and slower acting functions (see Table 4.4) through the secretion of hormones, i.e. substances which are secreted in one organ, carried in the bloodstream and then act on a distant tissue or organ. The major integrating centre of the endocrine system is the *hypothalamus* of the brain, which can respond to emotional states and external conditions through input from other parts of the brain, as well as taking account of the internal state of the body. The hypothalamus is the major point of interaction of the nervous and endocrine systems.

FEEDBACK – NEGATIVE AND POSITIVE

Feedback, in which the state of the situation being controlled or co-ordinated is relayed back to the integrating centre, is an essential characteristic of the

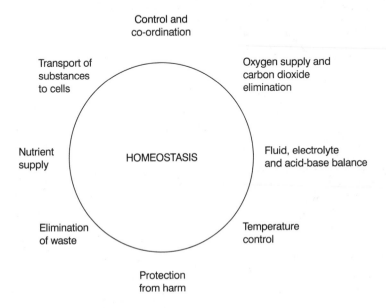

Figure 4.2   The contribution of body systems to homeostasis

Table. 4.3   Systems of the body with major involvement in bodily functions

Bodily functions	Systems of the body
Control and co-ordination	Nervous system Endocrine system
Transport of substances to cells Oxygen supply and carbon dioxide elimination	Cardiovascular system Respiratory system Blood
Nutrient supply	Gastrointestinal tract Liver and gall bladder
Fluid, electrolyte and acid-base balance	Renal system Respiratory system Blood (buffers)
Elimination of waste	Renal system Liver Gastrointestinal tract Skin Respiratory system
Temperature control	Skin Liver
Protection from harm	Immune system Skin Musculoskeletal system

Table. 4.4   Functions regulated by the endocrine system

Control of metabolic rate
Control of glucose metabolism
Growth and development
Fluid and electrolyte balance
Calcium and phosphorus balance
Response to environment
Reproduction and nurturing

activity of control and co-ordination, and operates in both the nervous system and the endocrine system. It enables the initiation of activity from the control systems to be adjusted according to the state of the condition being controlled.

Negative feedback describes the way in which the condition being controlled is brought back towards its normal level through the function of a biological control system (Figure 4.3). Figure 4.4 illustrates this in relation to activities that are controlled through the brain acting as the regulating centre. Blood pressure, temperature, electrolyte levels and many other body parameters are regulated by negative feedback, which is the most common form of feedback in regulation of homeostasis.

The central nervous system or integrating centre for nervous activity receives information through the sensory nervous system. This relays information about the external environment (e.g. from eyes and ears, and from smell, taste, and touch *receptors*), about the position and activity of the body (e.g. from *proprioceptors* in joints) and about the internal state of the body (e.g. from *baroreceptors* which sense blood pressure or *chemoreceptors* which sense carbon dioxide level). Sensors within the endocrine system similarly monitor information about the substance being regulated or the hormone being secreted, and adjust the level of hormone production accordingly.

Positive feedback occurs when the information being relayed results in increasing change occurring, and this form of feedback is much less common. Two important examples occur in blood clotting following injury

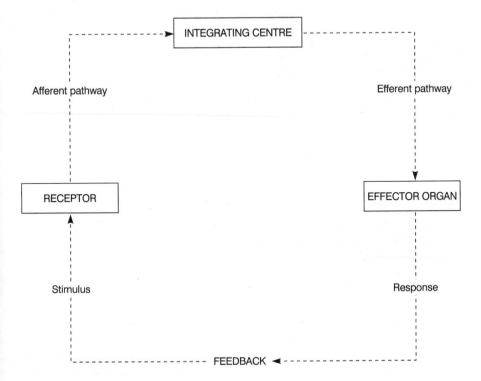

Figure 4.3   Biological control system (Boore, 1981)

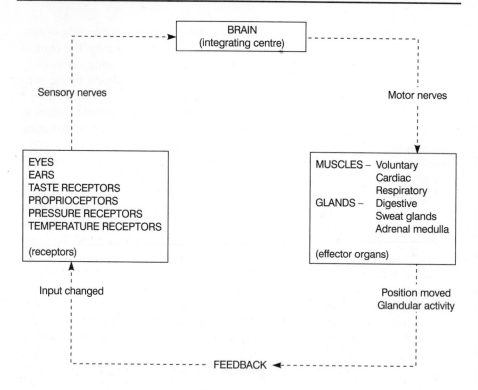

Figure 4.4   Negative feedback with brain as regulating centre (Boore, 1981)

and in uterine contractions during labour. In both situations an increase in activity is necessary for the fulfilment of the function concerned, i.e. prevention of further blood loss or birth of the baby.

The number of mechanisms involved in the regulation of any one factor tends to be related to the narrowness of the limits within which that factor must be maintained. For example, plasma calcium levels are closely regulated by the combined activities of three hormones, parathormone, calcitonin and vitamin D (following activation).

FEEDFORWARD AND BIOLOGICAL RHYTHMS

Feedforward regulation occurs in anticipation of changes which will occur, and activates homeostatic mechanisms to minimise fluctuation in the variable under consideration. For example, a fall in skin temperature activates mechanisms to retain body heat even before there has been any decrease in body temperature (Vander et al., 1994).

Rhythmical variation occurs in many of the functions of the body. *Circadian rhythms*, which are about 24 hours in length, are the commonest type, but monthly and other cycles also occur. One example of circadian rhythm variation is that of body temperature, which is low early in the morning and higher in the evening. Endocrine secretion also varies, e.g. with an increase in cortisol secretion shortly before it is time to rise in the morning, and then a gradual fall throughout the day (Passmore and Robson, 1986). These cycles can be considered as a 'feedforward' response in that they produce variation in different characteristics in preparation for likely activity (Vander *et al.*, 1994).

BALANCE

In regulating the levels of body constituents, the quantity present is related to the balance between input and output (Figure 4.5). In many circumstances it is the substance in its free form (i.e. not combined with any other substance) in the plasma that is important, and thus the amount in combination with other substances becomes part of the input–output balance equation, as illustrated.

In the normal adult healthy state, the input and output are usually equal in a state of stable equilibrium (Vander *et al.*, 1994). In a state of negative equilibrium the output is greater than the input, e.g. a negative nitrogen balance occurs in a patient with cachexia due to cancer. In a state of positive equilibrium the input is greater than the output, and this is the normal state for virtually all body constituents during growth.

Age-related change

Age-related change involves a consideration of growth, development and ageing from the time of conception until death. Growth and development

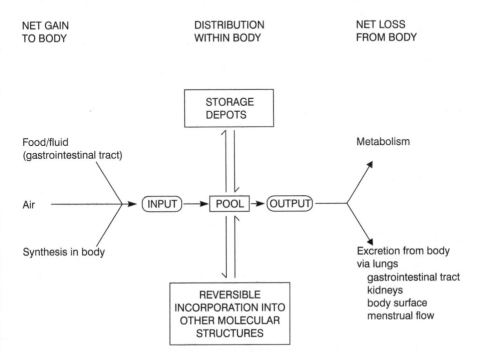

Figure 4.5   Input and output balance (Vander *et al.*, 1994)

consist of a highly complex series of events in which close control and co-ordination are essential. It begins with the fertilisation of an ovum by a sperm, and continues until the fully functioning mature adult is created (Tanner, 1978). Ageing can be regarded as a continuation of development during which functioning deteriorates and eventually is no longer able to maintain homeostasis.

The state of the individual at any point on this journey through life is the result of an interaction between *nature* and *nurture*, an issue which receives considerable attention in debates about influences on development (Bee, 1995). This debate is most commonly discussed in relation to psychological development of the child, but is also relevant in relation to biological development. Nature, in this context, is the genetic composition of the individual, resulting from the combination during fertilisation of 50 per cent of the genetic material from the mother with 50 per cent of the material from the father. The information carried in the genetic material in the form of *deoxyribonucleic acid* (DNA) determines the potential for growth, development and healthy ageing in that individual, but external influences (the nurture part of the equation) throughout life will determine the extent to which that potential is achieved.

GROWTH AND DEVELOPMENT

Co-ordinated progression through the life cycle from the newly formed embryo to old age is the result of a number of cellular and tissue activities that are regulated by the genetic material in the nucleus of the cell. Development of the embryo into an adult occurs through a closely co-ordinated combination of different activities, namely cell division, cell specialisation, tissue movement and programmed cell death. The requirements for these activities to occur in the correct sequence and at the correct time are the same as those for the maintenance of homeostasis, but their provision is through the maternal blood supply within the environment of the maternal uterus. At birth, anatomical and physiological changes occur which enable the infant to live outside its previous highly protective environment.

Co-ordination of the activities involved in growth and development takes place through the genetically determined endocrine and nervous activity (nature) initially of the mother, then of the pre-placental tissue, subsequently by the growing foetus in combination with the placenta, and finally of the physiologically independent growing infant. However, external factors (nurture) are equally important for normal development to occur and, in relation to foetal development, this includes conditions within the uterine environment. Changes in this environment can have deleterious effects. For example, a mother who smokes will reduce the oxygen content of her blood, and thus the oxygen supply to her infant, and is likely to have a smaller than average baby (Floyd *et al.*, 1993) who may also be disadvantaged in the longer term.

A key concept in relation to development is that of the *critical period*. Within normal growth and development there is considerable latitude for redressing deficiencies which have developed as a result of illness. For example, reduced height may be corrected by a period of increased growth rate. However, if normal development of a particular attribute does not occur during the critical period for that characteristic, then it will never be achieved. Critical periods for brain development are reported in the months after birth, during which the infant needs to receive specific types of experiences to allow normal development (Hirsch and Tieman, 1987). In the UK, growth and development are monitored throughout childhood, and divergence from the normal growth curve is investigated. Normally, a rapid rate of growth in the first couple of years of life is followed by a slower steady rate during childhood and by the dramatic growth spurt during adolescence, which slows to a halt as the adult height is reached.

AGEING

It is difficult to differentiate many of the effects of ageing from the effects of disease. However, it is clear that the large reserve in the functioning of most organs in the young adult is gradually lost throughout life (Passmore and Robson, 1980). The details of the physiological changes which occur during ageing cannot be dealt with here, but the key point is that the elderly person becomes less able to maintain homeostasis in the face of demands placed upon the body by environmental and other stressors (Vander *et al.*, 1994).

Theories of ageing fall into two groups, namely *deteriorative theories* and *programmed ageing theories*, although they tend to merge (Passmore and Robson, 1980), with some empirical support for both of these groups of theories. The deteriorative theories assert that ageing is largely due to cumulative deterioration of cells and of the mechanisms for the maintenance of homeostasis. On the other hand, the programmed theories suggest that ageing is determined by the genetic make-up of the individual mediated through mechanisms that come into play later on in life. It has been stated that 'the best way to achieve a long life is to choose long-lived grandparents' (Pearl, 1934, cited in Redfern, 1991).

The individual within the population

VARIATION

So far this chapter has considered only the individual, but individuals function within a population consisting of numerous individuals with varying characteristics. One of the factors of which nurses need to be aware is the range of variation which can be anticipated within a healthy population. Only with this knowledge can the measurement of characteristics be interpreted correctly.

Overfield (1985) has discussed some of the variation which occurs with ageing, with gender, between different races and in different climates, which is of relevance to nursing. The rate of development and the ages at which different stages are reached can vary between different races. For example,

Asian children grow more slowly than Caucasian children and have a more accelerated growth spurt at puberty; when using growth charts to assess their growth pattern, this needs to be taken into account. Anatomical differences are also important. For example, Negro women tend to have smaller pelvises than Caucasian women and also have smaller babies (compensating for the size of the pelvis) which are more mature than Caucasian babies of the same weight.

The norms (i.e. the values used for comparison) for many biochemical and physiological parameters have been determined on large samples of fit adults between 18 and 65 years of age (blood donors), and thus need to be used with caution in the case of children and older people. A study by Jernigan *et al.* (1980) found that 15 per cent of 73 healthy subjects between 74 and 94 years of age had at least one characteristic for which an abnormal value was found. So what do these findings mean? Do these subjects have some unknown illness, or is it normal for such parameters to be altered in the elderly? Of particular interest is the finding that studies cited by Overfield (1985) show that women have higher blood glucose levels than men and that this difference increases with age.

DETERMINATION OF CHARACTERISTICS

Much of the variation between individuals is determined by the genetic material carried on the 46 chromosomes (22 pairs plus 2 sex chromosomes) within each human cell. A female embryo carries two X chromosomes while a male has one X chromosome (from the mother) and one Y chromosome (from the father) as well as the 44 autosomes. Half of the chromosomes (one of each pair plus one sex chromosome) come from each parent, and the paired chromosomes carry paired genes, at identical locations, which code for specific proteins that result in particular characteristics. These paired genes may be identical, in which case the individual is *homozygous* for that characteristic, or the two chromosomes may carry different variants of the gene, in which case the individual is *heterozygous* for that characteristic.

Some of the variation in characteristics has no or minimal biological implications, e.g. brown or blue eyes. However, other characteristics may confer enhanced or diminished biological fitness in relation to the individual's particular environment. Biological fitness refers specifically to the ability to pass on one's genes through reproduction (Harrison *et al.*, 1988). Within certain populations enhanced biological fitness in the *heterozygote* appears to be the explanation for the high incidence of genes which, in the *homozygote*, cause considerable morbidity and mortality and would be expected to be lost from the population through reduced reproduction by those affected. An example of such a condition is sickle cell anaemia, which is common in some malaria-infested parts of the world. The heterozygote for this condition has a substantial degree of resistance to malaria and, although the homozygote has reduced fertility, the biological advantage to the heterozygote ensures that the gene is maintained in the population.

Some characteristics are *monogenic* in nature (i.e. determined by a single gene) while others are *polygenic* (i.e. involving several genes) or multifactorial in nature. Multifactorial characteristics are determined by the interaction of several gene sites together with environmental influences (Weatherall, 1991). Much normal variation, such as that in height, but also that in many clinical conditions, such as cardiac disease, has a multifactorial causation.

The chromosomes consist of DNA, a very large complex molecule in the form of a double helix, which codes for all of the proteins formed within the body – both those forming the structures of the body and those which, as enzymes or hormones, control the functions of the body (including the formation of other structural molecules). Through the intermediary of *ribonucleic acid* (RNA), each protein is formed as a chain consisting of a unique ordering of amino acids. Any alteration from the correct amino acid structure will reduce the ability of that protein to function normally, and thus it is essential that errors in the DNA structure of the cells are not transmitted in cell division. Such errors can be caused by certain environmental chemicals or by radiation, and they are considerably reduced by the action of the DNA repair mechanisms (Lindahl *et al.*, 1991).

During cell division, which occurs during growth and development but also continues throughout life in some tissues, the DNA is normally copied to produce two daughter cells which have exactly the same DNA composition. However, damage can occur. An alteration in the DNA occurring during the formation of the ovum or sperm (when the chromosome number is reduced to 23, i.e. one of each pair) or early in foetal development may result in a natural abortion or in a genetically determined disorder, such as achondroplasia. Damage to DNA later in life, which is not repaired by the DNA repair enzymes, is thought to be one of the causes of cancer, which can be considered to be a genetic disorder (Weatherall, 1991).

Knowledge about human genetics is rapidly increasing and is likely to impinge to a growing extent both on patient care (Weatherall, 1991) and on nursing. The Human Genome Project aims to map the structure of the entire DNA content of every chromosome within the human cell. It is already possible to identify a considerable number of genes which cause specific hereditary conditions, such as cystic fibrosis, but this project will greatly increase the amount of information which can be obtained about each individual. At present, information about a few relatively uncommon conditions can be provided but in future a predisposition to many more common conditions such as heart disease or cancer may be diagnosed. There are ethical and personal implications both for society and for individuals arising from these developments, which are already being discussed elsewhere (Müller-Hill, 1993).

It is essential to realise that, while someone may have a genetic predisposition to development of a particular condition, this does not mean that he or she will develop that disorder. However, it does make it possible to identify those individuals who need to pay particular attention to the environmental factors which, in a susceptible individual, may trigger development of a specific condition. Nursing intervention can then be focused to enable these people to take responsibility for minimising their risk through modifying the environmental trigger factors.

Environment (individual–environment)

Each individual exists in relation to his or her environment and there are a number of biological concepts within this area that are of particular relevance to nursing. In health one lives in a state of equilibrium with the external world and there are physiological mechanisms that maintain this balance within a changing environment.

Stress and adaptation

The environment imposes a number of stressors on the individual, who must be able to adapt in order to maintain health (see Chapter 5). *Stress* and *adaptation* are important concepts in nursing and are more usually considered from a behavioural point of view. However, it is equally important to understand the physiological changes which occur and are essential for healthy living, and the relationship between the mental and physiological state in stress. Stressors may include physical conditions such as heat or cold, physiological disturbances such as illness or altered circadian rhythm, social/environmental factors such as noise or overcrowding, or psychological states such as anxiety.

The *transactional model of stress* (Cox, 1978) identifies clearly that the key determinant of whether or not stress occurs is the way in which the individual involved interprets the situation. When the demand exerted on the individual is perceived as greater than that person's ability to cope, then stress exists. In this model the behavioural and emotional facets of the response to stress are identified as well as the biological response. The biological response is partly comparable to that originally described by Selye in 1956 *The Stress of Life* (second edition published in 1976) in the *general adaptation syndrome*, athough this has since been extended by further research.

The general adaptation syndrome described by Selye has three stages, namely the *alarm reaction*, the *stage of resistance* and the *stage of exhaustion* (see Figure 4.6). In the alarm reaction, when the individual is first exposed to the stressor, specific changes occur, including peptic ulceration, enlargement of the lymph glands and thymus gland, and shrinking of the adrenal cortex. If adaptation occurs, then in the second stage these changes are reversed in the stage of resistance. If exposure continues, then the individual may lose the ability to continue to resist the stressor, all of the changes of the alarm reaction reappear and the person dies. According to Selye, the changes of the general adaptation syndrome are the same for everyone and result from all types of stressor. However, the stress response is now known to be considerably more complex, with variation between individuals and in different situations (Ur, 1991).

There are two aspects of the stress response, namely the acute short-term response and the slower longer-lasting response which corresponds to that described by Selye (1976).

THE RAPID STRESS RESPONSE

This is also known as the 'fright, flight or fight' response, indicating the major physiological changes which enable the body to react swiftly and effectively to physical threat. It is initiated by the release of already formed *catecholamine hormones* (adrenaline and noradrenaline) from the adrenal medulla and the sympathetic nervous system. The oxygen and nutrient supply to the body tissues is increased, the nervous system becomes aroused, and the blood coagulates more rapidly. While these effects are important when dealing with a physical threat, the physiological changes which cause them can be deleterious if a physical response is not required. For example, prolonged and frequent release of catecholamines as a result of stress can result in hypertension in susceptible individuals (Groër and Shekleton, 1989).

THE SLOW STRESS RESPONSE

This occurs as a result of stimulation of the synthesis and secretion of *glucocorticoid hormones* (e.g. cortisol) from the adrenal cortex and the effect of these hormones on the formation of cellular enzymes. Thus the response takes longer to be initiated and lasts longer than the rapid response. This response also plays an important role in increasing the body's ability to cope with physical demand through the release of additional nutrients into the bloodstream for energy production and tissue repair, and by making the body better able to cope with blood loss by increasing the fluid volume of the body and enhancing the coagulability of the blood.

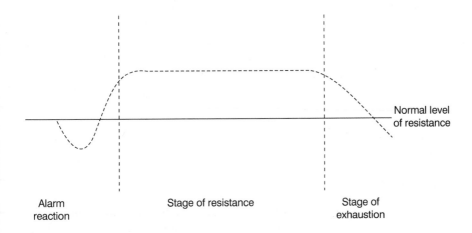

Normal level of resistance

Alarm reaction   Stage of resistance   Stage of exhaustion

Figure 4.6   The general adaptation syndrome (Selye, 1976)

The stress response is essential for adaptation, and those individuals who are unable to respond by increased secretion of glucocorticoid hormones are not able to adapt adequately within a stressful situation. Even relatively minor stressors may therefore result in death (Hubay *et al.*, 1975).

The stress response which is not utilised through physical action and which is prolonged can cause numerous maladaptive changes which can result in disease (Fletcher, 1991), including increased protein breakdown to form new glucose (*gluconeogenesis*) and a reduction in the immune response. However, it has been demonstrated that nursing interventions designed to minimise stress can cause a reduction in glucocorticoid hormone secretion and the resulting deleterious effects in post-operative patients (Boore, 1978).

The microbiological environment

People live within a biological environment which is teeming with micro-organisms, i.e. organisms that can only be observed with the aid of a micro-scope, and healthy individuals coexist in equilibrium with these organisms. There is a wide range of one-celled organisms within this range, some with the DNA circumscribed within a cell nucleus and the usual cell structures found in human cells, but others (including the bacteria) without a cell nucleus or distinct organelles. Even smaller in structure are the viruses, which contain merely a nucleic acid within a protein coat and can only repli-cate within a cell. Recently, structures even smaller and less complex than viruses have been identified. Known as prions, these have been associated with disorders of the central nervous system that progress slowly, such as Creutzfeldt-Jakob disease (Ellner and Neu, 1992) and possibly multiple sclerosis (Youmans *et al.*, 1985).

Many micro-organisms exist in association with animals or plants, and may be beneficial, harmless or harmful to the host, those that cause disease being known as pathogens. An equilibrium exists between the host defence mechanisms and the virulence of the micro-organism, such that the more virulent the micro-organism, the greater its potential for causing disease. Some organisms can cause disease even when present in small numbers within a healthy host, and these are known as primary pathogens (Ellner and Neu, 1992), while others, described as opportunistic, only result in dis-ease when present in large numbers or within a host whose defences are weakened. A number of organisms, known as commensals, exist in a healthy equilibrium in many parts of the human body and form an important part of the innate defence against infection. Some of these are capable of causing disease in a host if they gain access to a part of the body from which they are usually excluded.

IMMUNITY

The host's resistance to infection is due to two types of immunity, *innate immunity* and *adaptive immunity*. Innate immunity is produced by the differ-ent mechanisms present within the body which do not depend on previous exposure to the organism. The first line of defence consists of physical and chemical barriers to entry to the body, such as the skin, the acid environment of the stomach or the chemical *lysozyme* present in tears and other secretions. The presence of the indigenous flora of the skin, gut, upper respiratory tract and vagina plays an important role in reducing the opportunities for pathogenic organisms to gain entry to the body as the potential sites for colonisation are occupied. Innate immunity also includes the acute-phase response in which a number of changes occur, including activation of phagocytic cells which engulf and destroy bacteria, and the activation of other substances within the immune system which facilitate the action of the phagocytes.

Adaptive immunity is acquired through the response of the immune system to the presence of pathogens. It is mediated through two major groups of white blood cells, namely the B-lymphocytes and the T-lymphocytes. Although the two systems are interdependent, the B-lymphocytes are responsible for free antibody production, while the T-lymphocytes are responsible for cell-mediated immunity which directly damages foreign cells. Both the T-lymphocyte and B-lymphocyte systems exhibit three key characteristics: high specificity, memory (neither of these are found with innate immunity) and tolerance (shared with innate immunity).

Specificity

The immune response is stimulated by a small portion (the epitope) of the foreign antigen (the substance that stimulates the immune response) which interacts with a specific receptor on a lymphocyte. This interaction stimulates cell division and produces daughter cells which either form antibodies which combine with that specific antigen (and no other) or are able to interact physically with the foreign cell at the epitope and cause damage. The antigen-antibody complex triggers the events associated with inflammation and the actions already initiated through the innate immunity (Vander *et al.*, 1994), and is primarily associated with bacterial infection. Cell-mediated immunity is associated with the destruction of cells containing viruses that are presenting viral epitopes on the cell membrane, with the destruction of malignant cells, or with graft rejection. In both B- and T-lymphocyte-mediated immunity, a highly specific receptor on the lymphocyte or the antibody interacts with the epitope on the antigen foreign cell or particle. Each lymphocyte will recognise only one epitope, and the human body contains lymphocytes that are able to recognise many millions of different epitopes.

Receptors, in this context, are proteins within the cell membrane (or, in a few cases, within the cell itself) that will bind only with a complementary particle, similar to the matching of a lock and key. (These must be differentiated from those sensory receptors which respond to information received and transmit information to the nervous system.) The binding of a receptor to its complementary particle will alter activity within the cell in a way that is dependent on the particular type of substance with which it is interacting. The concept of receptors is important because it represents a general way in which body cells interact with molecules in the extracellular fluid, and has implications beyond immunity. The release of chemicals known as *neurotransmitters* from the end of one nerve fibre and their passage across the synapse (the space between adjacent nerve cells) to link with the receptor on the adjacent nerve, or on a muscle cell, is the method whereby nervous impulses are transmitted. It is also the way in which hormones alter cell activity, and the action of drugs (considered later in this chapter) is mediated through receptors as well.

Memory

Memory is the ability to remember antigens with which that lymphocyte's precursor has previously come into contact and it is the principle underlying immunisation. In the previous section, it was indicated that a particular antigen combining with the specific receptor on a lymphocyte will stimulate cell division. While the majority of the cells resulting from such division will become specialised either for production of antibodies to the particular antigen or for attacking foreign cells, some of the cells will act as memory cells. The memory cells will recognise the antigen on the next occasion when it is encountered and, through rapid cell division, will initiate the immune response.

On the first occasion when a particular antigen is encountered, a primary immune response occurs when antibodies are produced slowly and in fairly small amounts. On the second and subsequent occasions the immune response is rapid and of much greater intensity.

Tolerance

Tolerance indicates that, under normal conditions, the immune system does not respond to 'self' – it has become tolerant to 'self' antigens through exposure to massive amounts during foetal life. In autoimmune disorders, this tolerance is lost and certain body tissues are attacked by antibodies to themselves.

THE HOST–MICROBE RELATIONSHIP

Changes which influence any part of the host–microbe equilibrium may increase the risk of the individual (the host) developing an infection. Changes in the virulence of organisms can occur and alter the extent to which they cause infection. However, in the general nursing context (as opposed to the specialist infection-control nursing arena) there are other factors which are of greater significance.

Micro-organisms also adapt to their environment, and one of the factors to which those micro-organisms found in hospitals and on hospital staff adapt is the presence of antibiotics. Many disease-causing organisms have become resistant to some antibiotics, and some have become resistant to many anti-microbial drugs and are now a cause of great concern (Youmans *et al.*, 1985). Thus it is a duty of care (United Kingdom Central Council for Nursing, Midwifery and Health Visiting, 1992) to minimise the likelihood of transmitting these organisms to patients, and knowledge of the source and routes of transmission of micro-organisms is essential for safe practice; see, for example, Hare and Cooke (1991).

An infection caused by micro-organisms from outside the body is known as an *exogenous* infection, while one that results from the action of the indigenous flora, i.e. micro-organisms already in or on the body of the individual, is said to be *endogenous*. As the patient's own flora can be an important cause of infection, and any infection that does result will require treatment, it is important to prevent, so far as is possible, replacement of the normal flora by antibiotic-resistant microbes. Thus all possible precautions must be taken to minimise transmission of microbes that are normally resident on the skin of hospital staff, or within other sources in the hospital environment, to the patients. Keeping patients in hospital for the minimum possible length of time is one way of achieving this objective.

The strength of host defences is a key issue and nursing interventions with patients need to enhance these to maintain a satisfactory equilibrium with the microbial environment. The situations or medical conditions that reduce these defences are numerous and can be grouped as follows: those which enhance microbial access; those which generally reduce the functioning of body cells; and those which specifically reduce the immune response.

Microbial access is facilitated by any break in the natural defences of the body, such as an open wound caused by accidental trauma or surgery. Antibiotic therapy can, paradoxically, sometimes result in increased risk of infection by facilitating microbial access as a consequence of reducing the numbers of indigenous microbial flora, and thus allowing colonisation by pathogenic micro-organisms. The general ability of the body tissues to resist infection is reduced by any condition which causes a deterioration in the supply of oxygen or nutrients via the bloodstream to the tissues. The activity of the immune system itself is decreased by several conditions, including those in which there is increased secretion of glucocorticoid hormones (thus reducing the immune response), malnutrition (which reduces the ability to manufacture the protein antibodies) and AIDS (which specifically attacks particular lymphocytes) (Fan *et al.*, 1994).

Health (health–illness)

Health has been considered in different ways, many of them drawing on a wide social and psychological perspective (Davey *et al.*, 1995; see Chapters 3, 5 and 7), but in this chapter it is the biological perspective that will be considered. Details of the altered physiology in disease are not being addressed here. Rather, the aim is to examine briefly some of the principles involved.

Themes in pathophysiology

In the light of the discussion in this chapter, it is reasonable to consider that a state of health exists when an individual is able to adapt in order to maintain an equilibrium with the environment, and thus is able to maintain homeostasis in the presence of different types of stressors. The converse is true, that a state of ill health (or disease) exists when an individual is no longer able to maintain homeostasis and is not in equilibrium with the environment.

Spector (1989) identifies two ways in which failure of adaptation occurs. There may simply be a failure to respond adequately, e.g. to an overwhelming infection. On the other hand, disease may be partly due to a normal adaptive mechanism being turned against the individual concerned, e.g. antibody formation is a major defence mechanism against infection, but can also be a cause of disease in autoimmune disorders. In some circumstances, then, disease can be viewed as a distortion of a survival mechanism.

Failures of adaptation can be self-perpetuating and reinforcing (Spector, 1989). An example of this is the situation in a patient with congestive cardiac failure when the reduced pressure of the blood supplying the kidney triggers the renin–angiotensin–aldosterone system (Figure 4.7). This results in vasoconstriction and raised blood pressure, and increased sodium and water retention, and thus increased extracellular fluid volume. This increases the workload for the heart, and thus increases the extent to which it is unable to meet the demands placed on it. It is also the principle underlying the progressive physiological deterioration which can result in multiple organ failure.

Effects of disordered body function

Causes of disorder are numerous, and some have already been indicated in earlier sections of this chapter (e.g. micro-organisms), but in many ways it is

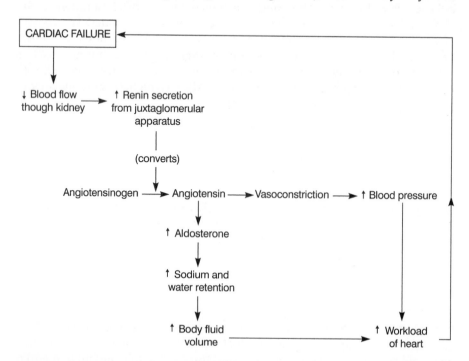

Figure 4.7   The renin–angiotensin–aldosterone system

the effect or response of the body which is most important for nurses. These effects have been identified by Spector (1989) as follows: inflammation, with the signs and symptoms of rubor (redness), calor (heat), dolor (pain), tumor (swelling) and loss of function; degeneration in which loss of normal structure and functioning occurs; and neoplasia (i.e. new growth), which can be benign, causing difficulties only by virtue of its size and/or position, or malignant, spreading throughout other parts of the body. In addition, there is a fourth group of conditions, which are congenital (present at birth) or genetically determined (inherited), and this category cuts across the first three types.

The effects of disorder on the functions of the body are often similar, although due to different causes, and relate to the altered functioning of the organ or system of the body that is affected. If cells are relatively deprived of oxygen or nutrients, or the pH is no longer within the normal range, or waste products are not being removed normally, then the cell enzymes will not work effectively and the functioning of those cells will be reduced. The functioning of the tissue and organ affected will also be impaired, with resulting effects on homeostasis due to the reduced contribution of that organ to the maintenance of the whole organism.

Thus disorders which cause such changes will affect all of the systems of the body. Examples of disorders that will all have similar effects on cell functioning include the following: respiratory disorders resulting in lowered oxygen supply; anaemia reducing the amount of oxygen transported to the tissues; cardiac disease decreasing the flow of blood to the tissues; renal, liver or cardiac disease which may cause oedema and thus increase the distance between capillaries and cells and, therefore, the amount of nutrients and oxygen that reaches the cells. The patient is likely to have reduced gastrointestinal functioning with anorexia and constipation, lowered skin resistance to pressure and reduced healing, impaired liver functioning and thus enhanced effects of drugs and hormones, lowered nervous activity and slowed reflexes, and generally reduced energy levels for all activity.

Identification of risk factors

There are a number of constellations of factors that place individuals at greater risk of developing particular conditions, and these need to be recognised if appropriate education is to be provided. Genetic predisposition has already been discussed, but two other major groups are factors associated with lifestyle and environmental factors.

LIFESTYLE AND DISEASE

For a considerable number of disorders, lifestyle factors are implicated in the aetiology. Smoking in particular seems to be the single factor which receives most attention, and with justification. It greatly increases the incidence of lung and several other cancers, and is the single major cause of chronic bronchitis and emphysema, causing considerable levels of morbidity. It also increases the risk of development of atherosclerosis, which can result in myocardial infarction (heart attack), cerebrovascular accident (stroke) or peripheral vascular disease leading to amputation (Nowak and Handford, 1994).

However, a diet high in fat or cholesterol, refined carbohydrates and salt, particularly in combination with lack of exercise, also increases the risk of development of atherosclerosis (Heller *et al.*, 1987). Stress, as discussed earlier, is an additional contributory factor. Many of the same factors also contribute to the development of hypertension which, if not treated adequately, can result in renal disease and eventually renal failure, and also in atherosclerosis with the effects indicated above. Changes towards the type of diet found in Mediterranean countries appear to result in a reduction in the risk of coronary heart disease (Kushi *et al.*, 1995).

Alcohol is another major lifestyle factor which has implications for health. There is some evidence that moderate drinking, particularly of red wine, reduces one of the risk factors for heart disease (Sharpe *et al.*, 1995), although the mortality rate from all causes increases progressively as alcohol consumption rises above the recommended amount (Doll *et al.*, 1994). There is evidence that excessive drinking can result in cirrhosis of the liver as well as a considerably increased risk of accidents and non-accidental injury to others (Anderson, 1991).

ENVIRONMENTAL FACTORS

In 1859, Florence Nightingale (cf. Skretkowicz, 1992) emphasised the importance of environmental factors in promoting recovery. Conversely, a wide range of conditions within the home, work or social environment can be aetiological factors in disease. Environmental factors are capable of contributing to the development of ill health by exposing the individual to micro-organisms, by the presence of harmful substances such as asbestos or cigarette smoke, or via the stressors inflicted by, for instance, overcrowding (Smith, 1991).

In this area, biological factors interact with social circumstances. The relationship between poverty and ill health has been demonstrated (Townsend *et al.*, 1988), with individuals in the higher social classes having lower morbidity and mortality (see Chapter 7). An understanding of the range of factors which can influence health is important if nurses are to help patients to cope with these conditions.

Nursing (treatment–care)

In this section, it is necessary first to define the role of nursing and thus to be able to begin to identify concepts that are relevant to nursing. Nursing has been described in numerous ways, including supporting *self-care* (Orem, 1995), promoting *adaptation* (Andrews and Roy, 1991) or assisting with *activities of daily living* (Roper *et al.*, 1990). Considering these from a biological perspective, they all implicitly include the support of homeostasis as a key concern. However, nursing care does not take place divorced from medical and other treatments being administered, and the support of homeostasis needs to include consideration of these other therapeutic activities. In order to provide effective care, the nurse needs to understand the key concepts that are relevant to the treatments being administered, and be able to incorporate their actions into the patient care provided.

In many medical treatments there is a balance to be struck between the benefits to be achieved and the possible side-effects or deleterious results of the treatment. Particularly important examples are radiotherapy and chemotherapy which can have severe and sometimes permanent adverse effects, but have the balancing potential to save life or to minimise the effects of malignant disease.

Some of the biological principles underpinning drug therapy and surgery are considered in some detail, because they are both forms of therapy in which the nurse has considerable scope to enhance the effectiveness and minimise the risks of treatment.

Drug therapy

Drug therapy carries both benefits and risks, and the decision to prescribe a drug should consider both sides of the equation. Drugs are used in three ways: to cure disease, such as infections; to suppress a disease condition or symptoms, as in disorders such as hypertension, asthma or congestive cardiac failure; or to prevent disease, as when antimalarial drugs are taken before, during and after one is staying in or visiting an area where malaria is endemic (Laurence and Bennett, 1992).

Drugs act by altering the normal control mechanisms of body function, either unselectively, e.g. general anaesthetics, or selectively by binding to a specific component of the cell and thus altering its functioning. The effectiveness of any drug depends on the level of the substance in the extracellular fluid which transports the active molecule to the cells. Here it will interact with the appropriate receptor on the cell membrane, or with some other structure. The principles involved in drug therapy revolve around an understanding of those factors which influence the level of the drug in the blood.

For any drug there is a therapeutic level at which the drug is active, and a toxic level at which the side-effects or toxic effects of the drug become excessive. The *therapeutic index* indicates the relationship between these two levels, neither of which will be an exact measure, and allows drugs to be considered in relation to the safety and efficacy of the substance concerned (Laurence and Bennett, 1992).

PHARMACOKINETICS

This topic deals with those factors related to the drug reaching its site of action and, specifically, the processes of absorption, distribution, metabolism and excretion. All of these processes are influenced by the chemical and physical properties of the drug molecule (Grahame-Smith and Aronson, 1992).

The rate and amount of drug that is absorbed into the general blood-stream is determined by the route of administration and by factors which influence absorption. The absorption of drugs from the gastrointestinal tract is modified by the presence or absence of food, or by altered motility of the gut, while the state of the circulation through the tissues influences the absorption of drugs administered by subcutaneous or intramuscular injection.

The active drug is that portion which exists in its free form within the extracellular fluid, but the processes involved in distribution will both reduce this level and maintain an adequate level over an extended period of time. Some of the drug, particularly if it is fat-soluble, will be distributed to the fat stores of the body, and some of it will be carried in combination with the plasma proteins. The free drug molecules in the extracellular fluid are available to combine with receptors on the cells and exert their action.

These free drug molecules are also exposed to the action of the drug-metabolising enzymes in the liver, which make the molecules water-soluble and thus capable of being eliminated from the body. Some drugs are administered in an inactive form and are activated by this metabolism, but the end-result of drug metabolism is inactivation. Elimination takes place mainly via the kidneys and the biliary tract.

Certain substances can inhibit or enhance the effectiveness of these drug-metabolising enzymes, and thus alter the effectiveness of therapy. One of the mechanisms whereby drug metabolism is increased is enzyme induction, i.e. stimulation by other substances of the amount of these enzymes produced by the liver cells. A considerable number of drugs have this effect, but so also do barbecued meats, brussels sprouts, cigarette smoke and insecticides. The significance of this action is that important drugs may be metabolised and removed from the bloodstream more readily than normal. The action of the drug will thus be reduced, and this can result in loss of effectiveness, e.g. anticoagulant/coagulant control may be lost (Laurence and Bennett, 1992).

The half-life of a drug is the time taken for its concentration in the blood to decrease by 50 per cent, and it is a crucial factor in determining the timing of doses if drugs are to be maintained at the therapeutic level within the bloodstream.

DRUG ADMINISTRATION

Drug doses are administered, as illustrated in Figure 4.8, in such a way as to build up to and maintain the therapeutic level. As can be seen, the timing of administration is important to ensure that the level of the drug does not fall below the concentration at which it will be active.

However, the timing of administration is also important in relation to food intake. Most drugs, including many antimicrobial drugs, will be absorbed most effectively on an empty stomach and, in order to maintain the necessary level in the blood, must be administered before food. Other substances can cause gastric irritation if administered on an empty stomach, and must

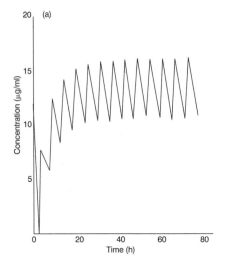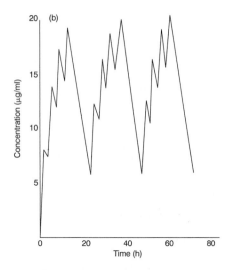

Figure 4.8 Half-life and dose regimen required to maintain a therapeutic level of a drug (Rogers *et al.*, 1981) (a) Dosing at 6-hourly intervals to achieve a therapeutic range between 10 and 16 μg/ml (b) Dosing at 10 a.m., 2 p.m., 6 p.m. and 10 p.m. instead of at strict 6-hourly intervals may produce both toxicity and lack of therapeutic effect

therefore be administered with or after food. In addition, drug–food interactions can result in the active drug molecule being removed from availability, e.g. the interaction of tetracycline with dairy products. A reduction in the serum levels of the drug by as much as 50 to 80 per cent has been reported, and this can totally abolish the effectiveness of the medication (Stockley, 1991). Administering the medication at the wrong time can have serious implications for the effectiveness of therapy.

The time of day at which some drugs are administered takes into account the normal circadian rhythm in order to minimise disruption of the normal homeostatic mechanisms. For example, corticosteroid hormones should be given in the morning, or divided between the morning and early afternoon, in order to minimise adrenal suppression (Grahame-Smith and Aronson, 1992).

RISKS OF DRUG ADMINISTRATION

The aim of treatment is to produce the beneficial effects of drug administration while minimising the risks. These risks increase as more drugs are prescribed and the risk of interaction grows. It must be recognised that, practically, all drugs are toxic if an overdose is taken due to the direct effect of the drug on the body tissues, e.g. liver damage is caused by paracetamol. The adverse reactions to drugs which can occur at normally therapeutic dosages have been classified into two major groups (Types A and B) and three minor groups (Types C, D and E) (Laurence and Bennett, 1992).

Type A (augmented reactions)

These reactions are the normal effects of the drug, which are related to the dose taken and will occur in all individuals if enough of the drug is taken. The aim is to minimise their extent by ensuring that the dose prescribed is the minimum that will be effective. An example of this type of reaction is postural hypotension.

Type B (bizarre reactions)

These reactions only occur in some individuals and are due to an unpredictable interaction between the drug and the patient, related to, for example, some inherited abnormality or an allergic reaction to the drug.

Type C (continuous reactions)

These reactions are due to long-term use of the drug, and include effects on the extrapyramidal motor system of such drugs as chlorpromazine, used in the treatment of schizophrenia.

Type D (delayed reactions)

These reactions are delayed in their manifestation, and include changes such as carcinogenesis or teratogenesis. One of the best-known examples is that of thalidomide.

Type E (ending-of-use reactions)

An example of these reactions is the adrenocortical insufficiency that can result at the end of treatment with corticosteroids.

Patients need to be aware of the types of adverse reactions that can occur with their medications, how to recognise them, and what actions to take. Thus the nurse has a major educative role with regard to all patients receiving drugs.

Surgical intervention

The details of surgical intervention are complex and it is not possible to examine them in detail here. However, an understanding of some of the principles underlying this form of management can be of considerable value in helping patients to cope with the experience.

An operation may be performed for any one or a combination of reasons, namely excision of diseased tissue, repair or reconstruction of a defect or deformity, drainage of infective lesions or cysts, modification of physiology, or investigation (Myers *et al.*, 1980). It may also be elective (in that it is not essential for survival but will enhance health and comfort), essential (in that it will remove a threat to life) or emergency (in that it needs to be carried out rapidly in order to prevent death). The reason for the surgery may considerably alter the patient's approach to the procedure and may also alter the focus of the pre-operative preparation required.

Developments in surgical techniques have been made possible by increased skill in management to prevent haemorrhage and infection, and by improvements in anaesthesia. All of these have considerable implications for nursing. Thus the four key areas for consideration are the following: the operation itself and the metabolic response to surgery; the risk of haemorrhage and haemostasis, and potential circulatory disturbances; the risk of infection and the necessity for asepsis; and anaesthesia and its complications, and the management of pain (Boore *et al.*, 1987). Many of the nursing activities before, during and after surgery are concerned with these areas.

THE OPERATION AND METABOLIC RESPONSE

It is only relatively recently that consideration has been given to the evaluation of surgical treatment and the comparative effectiveness of the various newly introduced surgical techniques. There has been a rapid growth in the use of laparoscopic techniques, in which operations are carried out by instruments inserted through small incisions in the abdominal wall and viewed through a telescope which is also inserted through a similar incision in the abdomen. Decreased post-operative pain and shorter hospital stays have been reported, compared to open surgery, for a number of conditions. However, long-term evaluation of the results is still needed (Donohue, 1994).

The physiological changes which occur during stress have been discussed briefly earlier. The effects on the immune system and on protein metabolism, which are enhanced by the similar changes that form part of the metabolic response to surgery, are potentially harmful. Pre-operative nursing interventions to minimise stress can enhance recovery (Boore, 1978), and nutritional care is also important. A reasonably well-nourished, healthy individual can tolerate the catabolic effects and fasting associated with surgery for about 1 week after a major operation. However, malnourished patients or those with severe infections need additional nourishment (Canizarro, 1981).

HAEMORRHAGE, HAEMOSTASIS AND CIRCULATORY DISTURBANCES

Blood clotting is essential for surgery to be successful, and enhanced haemostasis is a normal response to trauma. However, the converse aspect of this situation is that blood within the circulation elsewhere in the body is also more prone to clot. Adding to this the pressure on the legs during surgery and immobility, the three factors identified by Virchow in 1856 as being implicated in the development of deep vein thromboses (stasis, trauma and hypercoagulability) are all present. Precautions are now taken to minimise all of these factors.

INFECTION

Interaction with the microbial environment has been discussed earlier, and surgery will disturb the equilibrium between host and microbe for several reasons. The patient is admitted to an environment in which many of the micro-organisms will be antibiotic resistant, and he or she will be undergoing treatment that will increase exposure to those organisms. Secondly, the physical barrier of the skin is broken. Thirdly, the stress resulting from the physical and psychological effects of undergoing surgery and the metabolic response will reduce the effectiveness of the immune system.

Environmental management, including selection of theatre clothing so as to minimise dispersal of micro-organisms, is important. Wound care, and the selection and application of sterile dressings which will protect the wound from the environment and promote rapid healing by maintaining a high level of humidity, preventing cooling, and allowing gaseous exchange, will minimise the risk of infection (Westaby, 1985). Nursing interventions that enhance the circulation (adequate fluids, mobility), improve nutritional status and minimise stress will all promote recovery.

ANAESTHESIA AND PAIN

Improvements in anaesthetic techniques have enhanced the safety of patients and increased the scope of operations that can be performed. However, it is still true that the longer the period of anaesthesia and the greater the amount of anaesthetic needed, the greater the risk to the patient. Thus pre-operative preparation which minimises anxiety and so reduces the amount of analgesia and anaesthesia required (as well as promoting recovery more generally) is exceedingly important (Boore *et al.*, 1987; see Chapter 2).

Pain management is, of course, a much wider issue than that in relation to surgery, and is a topic that cannot be examined in the depth that it deserves within this chapter. The *gate control theory of pain* (Melzack and Wall, 1982) is helpful in demonstrating how the range of different nursing interventions (McCaffery and Beebe, 1994) can have a physiological basis.

Conclusion: application of biological sciences in nursing

This chapter has endeavoured to begin the process of identifying biological concepts of particular relevance to nursing within a structure that relates to a nursing framework. It has also indicated the broad range of knowledge that is relevant.

The importance of such knowledge lies in the way in which it influences the care provided for the sick or healthy individual in the promotion of health. Probably the most important area in which nurses use this knowledge is in the provision of care to support homeostasis in individuals with physiological disorders. Equally important is possession of the knowledge required to provide accurate information and teaching for patients in order to help them to understand their own condition and become as independent as possible of professional care. In addition, preventative care may be focused more effectively by identifying the personal and environmental circumstances which predispose individuals to development of ill health. Health monitoring or screening will take account of individual differences and thus allow more appropriate interpretation of findings. Early recognition of deviations from normal will increase the potential for treatment to cure or prevent further deterioration.

The greater task of determining the detail needed in relation to the different concepts considered here has yet to be undertaken.

References

Akinsanya, J. 1987a The life sciences in nurse education. In Davis, B. (ed.), *Nursing education, research and developments*. Beckenham: Croom Helm, 38–71.

Akinsanya, J. 1987b The life sciences in nursing: development of a theoretical model. *Journal of Advanced Nursing* **12**, 267-274.

Anderson, P. 1991 Alcohol as a key area. In Smith, R. (ed.), *The health of the nation: the BMJ view*. London: British Medical Journal.

Andrews, H. A. and Roy, C. 1991 *Essentials of the Roy adaptation model*, 2nd. edn. Norwalk: Appleton and Lange.

Bee, H. 1995 *The developing child*, 7th edn. New York: Harper Collins.

Boore, J. R. P. 1978 *Prescription for recovery*. London: Royal College of Nursing (reprinted in 1995 in Research Classics, Vol. 1. London: Scutari Press).

Boore, J. R. P. 1981 The physical sciences in nursing. In Smith, J. P. (ed.), *Nursing science in nursing practice*. London: Butterworths, 86–110.

Boore, J. R. P., Champion, R. and Ferguson, M. C. (eds) 1987 *Nursing the physically ill adult*. Edinburgh: Churchill Livingstone.

Canizarro, P. C. 1981 Methods of nutritional support in the surgical patient. In Yarborough, M. F. and Curreri, P. W. (eds), *Surgical nutrition*. Edinburgh: Churchill Livingstone, 13–37.

Cannon, W. B. 1939 *The wisdom of the body*. New York: Norton.

Carnevali, D. L. and Thomas, M. D. 1993 *Diagnostic reasoning and treatment: decision-making in nursing*. Philadelphia: Lippincott.

Chandler, J. 1991 Reforming nurse education 1 – the reorganisation of nursing knowledge. *Nurse Education Today* **11**, 83–8.

Clarke, M. 1995 Guest editorial. *Journal of Advanced Nursing* **22**, 405–6.

Courtney, M. 1991 A study of the teaching and learning of the biological sciences in nurse education. *Journal of Advanced Nursing* **16**, 1110–16.

Cox, T. 1978 *Stress*. London: Macmillan.

Davey, B., Gray, A. and Seale, C. (eds) 1995 *Health and disease: a reader,* 2nd edn. Buckingham: Open University Press.

Doll, R., Peto, R., Wheatley, K. and Gray, R. 1994 Mortality in relation to consumption of alcohol: 13 years' observations on male British doctors. *British Medical Journal* **309**, 911–18.

Donohue, J. H. 1994 Laparoscopic surgical procedures. *Mayo Clinic Proceedings* **69**, 758–62.

Ellner, P. D. and Neu, H. C. 1992 *Understanding infectious disease*. St Louis: Mosby.

Fan, H., Conner, R. F and Villarreal, L. P. 1994 *The biology of AIDS,* 3rd edn. Boston: Jones and Bartlett.

Fawcett, J. 1984 *Metaparadigm analysis and evaluation of conceptual models of nursing*. Philadelphia: F. A. Davis.

Fletcher, B. 1991 *Work, stress, disease and life expectancy*. Chichester: Wiley.

Floyd, R. L., Rimer, B. K., Giovino, G.A., Mullen, P. D. and Sullivan, S. E. 1993 A review of smoking in pregnancy: effects on pregnancy outcomes and cessation efforts. *Annual Review of Public Health* **14**, 379–411.

Grahame-Smith, D. G. and Aronson, J. K. (eds) 1992 *Oxford textbook of clinical pharmacology and drug therapy*, 2nd edn. Oxford: Oxford University Press.

Groër, M. W. and Shekleton, M. E. 1989 *Basic pathophysiology: a holistic approach*. 3rd edn. St Louis: Mosby.

Hare, R. and Cooke, E. M. 1991 *Bacteriology and immunity for nurses*, 7th edn. Edinburgh: Churchill Livingstone.

Harrison, G. A., Tanner, J. M., Tilbeam, D. R. and Baker, P. T. 1988 *Human biology: an introduction to human evolution, variation, growth and ecology*, 3rd edn. Oxford: Oxford University Press.

Heller, T., Bailey, L., Gott, M. and Howes, M. (eds) 1987 *Coronary heart disease: reducing the risk: a reader*. Chichester: Wiley.

Hinchliff, S. M. and Montague, S. E. 1988 *Physiology for nursing practice*. London: Baillière Tindall.

Hirsch, H. V. B. and Tieman, S. B. 1987 Perceptual development and experience-dependent changes in cat visual cortex. In Bornstein, M. H. (ed.), *Sensitive periods in development: interdisciplinary perspectives*. Hillsdale, NJ: Erlbaum, 39–80.

Hockey, L. 1973 Nursing research as a basis for nursing science (unpublished paper), University of Edinburgh. Cited in Smith, J. P. (ed.), *Nursing science in nursing practice*. London: Butterworths.

Hubay, C. A., Weckesser, E. C. and Levy, R. P. 1975 Occult adrenal insufficiency in surgical patients. *Annals of Surgery* **81**, 325–32.

Jernigan, J. A., Gudat, J. C., Blake, J. L., Bowen, L. and Lezotte, D. C. 1980 Reference values for blood findings in relatively fit elderly persons. *Journal of the American Geriatric Society* **28**, 308–14.

Jordan, S. 1994 Should nurses be studying bioscience? A discussion paper. *Nurse Education Today* **14**, 417–26.

Kushi, L. H., Lenart, E. B. and Willett, W. C. 1995 Health implications of Mediterranean diets in the light of contemporary knowledge. 2. Meat, wine, fats and oils. *American Journal of Clinical Nutrition* **61**, (Supplement) 1416S-1427S.

Laurence, D. R. and Bennett, P. N. 1992 *Clinical pharmacology*, 7th edn. Edinburgh: Churchill Livingstone.

Lindahl, T., Wood, R. D. and Karran, P. 1991 Molecular deficiencies in human cancer-prone syndromes associated with hypersensitivity to DNA-damaging agents. In Brugges, J., Curran, T., Harlow, E. and McCormick, F. (eds), *Origins of human cancer: a comprehensive review*. New York: Cold Spring Harbour Laboratory Press, 163–70.

McCaffery, M. and Beebe, A. 1994 *Pain: clinical manual for nursing practice* (edited by Latham, J. for the UK). London: Mosby.

Melzack, R. and Wall, P. D. 1982 *The challenge of pain*. Harmondsworth: Penguin.

Müller-Hill, B. 1993 The shadow of genetic injustice. *Nature* **362**, 491–2. Reprinted 1995 in Davey, B., Gray, A. and Seale, C. (eds), *Health and disease: a reader*, 2nd edn. Buckingham: Open University Press, 412–16.

Myers, K. A., Marshall, R. D. and Freidin, J. 1980 *Principles of pathology in surgery*. Oxford: Blackwell Scientific Publications.

Nowak, T. J. and Handford, A. G. 1994 *Essentials of pathophysiology: concepts and applications for health care professionals*. Dubuque: W. C. Brown.

Orem, D. E. 1995 *Nursing: concepts of practice*, 5th edn. New York: McGraw-Hill.

Overfield, T. 1985 *Biologic variation in health and illness*. Menlo Park: Addison-Wesley.

Passmore, R. and Robson, J. S. 1980 *A companion to medical studies. Vol. 2. Pharmacology, microbiology, general pathology and related subjects,* 2nd edn. Oxford: Blackwell Scientific Publications.

Passmore, R. and Robson, J. S. 1986 *A companion to medical studies. Vol. 1. Anatomy, biochemistry, physiology and related subjects,* 3rd edn. Oxford: Blackwell Scientific Publications.

Pearl, R. de W. 1934 The ancestry of the long-lived. London: Milford. Cited 1991 in Redfern, S.J. (ed.), *Nursing elderly people,* 2nd edn. Edinburgh: Churchill Livingstone.

Peplau, H. E. 1988 *Interpersonal relations in nursing.* Basingstoke: Macmillan (first published by Putman, New York, in 1952).

Redfern, S. J. (ed.) 1991 *Nursing elderly people,* 2nd edn. Edinburgh: Churchill Livingstone.

Rogers, M. E. 1989 Nursing: a science of unitary human beings. In Riehl-Sisca, J. P. (ed.), *Conceptual models for nursing practice,* 3rd edn. Norwalk: Appleton and Lange, 181–8.

Rogers, H. J., Spector, R. G. and Trounce, J. R. 1981 *A textbook of clinical pharmacology.* London: Hodder and Stoughton.

Roper, N., Logan, W. W. and Tierney, A. J. 1990 *The elements of nursing,* 3rd edn. Edinburgh: Churchill Livingstone.

Selye, H. 1976 *The stress of life,* 2nd Edn. New York: McGraw-Hill.

Sharpe, P. C., McGrath, L. T., McClean, E., Young, I. S. and Archbold, G. P. 1995 Effect of red wine consumption on lipoprotein(a) and other risk factors for atherosclerosis. *Quarterly Journal of Medicine* **88**, 101–8.

Skretkowicz, V. (ed.) 1992 *Florence Nightingale's notes on nursing.* London: Scutari.

Smith, J. P. (ed.) 1981 *Nursing science in nursing practice.* London: Butterworths.

Smith, R. (ed.) 1991 *The health of the nation: the BMJ view.* London: British Medical Journal.

Spector, W. G. 1989 *An introduction to general pathology,* 3rd edn (revised by Spector, T.D.). Edinburgh: Churchill Livingstone.

Stockley, I. H. 1991 *Drug interactions,* 2nd edn. Oxford: Blackwell Scientific Publications.

Tanner, J. M. 1978 *Fetus into man: physical growth from conception to maturity.* Cambridge, MA: Harvard University Press.

Tortora, G. J. and Grabowski, S. R. 1993 *Principles of anatomy and physiology,* 7th edn. New York: Harper Collins.

Townsend, P., Davidson, N. and Whitehead, M. 1988 *Inequalities in health: the Black Report 1980 and the Health Divide.* Harmondsworth: Penguin.

Trnobranski, P. H. 1993 Biological sciences and the nursing curriculum: a challenge for educationalists. *Journal of Advanced Nursing* **18**, 493–9.

United Kingdom Central Council for Nursing, Midwifery and Health Visiting (UKCC) 1992 *Code of professional conduct,* 3rd edn. London: UKCC.

United Kingdom Central Council for Nursing, Midwifery and Health Visiting (UKCC) 1994 *The future of professional practice – the council's standards for education and practice following registration.* London: UKCC.

Ur, E. 1991 Psychological aspects of hypothalamo-pituitary-adrenal activity. In Grossman, A. (ed.), *Psychoendocrinology: Baillière's clinical endocrinology and metabolism. Vol. 5.* London: Baillière Tindall, 79–96.

Vander, A. J., Sherman, J. H. and Luciano, D. S. 1994 *Human physiology: the mechanisms of body function,* 6th edn. New York: McGraw-Hill.

Virchow, R. 1856 Weitere Untersuchungen über die Verstopfung der Lungerarterie und ihre Folgen, In *Gesammelte Abhandlungen zur Wissenschaftlichen Medizin* **227**, from *Traube's Beitrs experiment Pathologie und Physiologie* **2**, 21.

Weatherall, D. J. 1991 *The new genetics and clinical practice,* 3rd edn. Oxford: Oxford University Press.

Westaby, S. (ed.) 1985 *Wound care.* London: Heinemann.

Wharrad, H. J., Allcock, N. and Chapple, M. 1994 A survey of the teaching and learning of biological sciences on undergraduate nursing courses. *Nurse Education Today* 14, 436–42.

Youmans, G. P., Paterson, P. Y. and Sommers, M. D. 1985 *The biological and clinical basis of infectious diseases,* 3rd edn. Philadelphia: W. B. Saunders.

Psychology – themes in nursing

5

Mary Watts and Andrzej Kuczmierczyk

The main aim of this chapter is to identify the relevance of psychology for enhancing nursing practice, and to familiarise the reader with a number of specific areas of psychology which are likely to have significance for all nurses, whatever their specialist field of activity. In an attempt to meet this broad aim, three forms of knowledge of specific relevance to nursing practice are identified: *implicit, experiential* and *empirical* knowledge. A psychological perspective is used to integrate and elaborate on these.

The focus of this text is nursing, an activity which is influenced by the three forms of knowledge outlined above. This chapter will start, therefore, by focusing on specific nursing activities, and will then introduce psychological themes in relation to those activities.

Research by Watts (1988, 1994) drew attention to nursing activities identified by student nurses as a significant part of their nursing role. Although a considerable number of specific activities emerged within the context of this research, these can be grouped according to certain themes. The overarching theme is of nursing as an activity involving communication and interpersonal relationships.

Those nursing activities identified by psychiatric nursing students (Watts, 1988) included 'therapeutic' activities, talking with and listening to patients, assessing patients, giving or receiving the ward handover report, physical caregiving, and activities involving relatives. Activities identified by general nursing students (Watts, 1994) included educating patients about their health and health problems, helping patients to cope with their worries, and either carrying out or assisting patients with a number of physical activities, e.g. helping a patient to maintain personal hygiene and comfort. One of the primary purposes of the research was to identify students' attitudes to, and perceptions of, those nursing activities which they identified as key features of their role.

The activities identified by students have psychological as well as physical dimensions, and require nurses to integrate psychosocial as well as physically related knowledge and skills (see Chapters 4 and 6). They are also activities that are likely to be influenced by nurses' own attitudes to, and perceptions of, their nursing role and health- and illness-related issues. Sundberg and Tyler (1963) suggested that the first task of the clinician should be to discover the conceptual framework under which he or she is operating. They, like Caine and Smail in 1969, recognised the link between impersonal theory and personal practice. Caine and Smail (1969) argued, in relation to the treatment of mental illness, that the basic assumptions of those who give and those who receive treatment significantly influence the course of treatment. However, it is not only in relation to mental illness that basic assumptions play a part. For instance, if a nurse believes that patients should passively receive without question whatever nursing care is provided for them, this is likely to be incompatible with the notion of a patient being actively involved in maintaining or promoting his or her own health. This in turn may have implications for health promotion activities (see Chapter 3). Marteau (1989) suggested that:

> As well as influencing the health outcomes of patients by determining the choice of treatment, staff cognitions may also influence health outcomes of patients by influencing patient cognitions and hence patient behaviour.
>
> (Marteau, 1989, p. 12)

Nursing is an interpersonal activity. The types of activities that nurses engage in, and the specific ways in which they engage in them, are influenced by nurses' self-awareness, including an awareness of the effect of self on others. Experience, knowledge and attitudes (often implicit) together combine to have a bearing on the interpersonal activity of nursing. This chapter will first focus on implicit psychology and the notion of the individual as a lay psychologist. It will then move on to the integration of experience into this perspective, and will finally focus in some detail on specific aspects of psychological knowledge that are of relevance to our understanding of health and illness.

Implicit psychology

Implicit psychology can be understood as the process of constructing theories about people and using the theories to predict behaviour (Wegner and Vallacher, 1977). We all act as lay psychologists when we try to make sense of our own behaviour or that of others. Often the sense we make of people and events is influenced by our implicit assumptions or theories. These are likely to have an effect on our own and others' behaviour, and it is for this reason that Sundberg and Tyler (1963) and Caine and Smail (1969) suggested that implicit assumptions should be made explicit. Implicit psychology is particularly relevant in relation to *beliefs*, *attitudes* and our *perceptions* of people and events, and these three all have a bearing on the interpersonal activity of nursing. Moss (1988) suggested that, although the nursing process provides, in theory at least, an effective framework for practice, nurses' attitudes are very significant determinants of patient care.

Attitudes

Definitions of attitudes vary considerably, although there is general agreement that a person's attitude to a specific object or situation represents a predisposition to respond to that object or situation in a particular way. Attitudes can be represented in terms of thoughts, feelings and behaviour. An attitude is more than just a belief or an opinion. A belief may not entail an emotional component. In practice, however, the distinction between beliefs and attitudes becomes fuzzy as feelings and emotions can accompany beliefs to a greater or lesser degree, and are not always clearly identifiable.

There is no precise relationship between the thought and feeling components of an attitude and behaviour. Behaviour can be influenced by external factors, such as positive or negative consequences of behaving in a particular way, by anticipation of these consequences, and also by an individual's perceptions of whether they feel capable of success if they behave in a particular way. This last point relates to Bandura's *theory of self-efficacy*, and is elaborated within the context of his *social learning theory* (Bandura, 1977). Social learning theory (SLT) attempts to provide a unified theoretical framework for analysing human thought and behaviour. It is based on the notion of a continuous reciprocal interaction between the individual and the environment. Central to this interaction are an individual's observations of events and behaviour, and their awareness of the relationship between behaviour and its consequences. Thus, nurses may have a positive attitude towards talking to patients and listening to their worries, and may believe that this aids recovery, but may modify their behaviour to make it compatible with the dominant ethos of the ward or clinical environment in which they are working, so as to avoid criticism from peers or seniors. Nurses may also modify their behaviour if they believe that they do not have the knowledge or skills necessary to be successful in what they do.

This may reflect a valid assessment of themselves or a lack of confidence in their effectiveness.

Behaviour, and thus nursing practice, is influenced by beliefs, attitudes, assumptions, and perceptions of ourselves and others, and by the nature of the relationship between these and environmental factors. Studies by Copp (1971) and Larson (1977), for example, suggested that nurses believe that people categorised as patients are dependent. Patients are vulnerable to the attitudes and role expectations of professional staff, and nurses form a very large and influential core of health care staff. Viney (1985) suggested that, even if communication between patients and staff is good, some *patient constructs* will receive more validation than others from staff, e.g. helplessness constructs receive more validation than competence constructs. (The notion of constructs will be addressed more fully later in the chapter in relation to *personal construct theory* [PCT].) Research also indicates that patients' descriptions of themselves contain many references to helplessness, and few to competence (Raps *et al.*, 1982; Westbrook and Viney, 1982).

Do nurses' perceptions and attitudes matter? The evidence would suggest that they do. A number of research studies supporting this position were cited by Moss (1988) who, following a review of these studies, stated that:

> While nurses today claim to be concerned with the whole patient, developing nurse–patient relationships, and individualised patient care, there is considerable evidence to suggest that nurses deal with types of people, types of behaviour and types of illness, rather than individual patients. That is, nurses' perceptions of, and the labels they or others apply to the patient, influence their behaviour towards that patient.
>
> (Moss, 1988, p. 619)

Moss quotes studies by De Vellis *et al.* (1984), Wallston *et al.* (1976, 1983) and Woods and Cullen (1983) to support this statement.

Learned helplessness and attribution theory

Several references have been made to 'helplessness', that is, to professional staff perceiving patients as helpless and patients perceiving themselves as helpless. Again the question can be asked, 'Do perceptions of helplessness matter?' Does it matter if a patient perceives himself or herself to be helpless, or if a nurse perceives either a patient or herself to be helpless? The basic question of interest is, 'What happens to people when they are not in control of their environment?' A study by Seligman (1975) demonstrated that cognitive deficit can occur when people experience helplessness. He found that individuals exposed to a *controllable* unpleasant event – a loud noise which could be turned off by pressing a button – were more successful at solving anagrams whilst exposed to the noise than individuals who were exposed to an *uncontrollable* unpleasant event – a loud noise which could not be turned off at will, but which stopped of its own accord. Hyland and Donaldson (1989) described four different psychological phenomena that can occur under conditions of helplessness. These are as follows:

1. *Cognitive deficit.* Problem-solving ability is reduced, people are less able to find solutions to new problems and less able to adapt to new situations. The cognitive deficit is a 'thinking' deficit.
2. *Motivational deficit.* Activity and the desire for action are reduced. The motivational deficit is a 'wanting' deficit.
3. *Sad affect.* People feel and appear depressed.
4. *Low self-esteem.* People feel worthless, of little value.

(Hyland and Donaldson, 1989, p.4)

Maier *et al.* (1969) described learned helplessness as the perception of independence between one's responses and the onset or termination of an aversive event. What is significant is an individual's perception of the controllability of an event, rather than its actual controllability. Hence *attribution theory* is crucial to an understanding of the learned helplessness situation.

Attribution theory focuses on how an ordinary person understands the causes of an event or behaviour. It stems from the work of Heider (1958), who was interested in what he called the 'naive psychology' of the 'man in the street'. Attribution research attempts to determine the rules that the average person follows when analysing the causes of events and behaviour. Clearly the average person does not analyse all behaviour, looking for its causes. The tendency is usually noted when an event is either important or unexpected. Nurses often observe that patients try to make sense of their illness by asking questions such as 'Why has this happened to me?' Or 'What is the cause of my illness?'

According to attribution theorists, the lay person acts as a scientist in trying to make sense of events, and uses a number of dimensions to explain them. Of particular significance are the dimensions concerning internality/externality, stability, controllability and globality. In relation to the experience of being ill, the sick person may make internal attributions, such as blaming himself or herself, or external attributions, that is, blaming someone or something else. The identified cause may be perceived as either stable and unchangeable, or unstable and thus changeable. An individual might perceive their illness as being caused by external factors which they have the power to change – those factors are thus controllable and unstable. Such a person is unlikely to feel helpless or to suffer from the psychological deficits outlined by Hyland and Donaldson (1989).

Other sick individuals may make internal attributions. They may blame themselves for their situation and believe that they cannot change it since it is uncontrollable, yet stable. They experience 'helplessness'. If, in addition, helplessness is perceived as global ('I am a helpless person'), lowered self-esteem is likely to follow. Abramson (1977) demonstrated that lowered self-esteem occurs only in personal helplessness. The longer the helplessness is experienced, the greater the psychological deficits that are likely to occur.

It is interesting to note a study by Marteau and Riordan (1992), which sought to investigate whether staff attitudes towards patients are affected by the causal attributions of ill health made by the staff. The results of the study suggested that information about a patient's health habits prior to illness affected staff attitudes to the patient. Staff had significantly more negative attitudes towards patients who had not engaged in preventative behaviour designed to reduce the likelihood of them developing their medical condition, than to those who had engaged in such behaviour. This research finding gives cause for concern when one considers that nurses are in a key position to influence or validate the attributions made by patients about the causes and subsequent resolution of their health problems. The attributional judgements made by patients are likely to have a bearing on both their mental state and their subsequent health-related behaviour.

A study by Johnston et al. (1992) demonstrated that it is possible to alter physiotherapy patients' perceptions of personal control over recovery during rehabilitation, via a psychological intervention involving the addition of a few paragraphs to the routine letter confirming the patient's appointment. On average, patients who received the routine appointment letter plus some additional paragraphs designed to increase their perceived control over the outcome of the rehabilitation, were found to have significantly higher levels of perceived control, and to be more satisfied with the information provided than the control group, 1 week after their appointment.

The findings of this study are significant when considered within the context of an earlier study (Partridge and Johnston, 1989), in which it was found that greater progress in recovery from disability was made by patients with a higher level of perceived personal control.

Self-blame attributions

A comprehensive review of the literature relevant to victims' attributions of and subsequent coping with disease, crime and accidents has been provided by Janoff-Bulman and Lang-Gunn (1988). Attributions consequent upon a search for meaning are likely to be made following life events of great personal intensity, personal meaning and negative outcome. Central to Janoff-Bulman and Lang-Gunn's analysis of this literature is their proposition that, although self-blame is commonly encountered in these victims, not all self-blame is maladaptive. These authors distinguish between *behavioural* and *characterological self-blame* for the cause of an event.

Where behavioural self-blame occurs, the cause of an event is considered to be associated with one's own behaviour, but the possibility still remains of controlling subsequent outcomes by changing or modifying one's behaviour.

In contrast, characterological self-blame consists of blaming enduring aspects of one's character for the occurrence of negative events. Personal control, such as that advocated by Johnston *et al.* (1992), requires an individual to accept an element of personal responsibility. However, it is important that attributions of the cause of negative events are perceived in behavioural rather than characterological terms.

The preceding discussion indicates that both nurses and patients make attributions, and that these have a bearing on the behaviour of each, thereby influencing the outcome of the helping relationship. The attributions made by an individual will reflect a combination of the values, attitudes and beliefs held by that individual. However, these are likely to be an implicit feature of the attributional judgements made by them.

The indications, therefore, are that perceptions of helplessness influence both staff and patient health-related behaviour, and may also have a signifi-cant bearing on a patient's psychological well-being. If helplessness is per-ceived by a patient to be short term, then the psychological phenomena outlined by Hyland and Donaldson (1989) might not occur. However, even if helplessness is likely to be short term, e.g. in the case of a short hospital admission, many people go through an initial stage of *reactance* when they try to regain control by fighting back. These people will probably present as hostile, angry and 'difficult', and they may fall into the unpopular patient category described by Stockwell (1972). Giving control back to these patients is likely to be a more effective way of helping them than being authoritarian and taking control away.

If helplessness is perceived to be long term, then reactance is likely to be followed by cognitive and motivational deficits, sadness and lowered self-esteem. This is a common phenomenon in institutionalised patients, and is well described by Goffman (1961) (see Chapter 7).

Under conditions of uncontrollability, internal attributions are more likely to lead to psychological deficits than are external attributions. On the other hand, external attributions can be associated with behavioural deficits. Eiser and Gossop (1979) demonstrated this in relation to drug dependency. They found that the addicts in their study had no confidence that they could con-trol their own behaviour and get better through their own efforts, and they tended to perceive their addiction as an illness requiring medical intervention to bring about a cure. These addicts were making external attributions for continuing their addictive behaviour, which had an ego enhancement effect, but this is likely to have reduced their attempts at self-control. Responsibility had been shifted to the professional. If this dependency is reinforced by pro-fessional staff, effective behaviour change is unlikely to occur.

Returning to the question, 'Do nurses' perceptions and attitudes matter?', the evidence indicates that they do, and that Caine and Smail (1969) and Sundberg and Tyler (1963) were correct in advocating that clinicians discover the conceptual framework under which they are operating. For this to occur, implicit assumptions and theories must become explicit. One psychologist who developed a theory and a methodology consistent with this goal was George Kelly.

Personal construct theory and repertory grid technique

Personal construct psychology was both a theoretical and an applied psychological perspective developed by George Kelly (1955). *Repertory grid techniques*, which are derived from the theory, represent a number of methods which have evolved from the theory for investigating the personal constructs of an individual or group of individuals. Put more simply, the method represents a way of exploring an individual's implicit or explicit view of the world, i.e. their personal psychology. Exploration of this kind is considered to be valid in *personal construct theory* (PCT) terms, since Kelly suggested in his theory that each person holds a representational model of the world which enables him or her to chart a course of behaviour in relation to that model. Kelly's theory focuses on the experiences of the individual and the way in which these experiences are construed. He believed that we all make sense of experiences by considering them in relation to our very personal system of construing. Personal constructs are mental constructions, or ideas of a bipolar kind, which represent a perception or thought relating to a specific object, event, person or behaviour.

Kelly's (1970) philosophical position of *constructive alternativism* reminds us that the unique meaning we make of our world is just one of an infinite number of personal realities available to us. However, as Kelly stated:

> This is not to say that one construction is as good as any other, nor is it to deny that at some infinite point in time human vision will behold reality out to the utmost reaches of existence. But it does remind us that all our present perceptions are open to question and reconsideration, and it does broadly suggest that even the most obvious occurrences of everyday life might appear utterly transformed if we were inventive enough to construe them differently.
>
> (Kelly, 1970, p.1)

Constructions of reality are constantly tested out and modified to allow better predictions in the future. A reciprocal and dynamic relationship exists between an individual and his or her experience which results in that individual's representational model of the world being subject to change. However, even that experience which does not support an individual's system of construing does not always result in modified constructions of reality.

Kelly believed that if we never alter our constructions, all that occurs during our life is a sequence of parallel events which have no psychological impact. In other words, the experience is not used to allow us to become more effective 'scientists' or to increase our personal knowledge and self-awareness.

Kelly construed the unit of experience as a cycle having five phases: anticipation, investment, encounter, confirmation or disconfirmation, and constructive revision (Kelly, 1970). This can be reproduced in diagrammatic form as shown in Figure 5.1. Within this theory, experience is not represented by the number of events in which an individual engages, 'but by the investments he has made in his anticipations and the revision of his constructions that have followed upon his facing up to consequences' (Kelly, 1970, p.19).

The theory of constructive alternativism states that we make sense of our world in an individual and personal way, and that there are always alternative constructions which can be explored, but that we do not always allow ourselves to do this, even if our experience disconfirms previously held constructions. When this occurs, we experience a sequence of parallel events with no psychological impact. Learning is restricted by the fact that it occurs within a closed system of personal construing.

Personal construct theory is reflexive, in other words, it applies equally to exploring and understanding ourselves and to understanding others. Returning to an earlier part of this chapter, it was suggested that a dominant feature of the nursing activities outlined by students was their interpersonal nature. This implies communication and relationships between people, e.g. between the nurse and the patient, between different professionals, and so on. Kelly believed that for interpersonal relationships to occur, one person construes the construction processes of another and is thereby able to play a role in a social process involving the other person. In order to form a relationship with another person we need to try to understand their perspective or outlook. That understanding does not have to be complete, or reciprocal, but the degree of understanding and reciprocity will influence the nature of the relationship (see Chapter 6).

Therapeutic relationships require 'stepping inside somebody else's shoes'. If a nurse construes a patient solely in terms of her own construct system,

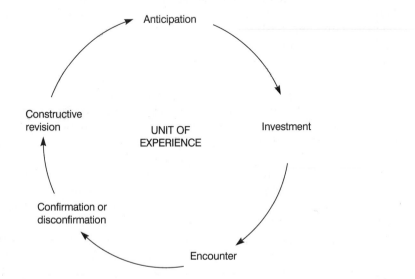

Figure 5.1   Diagrammatic representation of the five phases of the unit of experience (Watts, 1988; adapted from Kelly, 1970)

she is in danger of creating a reality to which the patient is expected to conform, and in many instances will conform. Patients who do not conform are in danger of being perceived as 'problem patients' and coming within the unpopular patient category identified by Stockwell (1972).

Following a review of the popular/unpopular patient research, Kelly and May (1982) concluded that the good patient is one who confirms the role of the nurse, whereas the bad patient denies that legitimation. Unfortunately, confirming the role of the nurse is often synonymous with letting the nurse take charge and the patient becoming dependent.

It was suggested earlier (Viney, 1985) that helplessness constructs receive more validation than others from staff (cf. section on 'Attitudes'). Helplessness is not compatible with self-determination, yet health maintenance and health promotion ultimately depend on individuals taking some degree of responsibility for themselves.

Kelly's theory provides a useful conceptual framework which can be applied to understanding ourselves and others. Repertory grid techniques – which have evolved from the application of Kelly's theory – are a useful tool for learning about the system of constructs held by an individual or a group of people, and can enable individuals to gain greater insight into their personal construing of situations and events. These techniques allow for exploration of the conceptual links between a person's ideas by demonstrating the nature of the relationship between them. PCT does not depend on the techniques to support it, but those techniques can provide a useful way of exploring the implicit psychology of an individual, monitoring change in this, and allowing the individual to learn more about himself or herself, including his or her reactions to situations and events and his or her anticipations about the future. Good reviews of the techniques and their applications have been provided by Fransella and Bannister (1977), Beail (1985), Button (1985) and Dunnett (1988). A detailed review of the application to nursing is provided by Watts (1988 and 1994).

At the start of this chapter it was suggested that nursing practice is influenced by implicit, experiential and empirical knowledge. An attempt has been made to identify some ways in which implicit knowledge can influence the experience of being nursed and of nursing. The way in which an individual reacts to an experience and the effect that an experience has on future experiences, are closely bound up with their attributions, beliefs and attitudes. Personal construct theory provides a theoretical framework for uniting implicit knowledge and personal experience. However, nurses are also influenced by what was referred to earlier as a third form of knowledge, namely that which stems from empirical evidence. This does not mean knowledge which has been empirically tested by each individual, but knowledge which is presented as grounded in some concrete and testable evidence (see Chapters 1 and 2). An example of this would be knowledge about the links between smoking and ill health, and between Type A personality and coronary heart disease. Nursing behaviour and patient behaviour are influenced by a combination of all three types of 'knowing', and these three also inevitably have a bearing on one another. For example, nurses' attitudes (implicit knowledge) are likely to influence their perceptions of their personal experience. In addition, aspects of empirically tested knowledge are likely to have an influence on nurses' attitudes. This was borne out by research (Watts, 1994) which demonstrated that nurses were far less sympathetic towards patients suffering from conditions which research had demonstrated were aetiologically linked to behavioural factors, than they were to patients for whom this was not considered to be the case.

In addition to the nurses' behaviour being influenced by the three forms of knowledge outlined above, so too will that of the patient. Furthermore, the nurse and the patient will inevitably be influenced by 'knowledge' of each other. However, as already indicated, the power relationship between the nurse and the patient is unlikely to be an equal one (cf. the previous section on 'Self-blame attributions').

Clearly the nurse and the patient are not only influenced by one another, as might be implied by Figure 5.2, since other individuals such as relatives and colleagues will feed into the system. The relative weight or power of any influence will also, in part, be situationally determined.

Behaviour is influenced not only by what people think or believe that they know, but also by environmental factors. Not all behaviour is actually thought about. Numerous examples can be found of learned behaviour which is carried out routinely or habitually within certain contexts or environments. Traditional learning theories of *classical* and *operant conditioning* (Pavlov, 1927; Skinner, 1938) can help us to understand these examples. However, they are significantly complemented by social learning theory (Bandura, 1977; Jarvis 1992).

Social learning theory (Bandura, 1977) draws attention to the reciprocal relationship which exists between the person and the environment. This relationship will inevitably be influenced by specific factors which relate to the environment. For example, 'Does the ward environment lend itself to patients being actively involved in self-care?' If it does not, then this environmental factor is likely to have a significant bearing on the behaviour of an individual nurse, even if that nurse has personal knowledge relating to the efficacy of promoting self-care.

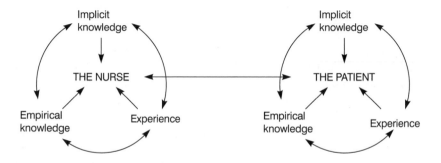

Figure 5.2   The relationship between implicit, experiential and empirical knowledge on nurse and patient behaviour

Today there is a large field of knowledge linking psychology, health and illness, of which both health professionals and the general public are becoming increasingly aware. Empirically supported knowledge is playing an increasingly significant part in determining nursing care and also patient behaviour. The following discussion will outline a number of areas in which research has increased our understanding of the nature of the relationship between health and illness.

Psychology and health

The twentieth century has seen a number of major health-related changes, one of which has been a shift from the prevalence of infectious diseases to chronic diseases with multiple causes. Pneumonia, tuberculosis and enteritis, once major killers, have been replaced by, among other diseases, heart disease, cancer, injuries, respiratory disease and diabetes mellitus. In recent years this picture has changed somewhat, with the rapid increase and spread of human immunodeficiency virus (HIV), and the concomitant number of AIDS cases. However, this does not change the picture of the major killers of today being associated with a combination of environmental and lifestyle factors (see Chapters 3 and 7). The fact that there is a relationship between behaviour and health has become increasingly clear. Factors such as diet, smoking, drug abuse, excessive drinking, unsafe driving, lack of exercise, working conditions and pollution all have a bearing on the health status both of the individual and of whole communities.

Recognition of the behaviourally linked nature of many illnesses makes health promotion and illness prevention more feasible. However, this does not imply that individuals suffering from ill health which is behaviourally linked should be considered personally responsible for their health status. Social and environmental conditions, for example, are significantly linked to health-related behaviours, both directly and indirectly. Unfortunately, not all illness is prevented, and the very nature of current health problems demands an approach to care which takes account of the multiple causation of ill health and the stress and anxiety associated with many of the medical interventions available.

Health and illness can be conceptualised and defined in a variety of ways. They can be identified as constructs, and thus by implication have an opposite pole. Individuals will have their own view of what constitutes the opposite end of the pole to healthy, and also what can be defined as either healthy or unhealthy. The opposite poles, e.g. healthy/unhealthy, can represent end-points on a continuum, and an individual's health state at any time will fall somewhere on that continuum. Where it falls will reflect many factors, including personal, social and medical definitions of health and illness, and the perception of the person or people making the judgement. It is possible for discrepancies to occur between an individual's own judgement about his or her health status, and the judgement of others, e.g. health professionals, friends and colleagues.

Age and sex factors are known to influence definitions of health. It has been suggested (Murray and Zentner, 1989) that children define health as feeling good and being able to participate in desired activities, while in contrast adults typically define health as a state enabling them to perform at least minimal daily activities, involving physical, mental, spiritual and social components. It would seem that an adult's perception, as well as their life situation, influences their definition of health.

Murray and Zentner (1989) summarised a number of definitions of health, the most marked contrast occurring between that provided by the World Health Organisation and that of Dunn (1961). The United Nations World Health Organisation define health as a 'state of complete physical, mental and social well-being, and not merely the absence of disease' (World Health Organisation, 1987). This definition makes no allowance for degrees of illness and health. By contrast, Dunn (1961) defined health and illness in terms of a continuum, representing a relative and ever changing state of being.

> Health–wellbeing and disease–illness are now thought of as complex, dynamic processes on a continuum that includes physical, psychological (emotional, cognitive, and developmental), spiritual and social components and adaptive behavioural responses to internal and external stimuli.
>
> (Murray and Zentner, 1989, p.5)

Final agreement as to what constitutes health is never likely to be reached. Despite this, it is possible to identify factors which have a bearing on an individual's health status, and the ways in which these interact to produce health change. A person's health status is in a constant state of flux. What is important is the direction of change and the processes involved in that change. The more we can understand the influential factors in the process, the better we are able to control it. This understanding has relevance for everyone, not just health care professionals. If it is confined to the professionals, then the general public and patients immediately become reliant on others for their health. To prevent this from happening, the sharing of knowledge becomes an important feature of health care.

Understanding the factors associated with the process of health change is of dual relevance for the nurse. On the one hand, it has significance in relation to their professional role, but on the other it also has personal significance. Health and ill health are experienced by all of us, and we can all play a role in promoting and maintaining our own health. It is only too easy as a health professional to focus exclusively on 'the patient' at the expense of caring for the self. What follows in this chapter is of equal significance both for the nurse and their own health, and for those in their care.

Before moving on to a number of specific psychological features associated with health, a model will be outlined which makes it possible to conceptualise health change in behavioural terms, and to demonstrate the relationship between environmental, social, psychological and biological influences on health (Figure 5.3). This model represents only one approach to conceptualising health change, but it provides a useful framework within which to place relevant aspects of psychological knowledge, and also to identify gaps in this knowledge.

Figure 5.3 demonstrates that an individual's state of health is influenced by a multiplicity of interrelating factors. Social learning theory centres on the reciprocal relationship which exists between the environment and the individual. When applying psychology to enhance our understanding of health and health-related behaviours, the relationship between the environment and the individual needs to be extended to include the relationship between psychology and physiology (see Chapter 4).

The term 'environment' is used to refer to both the people and the physical objects in one's life.

> The concept of environment encompasses the total surroundings of an individual's life and its relationship to the person's behaviour. We all live surrounded by air, which can be clean, smoggy or full of sulphur and carbon monoxide. We all drink water, which can be pure or contaminated. We are all affected by radiation. We all live in neighbourhoods that are safe or too dangerous to walk in. All these factors are a consequence of some human behaviour.
>
> (Goldstein and Krasner, 1987, p.39)

Not only are the above environmental features a consequence of human behaviour – they also have an effect on it. This effect may or may not be compatible with health promotion and the avoidance of negative health changes.

Stress

Central to our understanding of the environment/individual/health equation is the concept of *stress*. The notion that stress correlates with ill health is not new, but it is only in recent years that the interrelationships between

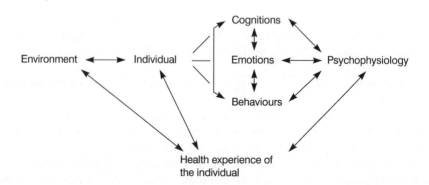

Figure 5.3 The reciprocal relationship between the environment, the individual, psychophysiology and health

environment, the individual and their appraisal of environmental stressors, and psychophysiology have been empirically investigated. Stress has been implicated in the development of a number of conditions, including coronary heart disease, hypertension, cancer, asthma, chronic pain, diabetes and psychological disorders (Frederickson and Matthews, 1990; Hammen *et al.*, 1985; Hatch *et al.*, 1992; Locke *et al.*, 1984; Treiber *et al.*, 1993).

Singer and Baum (1980) focused on three 'Cs' of environmental stress: crowding, commuting and cacophony (discordant sound or noise pollution). They emphasised that psychological and physiological responses to environmental threat were mediated by the cognitive appraisal of environmental stress factors by the individual.

This is consistent with the interactional approach to stress adopted by Lazarus (1976), Roskies and Lazarus (1980) and Cox and McKay (1978). Interactional models go beyond considering stress as a stimulus, e.g. overcrowded, noisy working conditions, or as a response, e.g. Selye's (1956) *general adaptation syndrome* (GAS), but propose that stress occurs through a particular relationship between the person and the environment. It is suggested that self-regulation of cognitive, emotional and behavioural coping strategies influences the impact of a stressor on the individual. The degree to which an event or situation is regarded as a stressor by an individual will be influenced by whether that individual perceives that he or she has the ability to cope with or control that situation.

Folkman and Lazarus (1980) identified two categories of coping. The first category involves actual behaviour which is *problem focused* and attempts to change the problematic aspects of the individual's relationship with his or her environment. The second category was described by Folkman and Lazarus as *palliative* or *emotion focused,* and is concerned with softening the impact of a stressor. An individual is thus allowed to detach himself or herself emotionally from a particular situation. A resultant problem may be that the potentially threatening aspects of that situation remain, and effective coping behaviour is not learned.

The way in which an individual perceives and copes with stress is significant both in relation to the development of ill health, and to the way in which that individual copes with ill health. The experience of ill health in itself becomes a potential stressor, to which an individual must respond and adapt and which, in turn, has a further cumulative effect on that individual's health state. We are all constantly having to adapt to external and internal stressors, and there are considerable individual differences in the ways in which we do this. Most people are probably unaware of their habitual methods of adapting, or the positive and negative consequences of those methods. However, an individual's stress response is intricately linked with his or her health experience and the process of health change.

Returning to Figure 5.3, each of the components can be viewed as a potential stressor or as a positive or negative response to a stressor, as indicated in Figure 5.4.

Change can be either a threat or a challenge to an individual. Environmental change can result in individuals experiencing stress if they

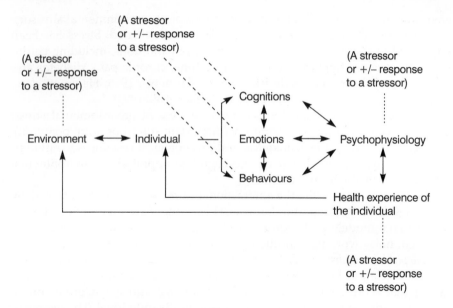

Figure 5.4 The interrelational model linking stress, the environment, the individual, psychophysiology and health

believe that the demands being made on them tax or exceed their adjustive resources (Lazarus and Folkman, 1984). Change thus becomes a threat leading to feelings of uncertainty, loss of control, and mental, physical and behavioural manifestations of stress. The linkage between stress and illness is not new. In recent years, however, a greater understanding of the physiological and neurochemical dimensions of stress has resulted in growing interest in mechanisms which could explain the links between stress and illness (see Chapter 4). Empirical data is now available which suggests that there is a relationship between the functioning of the immune system and stress (Herbert and Cohen, 1993; Jemmott and Locke, 1984).

In a study by Kiecolt-Glaser *et al.* (1986), a group of 35 volunteer medical students was assessed both before and during academic examinations. A number of measures of immunological function were monitored, including the percentage of various *T-lymphocytes* (some of the cells necessary to fight antigens) and the activity of *natural killer (NK) cells*. A decrease in T-lymphocytes or NK activity would reflect a reduction in the ability of the body's defences to fight off invasive agents.

The results showed that during the examination both the percentage of T-lymphocytes and the NK activity were reduced. However, this reduction was modified in 50 per cent of the subjects who had been instructed in a variety of relaxation procedures. This finding is consistent with the results of Arnetz *et al.* (1987) who, in an assessment of unemployed Swedish women, found that after 9 months of unemployment, they showed reduced *lymphocyte reactivity* to an antigen. However, this effect was not observed if the women were given a psychosocial support programme.

Anderson and Masur (1983) and Mathews and Ridgeway (1984) reviewed studies on the stress associated with hospitalisation, a number of which looked at procedures which teach and enhance coping strategies. They identified that a variety of techniques, including information-giving, *cognitive-behavioural* coping strategies and relaxation, can influence a patient's experience of hospitalisation and, to some extent, the results of that event. These and other studies have been reviewed by Harvey (1988), who concluded that 'it is reasonable to argue that stress (however defined) has measurable and serious effects on the body and on people's health ... . However ... there are enough data to show that intervention can alleviate the effects of the stressors' (Harvey, 1988, p.99).

Effective intervention can be relatively simple and economical, and can be taught by nurses in a number of settings. However, it is worth remembering that a threat to one person may be a challenge to another. Many people cope well with situations that others would find very stressful. There are individual differences in the ways in which people perceive change and manage stress, and an understanding of these differences can add to our understanding of the personality/ behaviour/health relationship, and be helpful in assisting the person who is not well or not coping.

Individual differences: Type A behaviour and heart disease

During the last quarter of 1986, half of all deaths in England and Wales – over 60 000 men and women – were due to diseases of the heart and its associated blood vessels (Harvey, 1988). The death rate from heart diseases is twice that from cancers, and in the USA it is calculated that it accounts for 1 620 219 years of potential lost life before the age of 65 years (Center for Disease Control, 1986). This represents enormous costs in human suffering and loss in economic terms.

In 1978, the Pooling Project Research Group was set up in the USA to co-ordinate and systematise data from eight prospective studies designed to identify factors which increase the likelihood that some people will develop coronary heart disease (CHD) compared to other individuals. A summary of the data from five of these studies confirmed that hypertension, cigarette-smoking and the amount of cholesterol in the blood are independent *risk factors* associated with the occurrence of CHD. A report by the American Heart Association (1993) further confirmed these findings and identified high blood pressure, diabetes, cigarette-smoking, obesity, high serum cholesterol levels and low levels of physical activity as risk factors for CHD.

In recent years, specific psychological factors have been associated with these risk factors and are postulated to play an aetiological role in the onset of CHD. For example, high levels of fats and dietary cholesterol have been linked to atherosclerosis resulting in CHD (Jeffery, 1992). Several studies have found that a reduction in cholesterol levels through dietary intervention or a combination of drug intervention and a low-cholesterol, low-fat diet reduces the incidence of CHD morbidity and mortality (Kushi *et al.*, 1985; Multiple Risk Factor Intervention Trial Research Group, 1982). In a more recent prospective randomised controlled trial to determine whether comprehensive lifestyle changes would affect coronary atherosclerosis after 1 year, Ornish *et al.* (1990) assigned 28 patients to an experimental group (low-fat vegetarian diet, stopping smoking, stress management training and moderate exercise) and 20 patients to a usual-care control group. In total, 195 coronary artery lesions were analysed by quantitative coronary angiography. After 1 year, 82 per cent of the patients from the experimental group showed an overall significant regression of coronary atherosclerosis, indicating the importance of lifestyle changes in reducing the risk of CHD.

The idea of a direct link between behaviour and heart disease is also the subject of considerable interest. As early as 1910, Osler described the sort of person likely to have angina as not being 'delicate or neurotic', but 'robust, the vigorous in mind and body, the keen and ambitious man, the indicator of whose engines is always at "full speed ahead"' (quoted in Harvey, 1988, p.11).

It was not until the 1950s, when Friedman and Rosenman noticed that many of their patients with heart disease had similar behavioural patterns, that systematic studies linking feelings, actions and cardiovascular disease were initiated. Friedman and Rosenman (1974) identified the *Type A behaviour pattern* (TABP), and found that it constituted an independent risk factor in the development of CHD. This finding has significant implications for the management and prevention of CHD, and also for the development of testable models that link physical and psychological factors in health and illness.

TABP refers to specific patterns of behaviour which occur in some individuals under specific circumstances. It is referred to by some authors as a *personality construct* (Taylor and Cooper, 1988) and by others as a *behaviour pattern* (Harvey, 1988). The notion that there are Type A individuals with a specific personality trait risks implying that certain characteristics are fundamental to the individual's psychological make-up and thus fixed. However, if certain individuals exhibit the Type A behavioural pattern, this implies the possibility for change.

Type A behaviour has been characterised (Jenkins, 1971) as exhibiting extreme competitiveness and an achievement orientation, aggressiveness (sometimes strongly repressed), haste, impatience, restlessness, hyperalertness, explosiveness of speech, tenseness of facial musculature and feelings of being under pressure of time and under the challenge of responsibility. Individuals who exhibit this behaviour often show an extreme commitment to their work, to the exclusion of other aspects of their life. Individuals who exhibit *Type B behaviour* are more relaxed, unhurried, and experience their drive as a steady confidence-building influence (Friedman and Rosenman, 1959).

Salient to the Type A construct is the consistent way in which individuals with TABP perceive demands, threats and challenges, and strive for control over people and events. The quest for control continues even when events are uncontrollable, and it is likely that this response is stress-inducing, maladaptive and detrimental to health. Strobe and Werner (1985) suggested that, through striving to remain in control, Type A individuals create their own stressful environment. However, we should note that Chesney and Rosenman (1980) observed that challenge and control are important factors for the well-being of Type A managers. These studies indicated both a positive and a negative aspect to TABP.

Further conflicting results emerge from the findings of the Western Collaborative Group study reported by Ragland and Brand (1988). It was observed that, following an initial heart attack, the numbers of Type A and Type B deaths were approximately equal, but over a longer period of time Type A survivors outnumbered Type B survivors. Taylor and Cooper (1988) suggested that a possible explanation for these findings might lie within the framework of the control concept. There is some evidence to suggest that individuals who are 'internally' oriented, i.e. who believe that they are controllers of their own destiny, engage in more generally adaptive health responses at both preventative and remedial levels (Strickland, 1978). Certain Type A individuals would possibly fall within this category. Therefore Type A behaviour might not always imply coronary-prone behaviour.

Studies that have identified a positive dimension to Type A behaviour suggest that TABP cannot be considered globally, and that global attempts to modify Type A behaviour could have negative consequences for some individuals.

Friedman et al. (1985) proposed two categories of both Type A and Type B individuals. They distinguished between charismatic and hostile Type A individuals, and relaxed and tense Type B individuals. They suggested that a charismatic Type A individual would be healthy, expressive, dominant, fast-moving, in control, coping well and sociable, and that such an individual would remain healthy under conditions of stress. In contrast, a hostile Type A individual would be competitive, expressive and dominant in a threatened and negative sense, and would be prone to coronary heart disease.

A relaxed Type B individual, who Friedman et al. (1985) suggested could be less prone to illness, would display quiet, unexpressive and submissive behaviour, whereas a tense Type B individual would be over-controlled, unexpressive and inhibited, but liable to explode under sufficient challenge, and could also be prone to illness.

Three of the negative components which exist within the Type A behaviour construct are anger, hostility and aggression, and these have been termed the *AHA syndrome* by Spielberger et al. (1985). It appears that some Type A individuals exhibit more of these behaviours than others (Check and Dyck, 1986), and that such behaviours ultimately undermine health. Cynical hostility characterised by suspiciousness, resentment, frequent anger, antagonism and distrust of others has in particular been implicated as the most significant behavioural component of the Type A behaviour syndrome, which both increases the likelihood of CHD (Barefoot et al., 1994; Miller et al., 1996) and is a risk factor for all-cause mortality (Smith, 1992).

Measuring the Type A behaviour pattern (TABP)

One of the problems associated with research has been the different methods used to assess the Type A/B construct. Assessment can be made by *structured interview* (SI) designed to elicit TABP responses, with both the content and manner of responses to questions being assessed. The SI needs to be performed by skilled personnel, and is thus time-consuming and costly as a measurement tool for large-scale research. A number of self-report questionnaires (Haynes *et al.*, 1980; Jenkins, 1971) have been developed which can be more easily administered, but which carry the risk of inaccurate reporting. The most commonly used self-report questionnaire is the *Jenkins Activity Survey* (JAS) (Jenkins *et al.*, 1979), which contains about 50 questions that ask the subject how he or she behaves in certain situations. Jenkins (1971) showed that the overall level of agreement in classification using the SI and the JAS was 73 per cent and thus acceptable. Other studies have found a much smaller margin of overlap (Chesney *et al.*, 1981; Matthews *et al.*, 1982). This indicates that caution must be exercised when comparing studies which have used different measures.

Intervention

The identification of a behaviour pattern found to be linked directly with CHD raises a number of important questions.

- Can the TABP be changed?
- If it is changed, does it lead to a reduction in CHD?
- What are the most effective procedures for change?
- What are the ethics of change?

A number of studies (Levenkron *et al.*, 1983; Roskies *et al.*, 1986) have shown that it is possible to alter aspects of TABP, and that these changes may parallel measures of physiological change. Some studies have used patients who already have CHD. Friedman *et al.* (1985) used a *group behaviour modification/cognitive behavioural* approach to help individuals who had already suffered a myocardial infarction to develop self-management techniques for reducing TABP. Their approach effectively reduced TABP, and the reinfarction rate was only 50 per cent of that in a control group. Similar subjects used in a study by Frasure-Smith and Prince (1985) were taught to self-monitor stress, and were given the opportunity to talk about this to a specially trained nurse. The death rate due to cardiac disease was found to be significantly lower in the experimental group compared to the control group.

The evidence so far is that TABP can be changed, and that this can lead to a reduction in CHD. However, since there are indications of positive as well as negative consequences of some aspects of TABP, global attempts to change TABP should be treated with caution. A careful assessment of the potential costs and benefits of change must be made, with patients/clients making their own decisions about what they believe is best for them, taking into account the many social, occupational and lifestyle factors that are likely to have a bearing on the decision.

Locus of control

A salient feature of research linking TABP to coronary heart disease is the role of control. Individuals with TABP strive for control over people and events. *Locus of control* is a personality variable which has its origins in social learning theory (Rotter, 1954). It defines a generalised expectancy concerning the extent to which an individual believes that reinforcements, rewards or success are either internally or externally controlled. An *internal* locus of control implies a belief in personal power, control and influence over the outcome of events. An *external* locus of control implies a belief that personal power has a minimal effect on the outcome of events, these being influenced by fate, chance and powerful others (Taylor and Cooper, 1988).

Extremes in either direction can be maladaptive (Rotter, 1966), and there is no such thing as *internality* without *externality*. To believe only in internality would be to deny the existence of any sources of external control (Reid, 1984). Externality has two components: 'fate/chance' and 'powerful others'. Jenner (1986) observed that a belief in the influence of powerful others correlated with a greater perception of organisational stress. This study also found a positive association between organisational stress and relationship stress. Oliver (1983) reported that employees in professional and managerial positions tended to be internally oriented. Lefcourt (1981) proposed that, whereas most individuals react to stress, *externals*, unlike *internals*, continue to carry and add to this stress over a prolonged period of time, and this ultimately has negative health consequences. In contrast, 'internals' seek to change situations as a means of increasing personal control and reducing stress. However, in situations where personal control is not possible, if continued attempts are made to assert control, as in the case of the extreme Type A individual, this is likely to be detrimental to health. An assessment of locus of control can be made using Rotter's *internality–externality (I–E) scale* (Rotter, 1966).

The notion of locus of control can be applied to the issue of who is responsible for an individual's health. Does the responsibility for one's health lie with the individual or with the professional, or is it dependent on luck or fate, with nobody ultimately responsible for it? Since the development of Rotter's I-E scale, health-specific measures of the construct have been developed and adopted by investigators in the health fields (Wallston and Wallston, 1981).

A measure of an individual's *health locus of control* (HLC) is a measure of their belief pattern at a particular point in time. It does not imply a fixed personality type. This distinction has significant therapeutic implications, as it allows for individual change.

Wallston and Wallston (1982) provide a detailed review of HLC research literature. They conclude that:

> most of the findings reported ... attest to the construct validity of the HLC scales. The most consistent relationship is between depressive affect and the belief that one's health is unpredictable (i.e. Chance Health Locus of Control (CHLC).
>
> (Wallston and Wallston, 1982, p.74)

Strickland (1978) summarised the research relating measures of locus of control to health knowledge and precautionary measures by suggesting that, with some minor exceptions, the bulk of the reported research on internality/externality and precautionary health practices supports the theoretical assumption that individuals who hold internal, as opposed to external, expectations are more likely to assume greater responsibility for their health. Those individuals who are identified as possessing an internal locus of control play an active role in guarding against accidents and minimising the risk of disease (Strickland, 1978).

Wallston and Wallston (1982) suggested that the ideal partnership between health care provider and consumer is one in which each believes that the other has something to bring to the relationship, and that they must work together to optimise outcomes. They considered that a consumer belief pattern consisting of high *Internal Health Locus of Control* (IHLC), high *Powerful Others Health Locus of Control* (PHLC) and low *Chance Health Locus of Control* (CHLC) is the most conducive to a positive therapeutic relationship. Research is still needed to determine the health locus of control beliefs of health care professionals, their expectations of their clients' HLC beliefs, and the significance of these for the client/carer relationship and therapeutic outcomes.

Unfortunately there are numerous examples within the health care system of an orientation towards removing control from patients and giving it to the professional. This is incompatible with the degree of responsibility for their health that many individuals find themselves expected to take once the acute phase of ill health has passed. In turn, this indicates the need for a partnership between the client and the professional, rather than a hierarchical relationship, and a role for health professionals in preparing their clients for responsibility and independence.

However, both therapeutic interventions and future research on control and health care delivery should take into account the potential for control, patients' perceptions and expectations regarding control, and the expectations of health care providers. Through the study of these complex interactions, more robust and predictive models of health behaviour and related interventions can be developed (Wallston and Wallston, 1982).

Hardy personality

The correlation between stressful events and illness is estimated to be only 0.30, and Kobasa (1979) demonstrated that many people are not becoming ill despite having quite stressful life experiences. There has been a shift in the emphasis in stress and illness research towards the study of *resistance resources* that can neutralise the negative effects of stressful life events. Such resources include constitutional strengths (e.g. unremarkable family history of illness), social supports (e.g. supportive social contacts), health practices (e.g. taking regular exercise and healthy eating) and personality dispositions (Kobasa *et al.*, 1982). A major question is how these apparently diverse resistance resources operate to maintain an individual's health during his or her encounter with stress. An integrating theme was suggested by Kobasa (1979) when she proposed the *hardiness concept* as a personality variable which combined several components and continued the theme of control.

Kobasa (1979) suggested that we look upon hardiness as a constellatory concept, consisting of a range of personality characteristics that function as a resistance force when the individual encounters stressful life events. The personality dispositions of hardiness include commitment, control and challenge (Kobasa *et al.*, 1982).

Commitment reflects a disposition to become involved in, rather than feel alienated from, whatever one is doing. Committed people have a sense of purpose and find meaning in their activities and experiences, and they do not give up easily under pressure. They demonstrate 'active approach' rather than 'passive avoidance' behaviours.

The control disposition reflects a tendency to feel and act as if one is influential rather than helpless with regard to life's events. This does not mean that such people believe they can determine all events and exercise total control, but that by exercising imagination, knowledge, skill and choice they will have a definite influence on outcomes and events. This increases the likelihood that events will be experienced as a logical outcome of one's actions and not as foreign, unexpected or overwhelming experiences. A sense of control is associated with actions considered to be consistent with an ongoing life plan, and thereby enhances an individual's sense of coping (Kobasa *et al.*, 1982). A feature of the challenge disposition is that change rather than stability is normal in life, and change represents a challenge rather than a threat to security. Events are perceived as stimulating rather than threatening, and lead to attempts to change oneself and 'grow', rather than clinging to a former way of being. Challenge fosters openness and flexibility, thus allowing for the effective appraisal of diverse and incongruent events.

Kobasa (1979) revealed that executives who experienced high levels of stressful events but low levels of illness displayed greater commitment, control and challenge than executives who experienced similar life events but high levels of illness. This lends support to the hypothesis that a combination of commitment, control and challenge, i.e. a 'hardy personality', keeps people healthy despite encounters with events that are generally regarded as stressful. Retrospective studies such as this leave open the possibility that personality data could be the result of illness and stress. However, a 5-year longitudinal study reported by Kobasa *et al.* (1982) suggests that the tendency towards commitment, control and challenge functions prospectively as a resistance resource, and that hardiness has its greatest health-preserving effect when stressful life events increase. Subsequent to Kobasa's (1979) initial study, several investigations have found that hardiness generally relates to good physical *and* mental health (Nowack, 1989; Wiebe and McCullum, 1986), and may also help to attenuate cardiovascular responses (Contrada, 1989). Furthermore, some researchers have observed that the effects of hardiness tend to be more beneficial for men, but not necessarily for women (Williams *et al.*, 1992).

Since hardiness has been identified as a significant resistance resource in buffering the effects of stressful life events, it is useful to consider first how hardiness develops, and secondly its role in relation to other resistance resources. With regard to the second point, Kobasa *et al.* (1982) made a number of suggestions relating to possible interactions between the resistance resources. They suggested that hardiness is especially effective in preserving health when constitutional strengths are low, and that the likely mediating mechanism could be health practices. Positive health practices such as adequate rest, exercise, and moderation in food and substance intake may offset constitutional predispositions to some extent. By virtue of their approach to life, hardy people might engage conscientiously and effectively in positive health practices, compared to people with low levels of hardiness, who might engage in more negative health practices and thereby exaggerate constitutional predispositions.

Another possible interaction suggested by Kobasa *et al.* is that social supports are more effective in preserving health when hardiness levels are high. When confronted with stressful events, hardy people may actively seek out the kinds of social contacts that could decrease the stressfulness of the events, and attempt to learn from and possibly alter what is happening. In contrast, people with low levels of hardiness might seek less support, or concentrate on blanket reassurances and distraction from the events.

If future research continues to indicate the importance of hardiness as a resistance resource, it will be important to learn more about how and why such a personality develops, and how people can be helped to acquire hardy personality characteristics. It is likely that *existential personality theory* and social learning theory will make a useful contribution to our understanding of such processes (see Chapter 6).

Implications of research

Research on the relationship between individual differences, stress and health has significant implications for all individuals, including nurses and patients, and also for organisations. The significance of control has been highlighted in much of the research. It is important at both an individual and an organisational level to identify ways of managing and coping with change so that it becomes a challenge rather than a threat. Change which leads to feelings of loss of control, threat and helplessness is associated with the experience of stress and negative health effects. These effects can occur in the health professional, the lay population and the patient population. They can occur as a result of changes brought about by ill health and slow down recovery, and they can occur in apparently healthy individuals and precipitate ill health.

Nurses can play a role in implementing programmes to ameliorate these negative effects at a number of levels – at the organisational and managerial level, and at the individual level with staff and patients. Taylor and Cooper (1988) proposed that three processes, namely communication, control and counselling, are of particular importance. They suggested that organisations need effective two-way communication systems, that good communications help to reduce high stress levels and decrease job dissatisfaction, and that, in return, the organisation is more readily able to pinpoint areas of potential pressure and dissatisfaction.

Good communication means that employees have a greater understanding of policies and reasons for change, experience less uncertainty, and have a greater perception of personal control. The provision of counselling services and the open acknowledgement that organisational structures and change can lead to stress could help to offset the *stigmatisation* associated with stress. Marshall and Cooper (1981) found that the provison of such services, combined with wellness programmes, including information on smoking, alcohol and drug abuse, and advice on diet and exercise, had beneficial effects for both the individual and the organisation.

Nursing management and organisation can be such that they generate stress and anxiety in both nurses and patients. Much of this could be prevented if its deleterious health effects were recognised and programmes focusing on communication, control and counselling were implemented. At the individual level, good communication reduces uncertainty and allows the open discussion of problems and more realistic identification of problem areas. This permits greater individual autonomy and control. It has already been identified that the perception of lack of control is associated with stress and ill health.

Individual counselling can increase self-awareness and understanding of how personality variables interact to affect the stress/health relationship. This awareness is equally valuable to the patient population, nurses and the general population for promoting health. If programmes to promote communication, control and counselling were implemented proactively to facilitate coping with the demands of life, rather than reactively, much ill health could be avoided.

Summary and conclusion

This chapter started by focusing on nursing activities which had emerged during research with student nurses, identifying that they all potentially involved psychological as well as physical dimensions, and that the overarching theme was of nursing as an interpersonal activity involving communication and relationships between people. It moved on to describe ways in which implicit knowledge and experience could influence the nature of communication, relationships and therapeutic outcomes. Control emerged as a theme in the early part of the chapter, and later in relation to empirical findings linking individual differences, stress and health.

Empirical evidence supports the position taken by Sundberg and Tyler (1963) that the first task of the clinician should be to discover the conceptual framework within which he or she is operating. A conceptual framework that ignores the importance of personal control and does not take into account the individual differences/stress/health relationship may be capable of ameliorating physical ill health in the short term, but will not effectively promote positive health in the long term.

Nursing is a complex activity requiring an immense range of knowledge and skills. The emphasis in this chapter has been on three forms of knowledge which can usefully be integrated to complement one another – implicit, experiential and empirical knowledge – and a psychological perspective has been taken with regard to each of these areas. Clearly the psychological perspective that is taken reflects inclusion of only a small selection of potentially relevant psychological knowledge. However, the material included demonstrates that the combination of these three forms of knowledge, together with a psychological perspective, can usefully be applied to inform nursing skills and attitudes, and to promote effective nursing practice.

Learning activities

The following is an exercise based on Personal Construct Theory (PCT). It can be carried out individually or in groups. Its main purpose is to increase the participants' awareness of their own and others' attitudes to nursing activities.

1. Write down a list of about 10 nursing activities in which you have recently engaged. (If the exercise is carried out with a group, the group together decides on 10 activities.)

   Examples of activities could be:

   assisting patients with personal hygiene;
   talking to patients;
   educating patients;
   giving medication.

   These activities are called *elements* in PCT language.

2. Take three activities at random from the list and think of a way in which two of the activities are similar and different to the third.

   For example, I enjoy this ... I do not enjoy this.

   This continuum is called a *construct*.

When this activity is carried out with a group, participants will identify a range of constructs relating to the same three elements (activities). There are no right or wrong constructs, and differences in construing can lead to interesting and useful discussion.

3. Select another three elements (nursing activities) from the list and follow the same procedure to produce further constructs.

For example, I felt well prepared for this ... I did not feel well prepared for this.

Patient centred ... nurse centred.

4. Continue this procedure until no new constructs can be produced. The final list of constructs is that which the participant(s) commonly use to judge nursing activities.

The discussion generated by this activity will have increased participants' awareness of their own and others' implicit assumptions about and attitudes to nursing. The implications (which are not the same as correctness) of construing elements in particular ways can be usefully discussed.

It is important that this activity is carried out within a non-judgemental and supportive environment.

References

Abramson, L. 1977 *Universal versus personal helplessness: an experimental test of the reformulated theory of learned helplessness and depression.* Unpublished PhD Thesis, University of Pennsylvania, Philadelphia.

American Heart Association 1993 *Heart and stroke facts.* Dallas, TX: American Heart Association.

Anderson, K. O. and Masur, F. T. 1983 Psychological preparation for invasive medical and dental procedures. *Journal of Behavioral Medicine,* **6**, 1–40.

Arnetz, B. B., Wasserman, J., Petrini, B. *et al.* 1987 Immune function in unemployed women. *Psychosomatic Medicine* **49**, 3–12.

Bandura, A. 1977 *Social learning theory.* Englewood Cliffs, NJ: Prentice-Hall.

Barefoot, J. C., Patterson, J. C., Haney, T. L., Cayton, T. G., Hickman, J. R. and Williams, R. B. 1994 Hostility in asymptomatic men with angiographically confirmed coronary artery disease. *American Journal of Cardiology* **74**, 439–42.

Beail, N. (ed.) 1985 *Repertory grid technique and personal constructs.* London: Croom Helm.

Button, E. (ed.) 1985 *Personal construct theory and mental health.* London: Croom Helm.

Caine, J. M. and Smail, D. J. 1969 *The treatment of mental illness: science, faith and the therapeutic personality.* London: University of London Press.

Center for Disease Control 1986 *Morbidity and Mortality Weekly Report* **35**, 653–68.

Check, J. V. P. and Dyck, D. G. 1986 Hostile aggression and type A behaviour. *Personality and Individual Differences* **7**, 819–27.

Chesney, M. A. and Rosenman, R. H. 1980 Type A behaviour in the work setting. In Cooper, C. L. and Payne, R. (eds), *Current concerns in occupational stress.* London: Wiley.

Chesney, M. A., Eagleston, J. R. and Rosenman, R. H. 1981 Type A behavior: assessment and intervention. In Prokop, C. K. and Bradley, L. A. (eds), *Medical psychology*. New York: Academic Press.

Contrada, R. J. 1989 Type A behaviour, personality hardiness, and cardiovascular responses to stress. *Journal of Personality and Social Psychology* **57**, 895–903.

Copp, L. 1971 A projective cartoon investigation of nurse–patient psychodramatic role perception and expectation. *Nursing Research* **20**, 100–12.

Cox, T. and McKay, C. 1978 Stress at work. In Cox, T. (ed.), *Stress*. Baltimore: University Park Press.

De Vellis, B. M., Adams, J. L. and De Vellis, R. F. 1984 Effects of information on patient stereotyping. *Research in Nursing and Health* **7**, 237–44.

Dunn, H. J. 1961 *High level wellness*. Washington: Mount Vernon Publishing Co.

Dunnett, G. (ed.) 1988 *Working with people: clinical uses of personal construct psychology*. London: Routledge.

Eiser, J. R. and Gossop, M. R. 1979 'Hooked' or 'sick': addicts' perceptions of their addiction. *Addictive Behaviors* **4**, 185–91.

Folkman, S. and Lazarus, R. S. 1980 An analysis of coping in a middle-aged community sample. *Journal of Health and Social Behaviour* **21**, 219–39.

Fransella, F. and Bannister, D. 1977 *A manual for repertory grid technique*. London: Academic Press.

Frasure-Smith, N. and Prince, R. 1985 The ischemic heart disease life stress monitoring program: impact on mortality. *Psychosomatic Medicine* **47**, 431–45.

Frederickson, M. and Matthews, K. A. 1990 Cardiovascular responses to behavioral stress and hypertension: a meta-analytic review. *Annals of Behavioral Medicine* **12**, 30–39.

Friedman, H. S., Hall, J. A. and Harris, M. J. 1985 Type 'A' behavior, non-verbal expressive style and health. *Journal of Personality and Social Psychology* **48**, 1299–315.

Friedman, M. and Rosenman, R. H. 1959 Association of specific overt behavior pattern with blood and cardiovascular findings: blood cholesterol level, blood clotting time, incidence of arcus senilis and clinical coronary artery disease. *Journal of the American Medical Association* **169**, 1286–96.

Friedman, M. and Rosenman, R. H. 1974 *Type A behavior and your heart*. New York: Fawcett.

Goffman, E. 1961 *Asylums: essays on the social situation of mental patients and other inmates*. Harmondsworth: Penguin.

Goldstein, A. P. and Krasner, L. 1987 *Modern applied psychology*. Oxford: Pergamon.

Hammen, C., Marks, T., Mayol, A. and DeMayo, R. 1985 Depressive self-schemes, life stress and vulnerability to depression. *Journal of Abnormal Psychology* **94**, 308–19.

Harvey, P. 1988 *Health psychology*. Harlow: Longman.

Hatch, J. P., Moore, P. J., Borcherding, S., Cyr-Provost, M., Boutros, N. N. and Seleshi, E. 1992 Electromyographic and affective response of episodic tension-type headache patients and headache-free controls during stressful task performance. *Journal of Behavioral Medicine* **15**, 89–112.

Haynes, S. G., Feinleib, M. and Kannel, W. B. 1980 The relationship of psychosocial factors to coronary heart disease in the Framingham study. 3. Eight years' incidence of coronary heart disease. *American Journal of Epidemiology* **111**, 37–58.

Heider, F. 1958 *The psychology of interpersonal relations*. New York: Wiley.

Herbert, T. B. and Cohen, S. 1993 Stress and immunity: a meta-analytic review. *Psychosomatic Medicine* **55**, 364–79.

Hyland, M. E. and Donaldson, M. L. 1989 *Psychological care in nursing practice*. Harrow: Scutari.

Janoff-Bulman, R. and Lang-Gunn, L. 1988 Coping with disease, crime and accidents: the role of self-blame attributions. In Abramson, L. (ed.), *Social cognitions and clinical psychology*. Surrey: Guildford Press, 116–47.

Jarvis, P. 1992 *Paradoxes of learning*. San Francisco: Jossey-Bass.

Jeffery, R. W. 1992 Is obesity a risk factor for cardiovascular disease? *Annals of Behavioral Medicine* **14,** 107-12.

Jemmott, J. B. and Locke, S. E. 1984 Psychosocial factors, immunologic mediation and human susceptibility to infectious diseases: how much do we know? *Psychosocial Bulletin* **95,** 78–108.

Jenkins, C. D. 1971 Psychological and social precursors of coronary disease. *New England Journal of Medicine* **284,** 244–55, 307–17.

Jenkins, C. D., Zyzanski, S. J. and Rosenman, R. H. 1979 *The Jenkins activity survey for health prediction*. New York: The Psychological Corporation.

Jenner, J. R. 1986 Powerful others, non-work factors and organizational stress. *Psychological Reports* **58,** 103–9.

Johnston, M., Gilbert, P. G., Partridge, C. and Collins, J. 1992 Changing perceived control in patients with physical disabilities: an intervention study with patients receiving rehabilitation. *British Journal of Clinical Psychology* **31,** 89–94.

Kelly, G. A. 1955 *The psychology of personal constructs, Vols 1 and 2*. New York: Norton.

Kelly, G. A. 1970 A brief introduction to personal construct theory. In Bannister, D. (ed.), *Perspectives in personal construct theory*. London: Academic Press, 1–30.

Kelly, M. P. and May, D. 1982 Good and bad patients: a review of the literature and a theoretical critique. *Journal of Advanced Nursing* **7,** 147–56.

Kiecolt-Glaser, J. K., Glaser, R., Strain, E. C. et al. 1986 Modulation of cellular immunity in medical students. *Journal of Behavioral Medicine* **9,** 5–22.

Kobasa, S. C. 1979 Stressful life events, personality and health: an inquiry into hardiness. *Journal of Personality and Social Psychology* **37,** 1–11.

Kobasa, S. C., Maddi, S. R. and Kahn, S. 1982 Hardiness and health: a prospective study. *Journal of Personality and Social Psychology* **42,** 168–77.

Kushi, L. H., Lew, R. W., Sture, F. J. et al. 1985 Diet and 20-year mortality from coronary heart disease: the Ireland-Boston diet heart study. *New England Journal of Medicine* **312,** 811–18,

Larson, P. 1977 Nurse perceptions of patient characteristics. *Nursing Research* **26,** 416–21.

Lazarus, R. S. 1976 *Patterns of adjustment*. New York: McGraw-Hill.

Lazarus, R. S. and Folkman, S. 1984 *Stress, appraisal and coping*. New York: Springer.

Lefcourt, H. M. (ed.) 1981 *Research with the locus of control construct. Vol. 1*. New York: Academic Press.

Levenkron, J. C., Cohen, J. D., Mueller, H. S. and Fisher, E. B. 1983 Modifying the type A coronary-prone behavior pattern. *Journal of Consulting and Clinical Psychology* **51,** 192–204.

Locke, S. E., Kraus, L. and Leserman, J. 1984 Life change, stress, psychiatric symptoms, and neural killer cell activity. *Psychosomatic Medicine* **46,** 441–53.

Maier, S. F., Seligman, M. E. P. and Solomon, R. L. 1969 Pavlovian fear conditioning and learned helplessness: effects of escape and avoidance behavior of (a) the CS-US contingency, and (b) the independence of the US and voluntary responding. In Campbell, B. A. and Church, R. M. (eds), *Punishment and aversive behavior*. New York: Appleton-Century-Crofts.

Marshall, J. and Cooper, C. L. (eds) 1981 *Coping with stress at work: case studies from industry*. Aldershot: Gower.

Marteau, T. M. 1989 Health beliefs and attributions. In Broome, A. K. (ed.), *Health psychology: processes and applications*. London: Chapman and Hall, 1–23.

Marteau, T. M. and Riordan, D.C. 1992 Staff attitudes towards patients: the influence of causal attributions for illness. *British Journal of Clinical Psychology* **31**, 107–10.

Mathews, A. and Ridgeway, V. 1984 Psychological preparation for surgery. In Steptoe, A. and Matthews, A. (eds), *Health care and human behaviour*. London: Academic Press, 231–59.

Matthews, K. A., Krantz, D. S., Dembroski, T. M. and MacDougall, J. M. 1982 Unique and common variance in structured interview and Kenin's activity survey measures of type A behavior pattern. *Journal of Personality and Social Psychology* **42**, 303–13.

Miller, T. Q., Smith, T. W., Turner, C. W., Cuijarro, M. L. and Hallett, A. J. 1996 A meta-analytic review of research on hostility and physical health. *Psychological Bulletin* **119**, 322-48.

Moss, A. R. 1988 Determinants of patient care: nursing process or nursing attitudes? *Journal of Advanced Nursing* **13**, 615–20.

Multiple Risk Factor Intervention Trial Research Group 1982 Multiple risk factor intervention trial: risk factor changes and mortality results. *Journal of the American Medical Association* **248**,1465–77.

Murray, R. B. and Zentner, J P. 1989 *Nursing concepts for health promotion* (adapted for the UK by C. Howells). New York: Prentice-Hall.

Nowack, K. M. 1989 Coping style, cognitive hardiness and health status. *Journal of Behavioral Medicine* **12**, 145–58.

Oliver, J. E. 1983 Job satisfaction and locus of control in two job types. *Psychological Reports* **52**, 425–6.

Ornish, D., Brown, S. E., Scherwitz, L. W. *et al.* 1990 Can lifestyle changes reverse coronary heart disease? *Lancet* **336**, 129–33.

Osler, W. 1910 The Lumleian lectures on angina pectoris. *Lancet* **1**, 839–44.

Partridge, C. J. and Johnston, M. 1989 Perceived control and recovery from stroke. *British Journal of Clinical Psychology* **28**, 53–60.

Pavlov, I. P. 1927 *Conditioned reflexes*. New York: Oxford University Press.

Pooling Project Research Group 1978 Relationship of blood pressure, serum cholesterol, smoking habit, relative weight and ECG abnormalities to incidence of major coronary events: final report of the pooling project. *Journal of Chronic Diseases* **31**, 201–306.

Ragland, D. R. and Brand, R. J. 1988 Type A behavior and mortality from coronary heart disease: a review. *Current Psychological Research and Reviews*, Winter Issue, 63–84.

Raps, C. S., Peterson, C., Jonas, M. and Seligman, M. E. P. 1982 Patient behavior in hospitals: helplessness, reactance or both? *Journal of Personality and Social Psychology* **42**, 1036–41.

Reid, D. W. 1984 Participatory control and chronic illness adjustment process. In Lefcourt, H. M. (ed.), *Research with locus of control construct. Vol. 3.* New York: Academic Press.

Roskies, R. and Lazarus, R. S. 1980 Coping theory and the teaching of coping skills. In Davidson, P. O. and Davidson, S. M. (eds), *Behavioral medicine: changing health lifestyles*. New York: Brunner/Mazel, 38–69.

Roskies, E., Seraganian, P., Oseasohn, R. *et al.* 1986 The Montreal Type A intervention project: major findings. *Health Psychology* **5**, 45–69.

Rotter, J. B. 1954 *Social learning and clinical psychology*. Englewood Cliffs: Prentice-Hall.

Rotter, J. B. 1966 Generalized expectancies for internal versus external control of reinforcement. *Psychological Monographs* **80**, 1–28.

Seligman, M. E. P. 1975 *Helplessness: on depression, development and death.* San Francisco: Freeman.

Selye, H. 1956 *The stress of life.* New York: McGraw-Hill.

Singer, J. E. and Baum, A. 1980 Stress, environment and environmental stress. In Feimer, N. R. and Geller, E. S. (eds), *Environmental psychology: directions and perspectives.* New York: Praeger.

Skinner, B. F. 1938 *The behavior of organisms.* New York: Appleton-Century-Crofts.

Spielberger, C. D., Johnson, E. H., Russell, S. F., Crane, R. S., Jacobs, G. A. and Worden, T. J. 1985 The experience and expression of anger: construction and validation of an anger expression scale. In Chesney, M. A. and Rosenman, R. H. (eds), *Anger and hostility in cardiovascular and behavioral disorders.* New York: Hemisphere McGraw-Hill, 5–30.

Smith, T. W. 1992 Hostility and health: current status of a psychosomatic hypothesis. *Health Psychology* **11**, 139–50.

Stockwell, F. 1972 *The unpopular patient.* London: Royal College of Nursing.

Strickland, B. R. 1978 Internal-external expectancies and health related behaviors. *Journal of Consulting and Clinical Psychology* **46**, 1192–211.

Strobe, M. J. and Werner, C. 1985 Relinquishment of control and type A behavior pattern. *Journal of Personality and Social Psychology* **48**, 688–701.

Sundberg, N. D. and Tyler, L. E. 1963 *Clinical psychology.* London: Methuen.

Taylor, H. and Cooper, C. L. 1988 Organizational change – threat or challenge? The role of individual differences in the management of stress. *Journal of Organization Change Management* **1**, 68–80.

Treiber, F. A., Davis, H., Musante, L. *et al.* 1993 Ethnicity, gender, family history of myocardial infarction and hemodynamic responses to laboratory stressors in children. *Health Psychology* **12**, 6–15.

Viney, L. L. 1985 Physical illness: a guidebook for the kingdom of the sick. In Button, E. (ed.), *Personal construct theory and mental health.* London: Croom Helm, 262–3.

Wallston, B., De Vellis, B. and Wallston, K. 1983 Licensed practical nurses' sex role stereotypes. *Psychology of Women Quarterly* **7**, 199–208.

Wallston K. A. and Wallston B. S. 1981 Health locus of control scales. In Lefcourt, H. M. (ed.), *Research with the locus of control construct.* Volume 1. New York: Academic Press.

Wallston, K. A. and Wallston, B. S. 1982 Who is responsible for your health? The construct of health locus of control. In Sanders, G. S. and Suls, J. M. (eds), *Social psychology of health and illness.* Hove: Lawrence Erlbaum, 65–95.

Wallston, K. A. Wallston, B. S. and De Vellis, B. 1976 Effect of negative stereotype on nurses' attitudes towards an alcoholic patient. *Journal of Studies on Alcohol* **37**, 659–65.

Watts, M. H. 1988 *Shared learning.* Harrow: Scutari.

Watts, M. H. 1994 *Professional education, ideology and learning: a study of student nurses' construing of patients and their care.* Unpublished PhD Thesis, City University, London.

Wegner, D. M. and Vallacher, R. R. 1977 *Implicit psychology: an introduction to cognition.* New York: Oxford University Press.

Westbrook, M. T. and Viney, L. L. 1982 Psychological reactions to the onset of chronic illness. *Social Science and Medicine* **16**, 899–905.

Wiebe, D. J. and McCullum, D. M. 1986 Health practices and hardiness as mediators in the stress–illness relationship. *Health Psychology* **5**, 425–38.

Williams, P. G., Wiebe, D. J. and Smith, T. W. 1992 Coping processes as mediators of the relationship between hardiness and health. *Journal of Behavioral Medicine* **15**, 237–56.

Woods, P. and Cullen, C. 1983 Determinants of staff behavior in long-term care. *Behavioral Psychotherapy* **11**, 4–17.

World Health Organisation 1987 *Evaluation of the strategy for Health For All by the year 2000: seventh report on the world health situation.* Geneva: World Health Organisation.

Caring – the nature of a therapeutic relationship

6

Paul Barber

Introduction

The author, a practising nurse educator and psychotherapist, examines his recent experience of hospitalisation and surgery for the purpose of analysing 'therapeutic' and 'non-therapeutic' influences in care. Events experienced as a patient provide the springboard to introduce those professional insights and interpersonal awareness that are necessary to the appreciation of a therapeutic relationship.

Much of this account is based on the author's observations of personal and social dynamics, skills and attitudes of direct care staff, the integrity of which has the power to maximise the therapeutic potential of the nurse–patient relationship.

Patient status, the clinical environment and the effects that carers can have on the sick are first reported, and then put under scrutiny and reflected upon, under the headings of 'Insights for carers'.

Finally, the author draws together his insights to form a comprehensive reference of the social dynamics, skills and awareness that contribute to a relationship becoming therapeutic, and makes suggestions as to how clinical practice and professional education may be harnessed to supervision to maximise the therapeutic potential of the nurse–patient relationship.

It is hoped that the following experience, gained at a time of intense emotional and intellectual growth, shared within a personal action research frame, will help to illuminate 'the client experience', provoke thoughtful reflection and enrich the reader's acceptance that *therapeutic relationing* cannot afford to be under-credited.

On being well: the nature of health

In December 1987, accompanied by my wife, Anna, I travelled to my mother's home for a couple of days prior to Christmas. The Autumn Term, having being particularly busy for both of us in our respective teaching careers, caused us to view this as a well earned trip where we might combine family reunion with a little diversionary fun.

After a light tea we went out for a drink. This outing had the feel of 'a treat', the more so as we called along the way to collect David, a younger cousin we had not seen for many months.

Following a short drive we alighted at an old beamed inn adjoining an ancient village churchyard. The sharp night air made the warmth of the interior all the more inviting.

A couple of hours – and a few pints – later, a troop of players resplendent in mediaeval costumes strolled in to offer entertainment, an impromptu mystery play of George and the Dragon. The main protagonists, a figure dressed as a jester, who gave a colloquial recitation, and two other fellows, dressed respectively as George and the dragon, frolicked around us. I joined with numerous other customers to become part of this fray, heckling and threatening George who, following each swipe of his sword, took a sup from the nearest pint to him – mine!

I had not felt so relaxed or had as much fun all year and was really starting to look forward to Christmas.

Over the course of the evening I drank three pints and, as Anna drove home, remembered feeling full and satisfied. It had been a good night with the family and Christmas had started well.

Insights for carers (1)

I am reminded in the above passage of just what the therapeutic relationship strives to achieve – *health*. Health is substantially more than a sanitised or symptom-free existence; it is rather 'for the sheer joy of it', a state of harmony between body, mind, spirit and our social community which permits us to live life adventurously. Health in this context relates to 'growth' and 'pleasure' and our ability to engage experientially with ourselves and to form intimate relations with others (see Chapter 3).

I am not alone in favouring an holistic definition. Other nurse theorists have observed health to be the following: an optimum level of energy when interpersonal and developmental activities are most productively performed (Peplau, 1988); the ability of an individual to meet his or her own needs (Henderson, 1969); one's position on a dynamic continuum of health–illness ever subject to change (Roy, 1979); a condition of personal integrity where all parts work to complement a whole (Orem, 1995); a value-laden word culturally denoting behaviours which are of high value (Rogers, 1970).

To be healthy is to have energy to play and self-actualise, to be at home in dynamic movement, organismically whole and socially able – in sum, to live life creatively with the confidence to experiment with new ways of being. Nurses, within the bond of a therapeutic relationship, must elicit and role model these qualities.

On becoming ill: regression and hospital symbolism

Back at my mother's home my sensation of fullness lingered on. At midnight, still feeling full I drank some water with Alka Seltzer. In bed the fullness persisted. At about 3 o'clock I started to retch.

Anna brought a bowl to the bedside and suggested that I saw a doctor – I refused. We were to drive back later that morning and I did not want to disturb my mother or make too much of a fuss. Lying in bed, occasionally retching but with nothing to show for it save an acidic taste in my mouth, I passed the night. I guessed the beer I had drunk had been off. Five o'clock came – still retching I now knew something was really wrong. At 7 o'clock I took up the offer of a doctor. My body felt hot to the touch and I felt dizzy and tremulous.

My breathing was by now laboured and, with my heart rate and temperature up, I realised I could no longer go home without seeking aid. From this time on events speeded up and I lost appreciation of time. A general practitioner came, examined me and diagnosed an ulcer. I queried this – 'I'm not the personality type' I said. An ambulance was called and in due time arrived. Not until I tried to get out of bed did I realise how weak I was.

In the ambulance, on a narrow bed with the cot sides up, earlier memories were triggered of a similar ride when I was seven and had broken my leg. I had spent a discomforting night then, too. I was surprised by how vivid these earlier memories were and how readily they had been restimulated by current events. It was difficult for a few moments to recollect if I was aged forty or seven. I made an effort to shake myself into present awareness, engaging the ambulance men in conversation to disengage from the past and a creeping sense of unreality.

I was by now feeling toxic; my mind swayed.

Insights for carers (2)

Distortions of time, memories of previous illness, unresolved fears relating to death and feelings of helplessness were all evoked in the acute onset described above. My being reminded of being seven again suggests that regressive influences were at work.

Regression is defined as a return to earlier less sophisticated adaptive behaviour. This may take the form of a client demonstrating dependence, avoiding responsibility, losing their initiative, enacting 'child-like' behaviours such as sulks or projecting 'parent-like' roles on those who care for them.

Folklore relating to 'The Hospital' compounds this process (Barber, 1996).

It is cautionary to remember that, to the public, 'hospitals' represent much more than a work-place; imaginative perception causes them to be seen as taboo places where the mysteries of life and death unfold and where 'special others' – such as doctors and nurses – 'fight' with death and disease.

Few people have a value-free view of hospital life. Many individuals naturally associate hospitals with the 'rites of passage' of birth and death, especially the latter – 'places where people go to die'.

When frightened or caught in the midst of a life-threatening event, it is all too easy to become haunted by fears of the worst possible outcome. Dramatic interpretation and symbolic communication are the common currency of acute illness and hospital care.

My observations offer a good deal of support for *symbolic interactionism* (see Chapter 7), a view of the world which states:

- individuals respond to those unique meanings they carry with them rather than concrete situations or events;
- the meaning and/or definition of a situation is determined via an individual's social interaction with others; and
- the symbolic meanings an individual attaches to life events are modified through ongoing reinterpretation.

(Blumer, 1969)

This has considerable implications for the therapeutic relationship and the performance of 'individualised care', for it suggests that care professionals, if they are to perform in research-minded and process-aware ways, must appreciate:

- that each client views the world uniquely;
- that there are as many definitions of reality as there are clients;
- that all behaviour has meaning;
- that they need to be wary of invalidating a client's meanings in favour of their own 'professionalised values' and biases; and
- that through the medium of their therapeutic relationship they have a particular potential for helping clients to redefine their experience in health-enhancing ways.

It is a tall order to ask nurses to attend to the subconscious symbolism they portray to clients; far better that they are exposed to professional preparation where their interactions are examined and to clinical supervision of a kind which feeds back to them 'how they are perceived'.

On entering hospital: establishing reality orientation and managing personal boundaries in the care relationship

On arrival at hospital, events felt real enough but happened twice as fast. I was examined – wheeled down a whirl of corridors to the X-ray department – fed what I took to be barium – and eventually told I had a hiatus hernia. Knowing this brought a degree of relief; it was something with which I could start to make sense of events.

Having a current diagnosis enabled me to speculate ahead; I envisaged bedrest, medical intervention and an early ride home. This was not to be. I was informed a nasogastric tube would be passed, after which I could expect to be conveyed to a hospital in Surrey, nearer my home. I swallowed the nasogastric tube – nothing came back. Several attempts later – with ever larger tubes – I began to cough up frothy blood. X-rays were taken. Eventually, it had to be admitted that my stomach was too distended and kinked to receive a gastric tube. All they could get were my lungs. Although the experience was uncomfortable I had not been anxious, but rather relieved and hopeful that a potential end might be in sight.

Insights for carers (3)

From a client's eyeview it was important to be told exactly what was happening to me and to be given a blow-by-blow account of investigations as they occurred. With my sensory world fragmented, fantasy started to predominate. Whenever a space of information was left amiss, I had a tendency to fill that space with anxiety. This suggests to me that:

- patients need as much information as possible to orientate to the crisis-ridden world around them;
- factual information removes a lot of unnecessary drama and helps clients to place their imagined fears on hold; and
- contact with a key worker – someone to provide consistency and to support the development of a relationship – is essential for psychological ease and reality orientation during admission.

Involvement and relationship with another is necessary for both the enactment of reality orientation (Glasser, 1965) and development of the therapeutic relationship (Peplau, 1988). Figure 6.1 indicates that maintaining orientation while keeping a relationship therapeutic also necessitates that 'personal boundaries' be effectively managed.

To remain 'separate', as opposed to 'emotionally distant', is a key skill if carers are to balance 'empathy' and 'friendliness' with 'intellectual clarity'. Therapeutic distance is important, for a client needs to perceive the carer as sympathetic, yet undamaged by the distress that they themselves are experiencing, and able to contain them emotionally.

On awaiting surgery: defence mechanisms in times of crisis

Now I prepared myself for the worst – surgery.

The physician gave way to a surgeon. I was informed that, as my stomach was pushing up through my diaphragm to embarrass my lung, an operation would have to be performed. This information, delivered in a matter-of-fact way, left little to discuss. Before this information had sunk in, or I was able to make enquiry, people had gone.

As evening fell I was wheeled into the surgical ward and my body was shaved and prepared for operation. The pre-medication stopped my retching and relieved most of my discomfort. I was alert and able to relay my medical history when asked.

A consultant anaesthetist now came to my bed. He was gentle, softly spoken, and for the first time I felt the busyness around me start to subside. His voice was slow and I felt supported and listened to.

I saw Anna and my mother again at this time, and stayed light and jokey while they wished me the best. No need to 'make a drama out of a crisis', I felt. I was resigned to what had to be. As there was no real choice to make, I felt little anxiety. I felt detached, witnessing events, and determined not to give in to hopelessness.

In the pre-operation room I met the anaesthetist again. His voice remained soft and unhurried and I felt myself relax. I remember saying to myself that if these were to be my final moments I was going to live them with dignity.

As the anaesthetic flowed into me and I drifted from consciousness I caught snatches of a dream of a canal bridge I played under in childhood. I remembered I had dreamt this dream under dental gas at the age of four.

(1) ORIENTATION

Carer and client meet as strangers, orientate to each other and establish rapport while working together to clarify and define existing problem. Carer notes personal reactions to client and seeks to avoid stereotypic responses that limit therapeutic potential.

(2) IDENTIFICATION

Client and carer clarify each other's perceptions and expectations, and examine past experiences that shade present meanings. Carer notes client's reaction to him/herself, sources of trust and mistrust, dependence upon them or rejection of their interventions.

(3) EXPLORATION

Carer encourages client to take an active responsible role in their own therapy, to self-explore and examine their feelings, thoughts and behaviour, and to trust to their own skills and resources. Carer seeks to convey acceptance, concern and trust to facilitate this process. Wellness becomes a goal in itself, carer listens and employs interpretive skills to enable client's understanding of all those avenues open to them and agencies available to help their self-adjustment.

(4) RESOLUTION

Termination of therapeutic relationship. Client encouraged to be less involved with helper. Carer also establishes independence from the client and works through issues of separation. Client's needs are met with regard to original problem and new goals orientated to enriching wellness. Occupational and leisure interests encouraged.

Figure 6.1   Phases of the therapeutic relationship (adapted from Peplau, 1988)

Insights for carers (4)

During the above period I drifted between internal sensations of discomfort within, and bewildering social relations without. If asked how I was, I said 'fine', as I could not or rather chose not to attend to the gravity of my situation. I believe I was engaging in defence mechanisms of *repression* and *denial*.

Defence mechanisms, i.e. coping strategies which give respite from anxiety, protect the self by enabling an individual to deny or distort a stressful event so as to restrict their awareness and emotional involvement with it. They are unconscious, and two or three may be combined together. When overused, such defences narrow down an individual's perception of reality. At times like these a carer may need to educate a client about the other behavioural options open to them.

Resolving and working through defence mechanisms is a salient task of the therapeutic relationship; it is therefore necessary for carers to acquaint themselves with the more common defensive behaviours.

REPRESSION

This involves the exclusion of a painful or stress-inducing thought, feeling, memory or impulse from awareness; it is the underlying basis of all mental defence mechanisms, and moulds much socialised and professional behaviour. Repressed feelings, commonly sexual or aggressive, although generally out of awareness, continue to exert pressure, and may be released in appropriate surroundings or expressed in times of extreme anxiety. Repression may also fail to function in febrile or toxic states.

DENIAL

Denial of reality shows itself when an individual discards or transforms an emotive event in such a way that it appears to be unrecognisable. Denial is typically present in the first minutes of an individual's adjustment to the death of a loved one. It may seduce the nurse into believing a client has less trauma or pain than is in fact experienced.

RATIONALISATION

Here reasoning is employed to deflect from the emotional significance of an event, i.e. the sudden death of a spouse may be rationalised as 'better than a long illness', although the hurt is just as acute. If carers take what a rationalising client says at face value, they may well see only half the clinical picture.

IDENTIFICATION

This is the wish to be like and/or assume the personality characteristics of another, so much so that the individual concerned becomes estranged from their own personality. Simply, it represents unconscious imitation, an integral part of socialisation and sexual programming. In the hospital such passive receptivity, in contrast to relational reciprocity, can lead to the client confirming all that we say and do. Such a client may validate all our biases, so causing us to be less exploratory than we might otherwise be.

PROJECTION

This is an unconscious means of dealing with unacceptable parts of ourselves by splitting them off and attributing them to others, i.e. others are blamed for one's own shortcomings. A client may project his or her own distress and self-absorption on to nursing staff and so view them as too busy or preoccupied to care for him or her.

DISPLACEMENT

This is the discharge of pent-up emotional energies on to objects or persons less threatening than the person or situation which caused them. I am reminded of the 'pecking-order' that may occur in families or work communities where anger is felt at the head but passed down among the ranks. The nurse whom a client feels safest with may receive the brunt of their emotional discharge. It is no accident that we show our tempers to those we trust or like the most.

REGRESSION

This involves reverting to an earlier, age-inappropriate level of behaviour in order to avoid responsibility and/or present environmental demands. This can be so easily compounded by patient status, bedrest and being placed at the mercy of a strange unfathomable clinical environment where people do things for you rather than with you.

Below, defences are related to their psychological roots and social use (modified from Kroeber, 1963). In this context they can be appreciated as exaggerated behavioural norms.

Psychological root	As a normal means of coping	As a defence
Impulse restraint	Appropriate suppression	Repression
Selective awareness	Concentration	Denial
Role modelling	Socialisation	Identification
Sensitivity	Empathy	Projection
Impulse diversion	Sublimation	Displacement
Time reversal	Playfulness	Regression

NOTE

Defence mechanisms are as common in the staff team as they are in the client population, and form a basis for much professional behaviour; their presence and/or overuse presents a powerful argument for clinical team supervision.

On extraordinary experiences: altered states of consciousness and psychospiritual aspects of the care relationship

My next conscious moment was filled with darkness. I tried to open my eyes and speak, but nothing moved or came out. 'Am I dead?' I wondered. Resigning myself to powerlessness, I reasoned I would just have to make the best of it.

I next heard a snatch of voices, seemingly far off, and felt myself being lifted and turned. I realised for the first time that I was not dead. Many questions surfaced: 'Has the anaesthesia worn off?', 'Is this before or after the operation?', 'Will I feel the surgeons cutting into me?'. This was all very matter of fact – I was not allowing myself the luxury of an emotion.

Gradually I explored my bodily sensations. I became aware it was not me breathing; something was inside doing this for me. I remembered a film, *The Alien*, in which a parasitic entity invades a human host; I smiled to myself, but nothing moved. Strange to say, I also felt free to take stock: 'I have had a full life – do I really want to go back?'. I weighed things up for some time, remembering and reflecting on my life and relationships.

Anna and Marc, my son, were foremost in my mind. I had lived a fatherless childhood, I would not inflict this on my own son. Similarly, I was determined not to leave the life I had with Anna in this way. In short, I contracted with myself to stay alive whatever it cost in terms of my personal resources. I never once during this time doubted that it was in my power to live – or to die.

This state of suspended existence lasted for some hours. Eventually my consciousness became hazy, I thought I heard Anna's voice – but could not tell how much was real and how much imagined before floating into unconsciousness again.

My awakening to conventional reality was blurred, but I was recognisably on a ward with a cardiac monitor and tubes around me. I was aware of Anna and mother but could not focus upon them; like in a dream, the more I tried to focus the harder it was to see. I felt as if I was suspended in thick syrup – all my movements and senses were out of synchronisation and my thoughts formed in slow motion. Occasionally this slow other world of heavy haze would suddenly rip apart and pockets of alertness and clarity would enter, to give way just as suddenly a little later to slow syrupy haze again. Even though my external world was fuzzy, my internal one stayed clear. It was as if an internal 'other-world' reality, one where I could witness myself – as in lucid dreaming – awoke, remained coherent and logical to its own laws and took over, to provide a venue where I could work things out in peace.

Insights for carers (5)

Lucid states, like the one described above, happen to clients more frequently than is imagined (Oakes, 1981; Orne, 1986; Trevelyan, 1989), but not enough time is given to attending to or processing them. Simply, there is often no heading for psychospiritual experiences in the nursing/medical records. Nevertheless, such experiences must be worked through for a return to full health; they are the meat of therapeutic relating in that they represent catalytic turning points. A little time spent in post-surgical counselling would do much to facilitate understanding and integration. Reintegration is the essential objective here. A counsellor who is attentive to spiritual aspects of care and the derivation of individualised meanings could do much in this area. If more clinical and managerial attention was directed towards balancing the view of 'client as an ailing body' with 'client as a spiritual being', I believe clinical environments would be much healthier places to live and work within.

As a nurse, I think I know what happened. While I was on the ventilator my anaesthesia wore off but my dose of muscle relaxant stayed effective; hence I could wake but not move.

On awakening from surgery: the case for individualised care

Gradually cohesion returned and I was able to glue my sensations back into a recognisable social world where I could start to relate to others. I checked my movement – I was stiff and full of heavy dull pain. Anna, my mother, and my son Marc were present. 'So I'm not dead after all', I thought. For the next 24 hours I slept, woke, passively received a blanket bath, drank 5 mls of water hourly and sucked lemon sticks. I looked forward to visiting, when I could sample a little of the 'normal me', but everything else ran together.

On my second conscious day I was brighter; it was also dawning on me how limited my movement was. A sudden intake of breath or a cough and my generalised dull pain focused into a sharp one at the site of my chest drain.

A taped dressing spiralled from my right hip to my left shoulder blade. I joked that I'd been mistaken for a potato. Joking, coping through displacement and denial, was the only means I had at my disposal to put things in perspective and relate in a more normal way.

During this period I tentatively explored the range of movement available to me. There were few comfortable positions and no pain-free ones. Sleep was a series of intermittent catnaps, and whenever my breathing relaxed to a sleeping rhythm I would cough and wake in pain. Talking also presented a problem; anything above a whisper caused my diaphragm to jump into spasms. Nights were long, and days were busy and tiring. I lived for those few lucid moment during visiting when I found the energy to feel really alive again.

The day staff kept busy, superficial and distant. By contrast, the night nurses drew close, chatted, took an interest in me and listened to the short whispered comments I could make. With them I felt a valued person first and a condition second. They answered my questions objectively, orientated me to what was going on and let a bond of friendship form. I felt that I really needed friends at this time.

Insights for carers (6)

As a 40-year-old I was used to an independent life; as a male my assertion was linked with my sexual identity; as a teacher and psychotherapist I was used to helping others from a position of strength. In the status of a patient these usual life roles were drastically reversed.

I felt myself becoming increasingly alienated from my previous sense of self-worth by the transient relationships of carers who came in to perform intimate 'tasks on me' with little more than a superficial 'good morning' or 'how are we?' and who left before I could answer.

I felt child-like and unimportant even though my body was being cared for. Being 'treated as an equal and valued in my own right' was an essential therapeutic need in this period. The day staff, in putting my condition first, failed to meet this need; the night staff, conversely, met it by attending to my person.

Rogers (1983) suggests person-centred care demands of practitioners that they:

- move away from facades, pretence and putting up a front;
- gain more self-direction and value this in others;
- cultivate a reduced need to pretend and hide real feelings;
- value honest communicative relationships;
- be open regarding their own inner reactions and feelings; and
- be aware and sensitive to external events.

Carers who give up their defences in favour of the above qualities are, I suggest, better able to:

- listen;
- demonstrate good contact with themselves and their own realities;

- stay open to and check out their perceptions;
- pay attention to those social processes that create fruitful interaction;
- share their own awareness and knowledge; and
- enable their clients to perform successfully without them (Barber, 1988).

Consequently, the therapeutic relationship they enact is more likely to:

- value the human condition;
- incorporate the client as a resource and cause them to feel valued;
- honour openness and honesty;
- volunteer information and invite questioning of the professional carer; and
- allow space for and encourage clients to express their fears.

A relationship founded upon such principles complements the nursing arts by creating a culture in which nurses may facilitate renewed energy via the medium of the nurse–patient relationship (Peplau, 1988), help patients meet components of basic care relating to breathing, eating and warmth (Henderson, 1969), analyse problems and potential problems while engaged in problem-directed activity (Roy, 1979), overcome the limitations of illness via supporting the patient's ability for self-care (Orem, 1995), while re-establishing and promoting the interactive balance of an individual and their environment (Rogers, 1970).

Nursing, in this account, is seen to be an interpersonal process that works best when relating insights from the care sciences to clients in a humanistic and person-valuing way, through the medium of an empathic relationship which incorporates the client as a care resource while facilitating them to ways of thinking, feeling and relating that maximise a potential for self-directed growth and health (see Chapter 5).

For care of this calibre to evolve, nurse educators must dovetail personal and professional development, and clinical managers need to make provision for peer support or supervision where the care practitioner may talk through those personal/professional distresses that emanate from the performance of care.

On the politics of experience: therapeutic and non-therapeutic intervention

On what I thought to be my third post operative day – but was in fact my fifth – I was approached just before visiting time by the Ward Sister, who told me she was going to give me a painkilling injection prior to getting me up and sitting me in a chair. As Anna was travelling up from Surrey to visit me, and as the injection cited made me sleepy, I enquired if this could be delayed so that I might remain alert during visiting time. This suggestion was not favourably received, and I was lectured on how important it was to get up. I agreed, but enquired whether 2 hours would make such a difference, and repeated my rationale. This did not go down well, and I was told that I must do as she asked.

The tempo now increased; we both had the bit between our teeth. I said that, with respect, as a client I had a right to be heard; it was important to my own well-being for me to fully contact my kin – they were my lifeline. She objected. Surely, I argued, in these days of the nursing process and client-centred care my request was a reasonable enough one to make. She stormed off. My visitors came and went.

With their departure I had my injection, was helped out of bed and sat in a chair. While attending to me the Sister said nothing. I did not feel forgiven for querying her instructions. A few hours later I heard laughter; the junior nurses and Sister were playing, flicking water at one another. When she realised I was watching, the Sister stopped. I seemed to represent a problem for her, and suspected I had been 'hit by a projection' (see 'Insights for carers (4)'). A little while after this a doctor was called and, following much flirtatious glancing, the Sister came out to tell me I was being transferred out from intensive care. I asked the Sister if this meant I was out of danger. She made no answer, but returned to the office where the doctor remained. More flirtatious glances ensued.

I checked myself – surely I was not becoming paranoid; I had earlier been told that I would be here for at least a week more. A change of environment felt quite daunting, especially separation from that meaningful contact forged with the night staff. Within the hour porters came to collect me. When a nurse came over to carry the intravenous drips, I asked her to relay to the Sister and doctor the message that I did not respect their professional cowardice; she looked embarrassed and I doubt if this message was relayed.

My move from intensive care felt ill prepared and emotive. On the positive side, I was aware that I had the resemblance of an emotion forming within me, a potential for anger – confirmation of my ability to experience emotions again.

Insights for carers (7)

A change of wards, a trivial thing for a healthy individual or nurse, can be a major event for a client emerging from a life crisis. Preparation is necessary. It felt like changing worlds, from a reality I knew to one I could not comprehend. The manner of this change put all my symbolic meanings in shift; those who pertained to care for me were now seemingly doing the most damage to my sense of orientation.

Attention to 'transitional periods', such as a change of ward, elevate care from a level of adequacy to one of excellence.

The need for carers to work through the 'resolution phase' of a therapeutic relationship, due to transfer or discharge, has been noted earlier (see Figure 6.1).

Although it is important for a nurse to relay accurate information to a client, as information is what we construct our reality from, this is but half the story. Consideration must also be given to the 'intervention style' employed. When nurses act as guardians of the ward and its formalised medical systems, there is a tendency for them to behave in a manner reminiscent of a critical or/and controlling parent. This occurred with the Sister described above, who made use of degenerative forms of authoritative intervention to:

- 'prescribe' what should happen;
- 'inform' me of her decision; and
- 'confront' me when my opinion differed from hers.

Authoritative interventions, when used in a therapeutic way, can set safe boundaries and complement care (Figure 6.2); when used in the defensive form described, they undergo degeneration.

In this phase of my illness, when I was attempting to rebuild myself and reorientate to the world, 'cathartic', 'catalytic' and 'supportive' interventions would have done much to release my emotional tensions, awareness, self-esteem and self-worth.

Traditionally, nursing has evolved in the shadow of medicine and adopted a similar 'controlling stance' to care; such behaviour, if untempered by the self-enabling interventions, perpetuates dependence, depersonalisation, categorisation and emotional detachment. Therapeutic relations need to be mindful of this.

Perhaps at the time described I was splitting off the 'good' night staff from the 'bad' day staff, idealising one and rejecting the other. Possibly this was regressive, emanating from an unconscious need to identify somebody to blame for my pain and distress (see 'Insights for carers (2) and (4)').

On supporting kin: humanistic values as a foundation for care

Anna and my mother arrived later than usual on the evening of my transfer. They had not been informed of my change of ward and had gone to the intensive-care unit. This aside, they did not seem at ease. Months later I heard the full story; they had initially sat outside the intensive-care unit hoping to catch sight of an available nurse. Eventually they wandered in to be confronted by my empty bed. This caused them to panic, a state from which they were just starting to recover when they met me. It was some time before they found a nurse to tell them where I was.

Insights for carers (8)

I am amazed that nurses could have overlooked informing my kin about my transfer, thus leaving them to be confronted in intensive-care by such a potent symbol of death as my empty bed. Possibly the Ward Sister was acting out an unconscious process of some kind (see 'Insight for carers (4)'), or was it that professional vision put more emphasis on the performance of 'instrumental tasks' than on 'interpersonal processes'?

AUTHORITATIVE INTERVENTIONS

Prescriptive: gives advice to, recommends behaviour to the client.
                 (Practitioner is prescriptive in a way that enhances self-determination in the client)

Informative: gives new knowledge and information to, interprets behaviour to, the client.
                 (Practitioner is informative in a way that enhances informed independent
                 thinking in the client)

Confronting: challenges the restrictive attitudes, beliefs and behaviours of the client.
                 (Practitioner is confronting in a way that enhances intentional growth in the client)

FACILITATIVE INTERVENTIONS

Cathartic: releases tensions in the client: elicits laughter, sobbing, trembling, storming (the
                 harmless and aware release of anger).
                 (Practitioner is cathartic in a way that enhances aware release of feelings in the
                 client)

Catalytic: elicits information and opinion from, self-directed problem-solving and self-discov-
                 ery in the client.
                 (Practitioner is catalytic in a way that enhances self-insight in the client)

Supportive: affirms the worth and value of, enhances the self-image of the client.
                 (Practitioner is supportive in a way that enhances a celebration of self in the client)

Figure 6.2   Six category intervention analysis (Heron, 1977)

As carers we need to realise and act on the premise that relatives suffer along-side clients. For example, Anna had much to contend with during my illness. She telephoned my work-place, friends and family, drove 200 miles every couple of days to visit me, supported my son and counselled my mother, all the while meeting the demands of full-time work and containing her own distress.

Next of kin are an integral part, once removed, of the therapeutic relationship. For instance, post-operatively, a singular act of kindness was performed by the surgeon who, following 7 hours in theatre and within the first hour of Christmas Eve, telephoned my kin to report that the operation was over and had been successful. This did much to relieve distress and cement the emergent therapeutic relationship.

The therapeutic relationship, when isolated from the support of an appropriate value-base, is at risk of degeneration. Throughout this chapter my own bias is one of 'humanism'; it is therefore only fair to alert the reader to what this implies, namely:

- that an individual's mind, intellectual and emotional being are indivisibly connected with their body;
- that given the resources, individuals have the potential to work towards resolution of their own problems;
- that it is important to maintain ongoing open-ended enquiry and to foster creative insight;
- that life experiences and relationships should be valued alongside freedom, growth and contentment as part of 'health'; and
- that there is a need to implement reason and the democratic processes into all social expression (Wilson and Kneisl, 1979).

Humanism puts the person at the centre of the care process, counters deper-sonalisation and instrumental task fixation and places the relational arts and humanistic philosophy alongside the medical sciences. It was missing from the Sister's actions and evident in those of the surgeon.

On stress: the clinical environment as antagonistic to health and therapeutic relating

On entry to my new ward I had been given the option of being in a side-room or the open dormitory. I chose the latter. After a few days this choice proved difficult to live with. I was in a 12-bedded subdivision of the ward, at a period just prior to New Year when only the most needy were retained. The nursing team was understaffed with few seniors to guide them. They were constantly engaged in ongoing physical maintenance tasks with an ever present eye upon the clock as to what must be done next. Observations of temperature, pulse and respirations, and blood and dextrose infusions all had to be attended to 'on time', and nurses appeared as emotion-ally unsupported as the rest of us. It was rare to see a qualified nurse in the open ward. Everything seemed to be pressurised and 'jobs were done' rather than care carried out; all the while the implied message behind ward activity was that 'time was running out'.

A poor soul to my left, demented, blind and deaf, regularly punctuated the night with loud tracts of disjointed dialogue. By the third day I asked if the offer of a side-room was still available. It was, and I was glad to make my escape. Originally I hoped I might be distracted and enjoy the company of my fellow patients, but I had failed to realise how little energy I had or how sapping the pain was when the injections wore off.

My sleep pattern was disrupted. I would be alert until around 5 o'clock, and I would then start to feel sleepy. From 6 o'clock onward care staff per-forming and charting observations, issuing drinks and collecting samples of blood broke my rest.

The ward seemed most antagonistic to my rest or biopsychological rhythms.

Insights for carers (9)

Stressors at any one time are patterned from three sources: our external environment (physical/social); our internal environment (psychological and emotional); and our physiological state or bodily needs. It is a sobering exercise to list those stressors at work in residential care settings.

ENVIRONMENTAL STRESSORS

- Sensory overload from constant noise, lights, people and constantly chang-ing events

- Sensory deprivation due to chemical blurring and immobility
- Close proximity to others and the bustle of an ongoing working environment that never rests
- Loss of usual belongings and routines
- Sudden appearance of unknown others to take samples and perform various personal services
- Estrangement from home and usual lifestyle
- Lack of choice and freedom

PSYCHOLOGICAL AND EMOTIONAL STRESSORS

- Constant fears of intrusion and/or being overwhelmed
- Fears of death and/or mutilation
- Depersonalisation and loss of self-identity
- Inability to meet needs in socially acceptable or accustomed ways
- Fears of nakedness and psychic exposure
- Experience of powerlessness and pain
- Lack of privacy or potential for relaxed retreat
- Separation from supportive others and sexual and community relationships
- Having to adapt to strange new routines

PHYSIOLOGICAL STRESSORS

- Being weakened through disease
- Suffering fever and/or metabolic changes
- Electrolyte imbalance
- The effects of anaesthesia and drugs
- Sleep deprivation
- Tensions/discomforts from investigative procedures
- An unfamiliar diet

To acclimatise to the clinical environment of the ward when healthy is challenge enough; to adjust to it when weakened through illness, let alone to get well, is nigh impossible.

Nursing takes into itself and perpetuates much stress. The folklore and symbolism of the hospital felt by patients and their relations ('Insights for carers (2)') comes out in complicated ways. One moment a nurse may be venerated, showered with affection and gratitude, and the next receive resentment and anger from the self-same folk who now feel frustrated by dependence, jealous of professional esteem and resentful of the care that nurses give to their loved ones:

> The hospital, particularly the nurses, must allow the projection into them of such feelings as depression and anxiety, fear of the patient and his illness and the necessary nursing tasks ... . Thus, to the nurse's own deep and intense anxieties are psychically added those of the other people concerned.
>
> (Menzies, 1960, p.7)

Clinical environments may be made tolerable through sympathetic management – but healthy, never.

The nursing profession has long recognised the stress it takes into itself, but
has been resistant to facing up to and dealing with its own client-like parts. I
believe a critique of nursing is called for here, for in its pursuit of professionalisation it has focused more attention on its 'status and tasks' than on its 'role and
processes'. Consequently, like a remote and defensive parent it has attempted to
ignore and distance itself from its own emotional vulnerability. Such a charge falls
squarely upon the shoulders of nursing education:

> Too often the nursing profession has bred in its practitioners an over strong
> degree of 'parenthood' along with such parental social fears as losing con-
> trol, losing self respect and the respect of others. As a consequence, nurses
> have tended to conform too rigidly. They have not been prepared in a way
> where fears may be voiced and worked through; their preparation is nearer
> one of 'papering over the cracks'; their superficial veneer is shallow and
> prone to fracture.
>
> Nurses are taught primarily to hide their vulnerabilities from others, and
> themselves, but in so doing they reduce their sensitivity.
>
> (Barber, 1993, p.358)

Burn-out is thus allowed to continue unabated. Perhaps denial and displacement (see 'Insight for carers (4)') have become bonded to nursing's professional psyche? It is well to remember that when anxiety-motivated behaviours
predominate over others, burn-out ensues. To survive such conditions, patients
need nurses trained as counsellors, and nurses require the support of supervision where they may be counselled and enjoy the benefits of a therapeutic
relationship themselves.

On advocacy: acting out as a form of unconscious communication

By the start of my third week post-operative depression had commenced.
The pain was still constant and I was attuned to sensation and had lost my
emotional 'highs'. With abdominal discomfort increasing I felt an increased
need to find out what had happened to me during surgery so that I might
understand those strange sensations I felt inside me.

Doctors and nurses came and went and were unable or unwilling to
explain the surgery performed. The nearest I got to an answer was from the
consultant, who said: 'You have had a fairly brutal operation; there is a lot of
bruising inside and you will feel like you have been in the boxing ring for a
few weeks; your diaphragm has now been stitched back together again and
you are making a remarkably good recovery. You are also lucky to escape
without any major complications.' It was impossible for me to extract any
more information than this.

Normally self-advocacy came easily to me, but the lack of energy I had available for any other than the basic functions of living at this time took it from me. Anna came to my aid at this time and served as an advocate for me. She queried nurses, consulted with the surgeons and fed back to me her findings. Her advocacy on my behalf helped me to feel cherished and valued; it also nourished me with information that I, as a patient, was denied. It was good to feel there was somebody on my side. As I had no key worker, and no care plan had been instituted, there was no single professional with whom to forge a therapeutic bond.

On the wall of the staff bay a chart of Roper's (Roper *et al.*, 1980) model of nursing was exhibited. I never ever saw it put into practice.

As a practising nurse, Anna was perplexed at this lack of care planning. On one of her visits she brought a publication of mine on nursing models to the staff's attention, and gave them a copy to read. The effect of this was to sensitise staff to my potential to be a resource or a critic. Those who saw me as a resource made more contact and asked questions of me; those who saw me as a critic gave me a wide berth and made less contact than before. As I improved I, too, became critical, the more so over a couple of days when:

- a staff nurse told me a friend had rung and sent me his best wishes but, yet again, she had forgotten the name of the person who rang!
- two nurses on different days said they would make arrangements for my stitches to come out, though these had been removed the week before!
- a doctor tried to remove my chest drain by pulling, before cutting the retaining stitch by which it was secured!
- I asked why I was syphoned daily of 10 mls of blood, and was told because I was anaemic!
- I was informed that I would have to stay on a gastric diet because of my ulcer repair!

Enough was enough. I walked down to the nursing bay, helped myself to my medical and nursing notes and sat down and read them.

My nursing notes made interesting reading:

- staff thought I was pain free, although they had not asked;
- because of the above, I had routinely been given a minimal level of analgesia, even though I had occasionally asked for more and it was indeed written up;
- although my blood haemoglobin was low no replacement therapy had begun, and 10 mls of blood continued to be taken daily for testing;
- no care plan was in evidence.

This was a great blow to my trust. From this time on, I reasoned, I would have to pay more attention to what happened around me, and examine ways in which I could take care of myself.

At root I was angry; after devoting so much of my working life to the nursing profession it felt so unfair that it could not be relied upon to do a decent job now.

Insights for carers (10)

My invasion of my medical and nursing notes demonstrates that I was caught up in behaviour symptomatic of *acting out*. Acting out, in the context of mental health, relates to the discharging of tension through physical acts, fuelled by emotional energies that an individual has failed to vent verbally. This may be due to:

- the impulse behind the acted out behaviour never having acquired verbal expression;
- the residual emotional energy being too intense for words;
- the individual concerned lacking the capacity for inhibition of his or her emotional energies (Rycroft, 1968).

Acting out has also been cited as the recreation of an individual's life experiences, an unconscious expression of their relationships with significant others, and as emanating from unresolved conflicts pertaining to their 'life script' or personal history (Wilson and Kneisl, 1983).

As a patient I had not been heard, I felt child-like and dismissed, and my emotional energy was at a level where words were insufficient; acting out, unconscious expression, was all that was left to me at the time.

Figure 6.3 illustrates the developmental phases of acting out, from the frustration of 'basic needs', the overwhelming of 'individual tolerance', through to a 'symbolic acting out of tensions'. At its extreme, acting out may lead to acts of violence against self and others. It is thus in the carer's interest to establish a relationship with a client, of an order where the energy behind acting out behaviour can be communicated.

Should this fail and acting out behaviours still be expressed, it is necessary to:

- bring the behaviour concerned to the client's attention;
- encourage the client to discuss their feelings and impulses;
- encourage the client to identify their feelings/needs prior to action;
- increase your frequency of contact with the client concerned;
- with repeated acting out, consider and state that you are considering withdrawing your support unless he or she sets limits on his or her behaviour (Carter, 1981).

Acting out is particularly destructive of the therapeutic relationship because it resists the building of rapport, and squanders energy which might otherwise enrich carer-client interaction.

On post-operative depression and the quest for purpose: a research-minded examination of pain

Nights on the ward felt interminably long and encouraged the negatives within me to surface. In the early hours, with nothing to divert me, I would often question my state and my future. At my most despondent I would

BASIC NEEDS
(To feel loved, trusted, a sense of belonging, autonomy and achievement)

↓

UNMET NEEDS
(Pain felt in the whole organism, and expressive outlets for sharing frustration blocked by parents, culture and fears of rejection)

↓

INDIVIDUAL TOLERANCE PASSED AND MIND OVERWHELMED
(Splitting of intellect and emotions from integrated action, and repression of painful experiences, with conflicts displaced into areas of sensation, emotion and relationships)

↓   ↓   ↓

DISTRESSING SENSATIONS
(Anxious excitation, physical tensions banished to various organs)

PAINFUL EMOTIONS
(Emotional tensions sealed off and repressed or expressed via mental defences)

RELATIONSHIP TENSIONS
(Idealised relations projected upon others, e.g. idealised other can do no wrong; role becomes self)

↓   ↓   ↓

SYMBOLIC ACTING OUT OF TENSIONS
(Tensions reappear in generalised form: 'mother hurt me' becomes 'women hurt me'; 'school crushed me' becomes 'life defeats me')

Prove there is nothing wrong with the body	Lust for sensations	Work off tensions	Fight bad with good works	Emotional thrill-seeking	Lust for knowledge
↓	↓	↓	↓	↓	↓
Fitness and health fanatics	Eroticised tensions	Professional workaholic	Ritual correctness	Drug and alcohol addiction	All is thought
↓	↓	↓	↓		↓
Obsessional body-building sports	Promiscuity	Work hero	Excitement about being righteous		Introverted intellectual-isation
		↓			↓
		Burn-out			Worship of intellect

Figure 6.3   Developmental phases of acting out (adapted from Kilty, 1982, 1989)

reflect 'Will the pain ever end?' and 'Will I ever get near to the health I enjoyed before?'. When more hopeful, I would reflect on 'What is the usual amount of pain to have following an operation such as mine?' and 'How might I facilitate my own advancement to a healthy recovery?'.

I also pondered my sexuality. I had no sex drive. 'Would it return?' and 'Would Anna ever find my scarred body sexually attractive?' and 'How much of a burden would I represent as a dependent, painfully preoccupied entity who could not care for himself let alone for her?'

Depersonalisation and *anomie* were highly charged issues for me at this time. My life seemed purposeless and I felt myself slipping further into apathy. Anna broke through this with a simple intervention on her next visit; she brought along a notepad and pens. I was accustomed to writing and researching and now had tools to do this. I had also begun to realise that I would have to self-facilitate myself to health.

Over the next few days I examined the major focus of my hospital life – 'pain' – and kept a journal to this end. Every so often I would appraise my situation by attending to my 'thoughts', 'feelings', 'senses' and 'intuitions'. This tool, generated from Jungian concepts I had earlier forged in discussion (Kilty, 1989) and written for publication a little before my illness (Barber, 1988), now came into its own as a means of purging the remaining confusion within me.

THOUGHTS

As I start off this reflective process I am aware of considering how best to make sense of my experiences and fit them into a cohesive structure I can understand. Intellectually, I am aware of housing a 'structure hunger' and a need for information so that I may work things out for myself. I am also aware of how hard I have to concentrate to move.

FEELINGS

Depressed and apathetic until aroused by fleeting bursts of thrill and emotional energy as my interest is mobilised by the immediacy of this task.

SENSES

Special senses blurred by dull pain which motivates me to experiment with my postural alignment in an effort to achieve greater comfort. Aware of a sensation of stiffness in my thorax, the quickness of my eyes to spot potential hazards, the shallowness of my breath, and hiccoughs when changing posture, I note that tension and discomfort seem to be my present bodily norm. When I close my eyes I see colourful three-dimensional geometric patterns flickering about me.

INTUITIONS

Visualise myself as a balloon with a slow puncture gradually losing its buoyancy and air and needing to replenish itself with more energy. I suspect that as my energy returns I shall be able to screen my crushing sense of vulnerability with anger. I am aware of an intuition that I will survive this time no matter what it takes.

The more I engaged in the above exercise the more fluid my thinking became. I also improved my concentration span, self-awareness and appreciation of my needs.

There was also another interesting discovery: when involved in activities which energised me with positive emotion, I felt less pain. Possibly 'involvement', 'love' and 'joy' countered pain? This was in some way confirmed for me in that I reported less pain during visiting and when engaged in humorous conversation.

As I continued to sift through my perceptions, a five-point pain scale emerged.

Level 1 +

Moderate discomfort, dull ache, attention can be displaced via concentration on sensory stimuli such as television and renewed energy conquested.

Level 2 + +

Constant discomfort thwarts concentration, displaced attention helps but does not solicit more energy or override residual feelings of dull heaviness, creativity lost, thinking an effort.

Level 3 + + +

Greatly interferes with perception and continually drains energy and interferes with other activities, attention drawn inward, begins to consume consciousness, thinking impossible.

Level 4 + + + +

Sharp focused pain overwhelms the individual's sense of self, little attention available for external world, fleeting glimpses of objective reality, disorientation and absorption in pain, responses instinctive.

Level 5 + + + + +

Individual powerless to communicate in grip of painful stimuli, no contact with external world as consciousness replaced by a twilight state attuned to pain-inducing stimuli.

When in 'Level 1', I could still work, write and watch television with a degree of enjoyment; this was my baseline, a point at which I could doze, think, feel and fantasise. At 'Level 2', with concentrated effort I could switch attention from pain to visual stimuli, that is, override one sensory stimulus with another. At 'Level 3', my thoughts, feelings and imagination were drawn to the field of pain. At 'Level 4', painful sensation permeated the whole and perception of reality came only in fleeting glimpses. At 'Level 5', there was a non-appreciation of everything; it was as if pain filled the universe.

'Level 2' pain was tolerable, but if allowed to develop to 'Level 3', life felt pointless. With this scale to hand I knew when it was necessary to request further painkillers.

I speculated upon relaxation as a means by which pain might be reduced, and to this end experimented with prolonged hot baths. These I found relaxed the muscle spasms I associated with stimuli at 'Level 3' and above, and if persevered with could reverse the pain spiral and cause 'Level 3' pain to transmute back to 'Level 2'. With this information to hand my environment felt less muddled and helpless.

I had used my research-mindedness to provide me with purpose and power, and was beginning to exorcise the apathy within me.

Insights for carers (11)

My research freed me from the idiocy of ward life and gave me purpose and meaning; it also displaced my perception of pain and served as occupational therapy.

By keeping patients passively awaiting the next care intervention, clinicians retain much power. Ward life generally felt like one long wet Sunday when everything has closed down and when the only respite available is to read the papers or turn on the television. Periodically into this sheltered climate someone dropped to perform tasks upon you and awaken your interest; less often your false sense of security is shattered by the sudden drama of an unforeseen crisis. Simply, clinical settings need to be normalised.

The *Normalisation Principle* (Nirje, 1976) suggests that individuals who are undergoing a crisis of living and/or state of ill health have the right to be treated as any other valued member of society and to receive care in an environment which preserves their dignity. If nurses are to act on this and preserve the dignity of those they care for, they will have to share their power base and avoid devaluing responses such as those listed here:

DEHUMANISATION

Treating clients as if they are less worthy than those who are healthy and gainfully employed; referring to clients as conditions, e.g. 'the dement in bed 10'; seeing clients as objects upon which instrumental tasks are performed, or paying so much attention to 'routines' that more care is lavished on the ward than on the clients within.

AGE-INAPPROPRIATE RESPONSES

Becoming over-familiar with clients or calling them by nicknames such as 'Pops', 'Granny' or 'Grandad'; parenting and making decisions for patients so as to reinforce parent–child aspects of the nurse–patient relationship, or with-holding information from patients and acting on their behalf.

FOSTERING ISOLATION

Attitudinally segregating patients from their civil rights and community – a legacy of the Victorian view of hospitals as places where the sick were to be iso-lated from the working well; keeping distant from clients and leaving them unsupported and unoccupied (adapted from Gunner, 1987; Tyne, 1978).

Nurses need to pay attention to the gap between 'what they believe they do' and 'what the consequences of their actions actually are'. They have great potential to serve as advocates, to offer support and counsel, or to damage their clients by doing the reverse of these things. Interestingly, my account sug-gests that when such positive feelings as humour, love and joy enter the care relationship, its therapeutic potential grows. It might be well, therefore, if nurses as a norm in therapeutic relating:

- resisted entering into negative social collusions, such as exchanging gripes or feeding into such negative emotional games as 'nothing will change'; 'there's nothing anyone can do about it'; or 'you mustn't take life seriously';
- rewarded all positive behaviour, no matter how small or fleeting it may be;
- paid attention to their own emotional show, and how this influences clients and the feeling tone of the therapeutic relationship;
- acknowledged the role they have as culture carriers, and all that this implies in terms of their influence on what they create around them.

Culture includes all those ideas and beliefs people hold about themselves, plus all those meanings which make life all the more worthwhile. In this context the nurse's clinical role as a 'culture carrier' and positive force for health is second to none.

On massage: the contribution of alternative therapies to nursing care

Since the operation my shoulders and thorax had remained rigid. It was as if I had armoured myself to protect the site of surgical intrusion. My shoulders were high, neck tight and I breathed shallowly. I looked and felt as if I was encased in metal.

Anna and I had always exchanged therapeutic massage, and this now came into its own. We contracted that on each of her visits she would mas-sage my back and neck.

The first time she massaged me it was difficult to take; my body had for-gotten how to receive touch. In the night following this massage, I awoke to feel my whole body pulsating with a warm tingling sensation that bubbled up through my skin. It felt as if life was flowing back into me. I also started to yawn. I evoked more yawns. The more I yawned, the easier my breathing became. Over the next few days my thoracic flexibility began to return. I now found I was able to stretch, breathe in deeply without coughing and, for the first time, could stand erect when walking. Trusting myself more to unconsciousness, I was now awoken less by sudden pain due to involuntary movements or coughs. As I now breathed and slept better, my energy returned and consequently my apathy began to lift.

Insights for carers (12)

Although alternative and body therapies are rarely taught in the formal curriculum, they have much to offer nurses. Note that the massage described above was the single most effective post-operative intervention I received.

As physiological organisms who psychologically determine their world and socially define it, clients need an approach to care which recognises and integrates all of these dimensions (see 'Insights for carers (6) and (8)'). Alternative therapies do this. Some, such as *Transactional Analysis* and *Gestalt*, elicit how we make sense and relate to the world; others, such as the *Alexander Method* and *Rolfing*, help us to understand how postural integration can balance our internal and external energy flows, while *Therapeutic Massage*, *Aromatherapy* and *Bioenergetics* provide us with modes of physical reintegration. Holistic approaches attend to the 'whole person' and experiential integration, areas of concern that are often missed by more orthodox systems of care.

The approaches below are recommended to nurses who wish to develop further their therapeutic potential.

THERAPEUTIC MASSAGE

Not to be confused with massage of the type associated with physiotherapy and sports, this form attempts holistically to reintegrate a client's body sense and to release feelings laid up through life in the various muscle groups. The effects of this are described in the text above.

AROMATHERAPY

This seeks to alleviate mental and emotional stresses via recourse to aromatic massage. Differing fragrancies are suggested to evoke differing reactions and are used to move a client in the direction of harmony and balance. Scented oils, incense and lotions are applied for the purposes described.

Aromatherapy combined with therapeutic massage was for me a very powerful relaxing agent post-operatively, at a time when my body was most resistant to relaxation.

BIOENERGETICS

After Alexander Lowen (1967, 1972), this offers techniques for reducing muscular tension through the conscious release of feelings. It makes less use of direct body contact (therapist-client) than other therapies, in that it offers a series of exercises and verbal techniques, and sensor and releasor exercises in order to increase the client's appreciation of his or her body defences. Deep breathing, stretching, and rigorous movement may be used to break through muscle rigidity and to express feelings blocked and/or trapped in postural armouring which restricts the flow and free exchange of energy.

GESTALT THERAPY

As a practitioner of gestalt psychotherapy I must declare a bias to this approach. Gestalt is for me the quintessence of an integrated research-minded holistic therapy. Originally evolved by Perls (1969) and later refined by Zinker (1977) and Polster and Polster (1974), gestalt therapists invite us to join with them in a series of experiential experiments to evaluate that store of conflicting emotions, frustrated needs and false perceptions which interfere with our ability to contact meaningfully ourselves and reality. In this sense the client is both a 'subject' and 'experimenter'. Via working through this bank of 'unfinished situations' we are enabled to assume responsibility for ourselves, to appreciate the choices before us, and to experiment with living life as a self-regulating, contactful and aware being. 'In this way people can let themselves become totally what they already are, and what they potentially can become' (Clarkson, 1989; Clarkson, personal communication). Awareness is thus the process and the goal of a gestalt approach.

THE ALEXANDER METHOD

Developed by F. A. Alexander (1976), this focuses primarily upon incorrect alignments of the head, neck and shoulders which cause stress throughout the whole body. Intervention is mainly via massage, manipulation and postural re-education.

TRANSACTIONAL ANALYSIS (TA)

Originated by Eric Berne (1964) and developed by Harris (1973), this approach presents a model for understanding socio-analytic influences within human development, role formation and interaction. Three ego states are commonly employed to explain personality and social functioning: the Parent – that part of ourselves formed by our own parents in childhood and the focus of 'the world as we are socially taught it to be'; the Adult – which is the part of our personality that deals with the objective sensory world and facts, and gives us our orientation to 'the world as we have found it and checked it out to be'; and the Child – the source of our free emotional energies, creativity and fantasies, and our reference for 'the world as we feel, intuitively create, or desire it to be'. Through analysis of our social 'scripts' and roles, TA enables us to understand ourselves and our conflicting social motivations. I have found TA to be an excellent vehicle for the transmission of relational insights.

ROLFING

Otherwise known as structural reintegration, this approach is based upon the premise that psychological conflicts are recorded and perpetuated in the body frame. Evolved by Ida Rolf (1977), Rolfing addresses the myofascia and connective tissue which supports the body weight; this, it cites, undergoes shortening and metabolic change that hampers energy flow and interferes with free movement. With age the body becomes a reflection of accumulated unresolved feelings. It is these that Rolfing attempts to undo.

Personally, I found increased energy, bodily awareness and the ability to unpack my own build-up of physical and emotional stress emanated from my exposure to Rolfing.

The above approaches, through development of 'the person', serve to enhance interpersonal sensitivity. As a nurse's interpersonal awareness increases so does the professional skill which, in turn, enhances the ability to form therapeutic relationships.

On the clinical environment: the need for research-minded care

With the new lease of energy obtained from massage, I returned afresh to my role as researcher. I had 'looked within' to examine pain 'experientially'. Now I chose to 'look without' to evaluate 'objectively' the clinical environment.

In order to clarify progress to date, I set about reviewing 'progress markers', i.e. events that enriched my quality of life and/or restored hope and caused me to feel glad to be alive.

1st day – Relief at being alive/seeing Marc and Anna/sucking ice
2nd day – First taste (a lemon stick)/talking with night staff
3rd day – My first recognisable catnap
4th day – First time standing up
5th day – First clear hour with visitors (no haze)/first hour's sleep/a taste of soup/first taste of orange barley squash
6th day – First comfortable time sitting in chair/walking without support/TV film appreciated/first bowel movement/first day I can write a little/first yawn
7th day – First walk from ward/a short period of deep sleep
8th day – First transient pain-free period/first pain-free cough/first bath/a clear un-drug-hazed day
10th day – First time I can take in what I read
14th day – Massage from Anna
15th day – Walked to hospital entrance
18th day – First day painkillers really relieve pain.

Such mundane events are very different from those medical nurses and doctors report in their notes.

After reviewing my past, I next turned my attention to what was happening 'now'.

Starting from the premise that a major nursing function is to nurture a safe environment in which clients may be observed and monitored, and speedily contacted when crises arise, I commenced one particularly sleepless night to check the time it took nurses to respond to the call bell over a 24-hour period.

A bell push operated in the 14-bedded section of the ward in which I was placed caused a red light to illuminate above the door of my room. Secure in the observation that nurses on answering a call had invariably in the past cancelled the summoning light before attending to clients, I used this light for the data collection of my survey. For brevity I chose to round up or down times of a minute or more to the nearest whole. Before this brief piece of research I thought that 30 seconds to 1 minute would be the average time it took to answer a call. I was some way out in my estimation.

Time of call (light on)	Answer of call (light off)	Waiting time
8.38 p.m.	8.54 p.m.	16 minutes
9.45 p.m.	9.48 p.m.	3 minutes
10.07 p.m.	10.09 p.m.	2 minutes
10.20 p.m.	10.22 p.m.	2 minutes
10.23 p.m.	10.25 p.m.	2 minutes
10.37 p.m.	10.39 p.m.	2 minutes
11.26 p.m.	11.26 p.m.	½ minute
12.49 a.m.	12.53 a.m.	4 minutes
1.25 a.m.	1.26 a.m.	1 minute
1.26 a.m.	1.26 a.m.	½ minute
6.25 a.m.	6.32 a.m.	7 minutes
6.38 a.m.	6.43 a.m.	5 minutes
8.45 a.m.	9.10 a.m.	25 minutes
9.12 a.m.	9.13 a.m.	1 minute
9.15 a.m.	9.20 a.m.	5 minutes
11.10 a.m.	11.12 a.m.	2 minutes
11.20 a.m.	11.23 a.m.	3 minutes
3.20 p.m.	3.25 p.m.	5 minutes
4.47 p.m.	4.51 p.m.	4 minutes
5.30 p.m.	5.32 p.m.	2 minutes
6.15 p.m.	6.18 p.m.	3 minutes
6.25 p.m.	6.29 p.m.	4 minutes
6.43 p.m.	6.49 p.m.	6 minutes
7.34 p.m.	7.36 p.m.	2 minutes
7.52 p.m.	7.53 p.m.	1 minute
8.20 p.m.	8.21 p.m.	1 minute
8.25 p.m.	8.28 p.m.	3 minutes

As a client I felt lucky to receive whatever I got; as a senior clinician my findings disturbed me. Out of every 27 calls I could expect to wait upwards of 2 minutes for some 14 calls and, of these, ten could involve 4 minutes' wait or more. On the outside I could expect a 25-minute wait.

In a crisis, a common occurrence on a surgical ward, a minute seems a very long time. I concluded from this that the ward was a very dangerous place indeed. I could be better served for the most part at home with a telephone by my bed.

Insights for carers (13)

At any one time the ward had an occupancy of 24 beds. Most of the work-force were students or pupils in training complemented by nursing auxiliaries. On an average night there was one senior student, one pupil nurse and one auxiliary, plus a roving night sister shared between other wards. During the days this tripartite work-force was supplemented by a ward sister or staff nurse who acted as team leader. Having worked as a student on the night and day shifts of a busy surgical ward, I can appreciate the work involved. As my sample represented one-third of the ward population, during a 24-hour shift 70 to 80 calls might be expected. Besides these regular 4-hourly observations of pulse, temperature and respirations have also to be made, 4-hourly drinks to be given and input and output charts maintained, numerous drips and blood monitored, medication given and recorded, incumbent clients bathed, pressure areas rubbed, bowls for washing and drinks ferried around, and all this without the emergency admissions and pre-operation procedures that form a regular part of clinical life. As three to four staff are not always sufficient for this, it is little wonder that crisis management thus becomes the norm.

Quality not quantity defines good care, but as successive governments apply profit and growth motives to the health service and ask hospitals in the public sector to run as if they were factories, care managers are driven to forsake qualitative aspects of care in favour of expediency. It is therefore essential that the effects of this are researched, for reduction of a ward's staff ratio may possibly correlate with higher levels of infection and other complications which necessitate an extended spell in hospital and in the long run cost more.

Nurses have little time, but ample data to research. As researchers they have the potential to act as participant observers, to chronicle clinical events and to process record the interactions they engage in with their clients. The qualitative research tools for this have already been refined (see Reason and Rowan, 1981), and the skilful use of these can now be taught in nursing education.

Those simple research enquiries I performed could so easily be facilitated by a clinical manager, or a key worker alongside the client. The awareness that accrues from such activity would no doubt prove beneficial to clinician and client alike.

It is beyond the scope of this account to reiterate ways in which a nurse may perform research, but the point must be made that it is essential that research-minded care is enacted within the therapeutic relationship (see Chapters 1 and 2).

On professional relationships: research-mindedness and supervision

Besides the restrictions of staff and time, other factors appeared to contribute to 'crisis management' and the disruption of therapeutic relationships within the ward, namely, nurses seemed locked into person-denying behavioural sets. Even when there were few patients within the ward, therapeutic relationships remained unformed. This awareness caused me to recollect a study some 30 years ago in which Isabel Menzies (1960), researching into low morale, had identified ways in which nurses structured their professional relationships to protect themselves from stress. Such defences, which were noted to interfere with self and person perception, could, if linked to my present environment, do much to explain how seemingly conscientious and busy nurses could overlook their patients' needs. Initially I set about simplifying Menzies' finding. Sifting through the main themes left me with seven categories:

1. splitting up the nurse–patient relationship: tasks emphasised rather than personal processes, little opportunity provided for development of one-to-one relationships;
2. depersonalisation and categorisation: patients described by their medical conditions, individuality and creativity discouraged, and all patients treated the same;
3. ritual task performance: instrumental activity encouraged and questioning discouraged; professionals let policies do their thinking for them;
4. feelings denied and controlled: emotional expression discouraged and/or ignored, staff disciplined rather than counselled;
5. avoidance of decisions – control pushed upwards to seniors and blame pushed downwards on juniors; personal and professional power unused;
6. avoidance of change – problem confrontation avoided, and fear of facing new situations without prescribed procedures;
7. checks and counter-checks – individual action discouraged, trust rare and fears of failure commonplace.

In order to evaluate the frequency of the above behaviours within the ward, I devised a five-point scale:

- **Rare** (+), when a behaviour is rarely glimpsed;
- **Emerges** (++), when a behaviour draws my attention;
- **Frequent** (+++), when a behaviour is a usual feature of interaction;
- **Very common** (++++), when a behaviour is a major characteristic;
- **Constant** (+++++), when a behaviour is ever present.

With the above constructs established, I now had an impressionable rating scale with which to profile clinical behaviour. As a participant observer, I attributed to nurses over an observational period of 2 weeks the following responses:

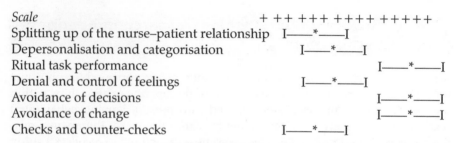

Scale

Note '*' shows the central position of my observations and 'I——I' the range of variability into which each behaviour fell

Balancing my expertise as an experienced practitioner/researcher with the subjective nature and obvious limitations of my approach, the results give interesting cues to the clinical culture.

'Ritual task performance', 'Avoidance of decisions' and 'Avoidance of change' figured predominantly, with 'Depersonalisation and categorisation' and 'Denial and control of feelings' following closely behind. Surprisingly, 'Splitting of the nurse–patient relationship', a central theme of this chapter, comes less to the fore than I expected, and as a patient I was less aware of 'checks and counter-checks'.

In sum, if this small sample – from the client's eyeview – is in any way representative, it might be suggested that research-mindedness is still very much absent from practice and that feelings are still very much avoided. Certainly it appears that those social defensive behaviours first identified some 30 years ago are very much alive and well in a modern provincial hospital.

Insight for carers (14)

My enquiry, first 'looking in' on my own condition, then 'looking out' to the clinical environment, suggests a frame from which clinical research-mindedness might emanate within the therapeutic relationship, namely the following:

LOOKING IN (FEELING/INTUITION)

Energies I feel emotionally within me, those creative meanings which intuitively arise from within, my ability to express and empathise.

LOOKING OUT (SENSING/ANALYSING)

Those external objects I sense – see, hear, taste, smell and touch – and use to intellectually structure reality with, my scientific biases.

Although models of nursing and knowledge of the 'care sciences' may be acquired by reading, facilitation skill and the 'caring arts' are only acquired through quality supervision and experiential reflection during practice.

The above diagram offers a frame for experiential reflection. It asks carers to be sensitive to and monitor their own internal processes, to attend to the 'emotional energy field' they share with a client and to pay attention to their biases and how they make sense of their clinical practice.

Figure 6.4 applies the above perceptual frame – 'looking-in' and 'looking-out' to the observation of 'self' and 'other' within the therapeutic relationship, where internal and external reflections are shared in relation to 'Examining social processes', 'Applying/sharing theoretical insights and models' and 'Owning emotional and intuitive meanings of relationship'.

When carers can witness themselves and their clients without the clutter of intellectual and professional labels, they will have achieved one of the goals of this research-minded relational process.

On integrating the whole: insights into therapeutic relations in nursing care and professional supervision

As I finish this account I am 18 months post surgery and am much healed. I also gained a great many insights from the trauma described. Much of my enquiry, post hospitalisation, was performed in psychotherapeutic settings in personal therapy. As a student and practitioner of gestalt psychotherapy, I had access to a therapy group and regular supervision (Clarkson, 1989; Clarkson, personal communication; Parlett, personal communication) in which to further enquire into my experience of the client's side of the therapeutic relationship; intuitive insights from this are shared below.

PRECOGNITION

I am aware that at the end of the Autumn Term, prior to commencing my Christmas vacation, I was acutely conscious of a strong desire to order my affairs and a sense that I would not return the following term. My intuition is that at an unconscious physiological level of functioning I was receiving biological cues to the internal physiological processes that were starting to come adrift. My dreams prior to the illness were likewise disturbed with imagery of being stabbed in the abdomen.

SYMBOLIC REGRESSION

With my academic year's work done, I started to relax, went back to my birthplace and, in a primitive symbolic way, returned to my mother to experience a life-threatening illness. At an organismic level I suspect I may have chosen when to experience my illness, where to enact it and with whom.

GESTALT COMPLETION

Post surgery I feel in one way completed. As if nothing is left to instil such fear in me again, I know I can stand pain and work my way through it. Likewise I can rely on my own store of courage; I feel tested and somehow

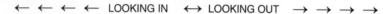

$\leftarrow \quad \leftarrow \quad \leftarrow \quad \leftarrow \quad$ LOOKING IN $\quad \leftrightarrow$ LOOKING OUT $\quad \rightarrow \quad \rightarrow \quad \rightarrow \quad \rightarrow$

(Examining social processes)

Questioning self		**Observing other**
What am I experiencing now – my feelings/intuitions/thoughts?	$\leftrightarrow$	Observing the environment and the evidence of my senses, the other's response to me
How might I facilitate or be of use?	$\leftrightarrow$	Attending to what is asked of me, sharing information and expertise, experimenting with interventions
How do I feel in this relationship?	$\leftrightarrow$	Focusing upon how I am relating and being related to in return
How is this relationship like and different to a therapeutic one?	$\leftrightarrow$	Differentiating how I am meeting my needs and meeting the needs of others
How much empathy do I feel for the person before me?	$\leftrightarrow$	Examining what is mutually accepted and supported, and issues and ways in which we differ

(Applying/sharing theoretical insights and models)

Reflecting upon		**Sharing/enacting**
The therapeutic relationship	$\leftrightarrow$	The phase of our relationship
Therapeutic factors	$\leftrightarrow$	Reality orientation, trust-building
Supervision strategies	$\leftrightarrow$	Forming a contract
Transactional analysis	$\leftrightarrow$	Ongoing analysis of the relationship process and transactions available
Models of care	$\leftrightarrow$	Care strategies and evaluation modes
Research approaches	$\leftrightarrow$	Illuminative/collaborative enquiries to assess effects of therapy
Mental defences	$\leftrightarrow$	Exploring blocks to communication
Invervention analysis	$\leftrightarrow$	Testing appropriate interventions

(Owning emotional and intuitive meanings in relationship)

Examining own		**Speculating upon**
Emotions and fantasies received	$\leftrightarrow$	Projections on to other
Current awareness of self	$\leftrightarrow$	Current sensitivity to other
Memories evoked by relationship	$\leftrightarrow$	Projections acted upon by other
Staying sensitive to own defences	$\leftrightarrow$	Attending to defences of other
Own unsaid material	$\leftrightarrow$	Attending to what is unsaid by other
Personal fears	$\leftrightarrow$	Fears of other

Figure 6.4 Research-mindedness in therapeutic relating

relieved. I am no longer the least bit afraid of death and, in my saying of this, conversely, feel I love life the more – as if this time 'I choose to be here' rather than 'find myself born'.

PERSONAL GAINS

I know I can trust to my courage and no longer need to prove or test myself. As a consequence, I am more self-caring. I have also gained a positive sense of vulnerability and feel more sensitive, and strangely stronger because of this.

In a Maslovian sense (Maslow, 1970) I feel I have stretched my boundaries and goals and integrated a new dimension of growth. The crisis of my illness plunged me from 'self-confidence and self-esteem' born of mastery of my environment and the affection of others towards consideration of 'how best to survive and get safe' again (see Figure 6.5). (Note: in the context of Figure 6.5, it occurs to me that the ward environment functioned very much at level 4.)

REINTEGRATING THE WHOLE

Reviewing my illness and convalescence, I am aware of having relived psychosocial crises of my childhood all over again – but this time, with a degree of consciousness and a sense of having been there before. Simply, I have gained greater reintegration. In a sense I have re-experienced crises of 'drive and hope' through to 'renunciation and wisdom' (Erikson, 1965) (Figure 6.6).

Interpersonally, Anna, Marc and myself have emerged from the experience closer, more loving and more appreciative of one another. I am also more tolerant and at peace within myself.

Insights for carers (15)

A carer's ability to forge a successful therapeutic relationship relates directly to their own degree of self-insight and understanding. Unaware carers give unaware care.

The quality of the therapeutic relationship is dependent upon the degree to which a nurse is able to experience and positively use his or her own qualities of 'self' (Barber, 1993). Such awareness requires specialist facilitation. Clinical supervision can supply this level of development (Barber and Norman, 1987), and develop 'the self' when seeking to:

- combine personal with professional development;
- be attentive to the social dynamics that develop between the supervisor and supervisee;
- provide first-hand experience of what it is like to be supported and cared for and enact a 'caring for carers';
- facilitate research-aware practice and role model relational skills;
- work towards those higher levels of functioning described in Figures 6.5 and 6.6.

MASLOW	KOHLBERG	LOEVINGER
	6	
Self-actualisation Being that self which I truly am and have it in me to be. Fully functioning person	Individual principles True personal consciousness, universal principles fully internalised. Genuinely autonomous, selfishness (B)	Autonomous Integrated: Flexible and creative, internal conflicts faced and recognised. Ambiguity tolerated and feelings expressed
	5	
Self-esteem 2 Goals founded upon self-evaluated standards, self-confidence/respect	Social contract Utilitarian law-making, principles of general welfare, long-term goals	Conscientious Bound by self-imposed rules, differential thinking, self-aware
	4	
Self-esteem 1 Respect from others, social status, recognition	Law and order Authority maintenance, fixed social rules – finds duty and does it	Conformist 2 Seeks general rules of social conformity, justifies conformity
	3	
Love and belonging Wish for affection and a place in the group, tenderness	Personal concordance Good-boy mentality, seeking social approval, majority as right	Conformist 1 Going along with the crowd, anxiety about rejection, needing support
	2	
Effectence Mastery, personal power, imposed control, blame and retaliation, domination	Instrumental hedonism Naive egocentrism, horse-trading approach, profit and loss calculation, selfishness (A)	Self-protective/manipulative Wary, exploitative, people are means to ends, competitive stance, fear of being caught, stereotypes ++
	1	
Safety Defence against danger, flight or fight, fear – world as a scary place	Obedience/punishment Deference to superior power, rules are external and eternal	Impulsive Domination by immediate cue, body feelings, no reflection, retaliation fears

Figure 6.5 Developmental spiral (adapted from Wright, 1974; as reported by Rowan, 1983)

Simply, the supervisor and supervisee, while remaining alert to the evolved behavioural levels of Figures 6.5 and 6.6, and facilitating the research-mindedness of Figure 6.4, can be managed in such a way as to illustrate social processes which are paralleled in carer-client relations. Supervision of this type sets up an experiential climate in which practitioners can explore themselves along with their responses and skills. Supervisions of this kind can start in experiential groupwork via social analysis of the student-teacher relationship. Fears, social expectations, learner resistances and group defences are all present in the educational group, and the resolution and working through of these may elicit immense personal and interpersonal learning, especially when approached in a psychodynamic way. Figure 6.7 illustrates what is available to a sensitive teacher in non-conspiratorial educational settings when the teacher/facilitator stops playing conventional classroom games (Barber, 1986).

Age-appropriate stages	Psychosocial crises	Significant relationship	Favourable outcome
Birth–first year	Trust vs. mistrust	Mother	Drive and hope
Second year	Autonomy vs. shame	Parents	Self-control and will-power
Third–fifth year	Initiative vs. guilt	Family	Direction and purpose
Six year–puberty	Industry vs. inferiority	Neighbourhood/ school	Method and competence
Adolescence	Identity vs. diffusion	Peer groups/ leadership	Devotion and fidelity
Early adulthood	Intimacy vs. isolation	Partners/co-operation	Affiliation and love
Young–middle adulthood	Generativity vs. self-absorption	Divided labour/ shared household	Production and care
Later adulthood	Integrity vs. despair	'Mankind my kind'	Renunciation and wisdom

Figure 6.6 Erikson's stages of psychosocial development (after Erikson, 1965; modified from original)

Summary

In this chapter I have attempted to interweave client-generated awarenesses and professional insights. To this end I have considered under respective headings of 'Insights for carers': (1) the nature of health; (2) symbolic interactionism; (3) nursing and reality orientation; (4) defence mechanisms; (5) spiritual meanings; (6) client-centred care; (7) intervention styles; (8) humanism; (9) clinical stressors; (10) acting out; (11) normalisation and clinical culture; (12) alternative therapies; (13) clinical research; (14) experiential reflection and (15) research-minded intervention and supervision. Finally, I will share how I weave my gestalt and psychodynamic vision to a conceptual frame where such insights can be therapeutically enacted.

Within the life of the therapeutic relationship, as described by Peplau (Figure 6.1, p.177), are acted through other cycles of therapeutic relating. These cycles (Figure 6.8) demonstrate the application of a therapeutic experiential research process, in which a nurse facilitates the awareness and resources of a client within the medium of a collaborative relationship. Many such cycles will be in operation at any time, and proceed at differing speeds. The cycle relating to hospitalisation and recovery will obviously move at a slower pace than the cycle enacted by an investigation such as an electrocardiogram.

As soon as one mini-cycle relating to something such as hunger is complete, another relating to physical or emotional comfort might arise. This goes a little way to explaining burn-out – when too many cycles are in operation and demand completion, unremitting stress will occur. A skilled intuitive nurse, by this same token, may be able to differentiate which cycle is on top for a particular client at any one time.

Fears	Learner/client expectation	Non-compliant facilitative behaviour	Learner resistances
Fears of being unable to control others	Facilitator will lead and initiate happenings		**Collusive resistances**
		Facilitator	Group conspires to be jocular and mildly cynical (cocktail party)
	Facilitator will adopt role of expert and impart information	resists	Retreat of two or more members into whispers, emotional (subgroups/pairing)
Fears of losing control		collusion to	
			Passive resistances
		be a	'Lost' silence (please rescue us)
	Facilitator will act as authority figure to be blamed if things go wrong	parenting	Waiting to be led (dependency)
Fears of being rejected		figure and	Day-dreaming (fantasy)
	Facilitator will assume responsibility for group and learning process	structure	**Active resistances**
Fears of failing		reality for	Criticism and blame of persons or systems, authority chastised (scapegoating/stereotyping)
		the group	
	Facilitator will acknowledge status barriers and stay emotionally remote		Teacher's credibility/contributions attacked (counter-dependency)

Figure 6.7 Group fears – expectations and resistances

I am mindful, when enacting a therapeutic relationship and addressing a client's experiential cycle, of certain qualities – after Yalom (1970) – which facilitate the working through of unfinished gestalts and successful reintegration.

1. **Imparting of information** – instruction, comments on psychodynamics, advice and suggestions about life problems.
2. **Instillation of hope** – faith in the caregivers and their approach.
3. **Universality** – becoming aware of others feeling as you do, learning you are not alone and that others share your problem.
4. **Altruism** – learning that you can help and be helped by others in return.
5. **Corrective recapitulation** – being able to relive and rework old problems, and in so doing to discover new ways of coping.
6. **Development of socialising techniques** – enhancing and learning new social skills and social behaviours.
7. **Imitative behaviour** – role modelling, trying on the behaviours of others to find out if they can also work for you.

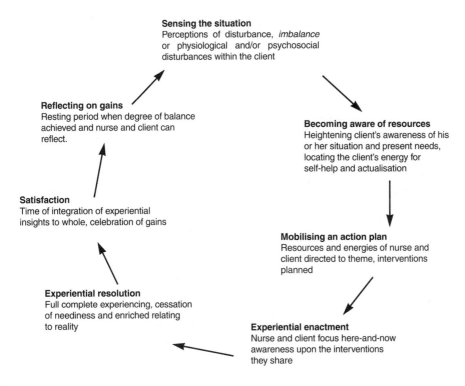

Sensing the situation
Perceptions of disturbance, *imbalance*
or physiological and/or psychosocial
disturbances within the client

Reflecting on gains
Resting period when degree of balance
achieved and nurse and client can
reflect.

Becoming aware of resources
Heightening client's awareness of his
or her situation and present needs,
locating the client's energy for
self-help and actualisation

Satisfaction
Time of integration of experiential
insights to whole, celebration of gains

Mobilising an action plan
Resources and energies of nurse and
client directed to theme, interventions
planned

Experiential resolution
Full complete experiencing, cessation
of neediness and enriched relating
to reality

Experiential enactment
Nurse and client focus here-and-now
awareness upon the interventions
they share

Figure 6.8   Experiential research cycles
Note that healthy movement is in the direction described, although an individual may be at
any stage in the cycle at any one time

8. **Interpersonal learning** – working through projections and correcting emotional experience.
9. **Group cohesiveness** – being nourished via accurate empathy, non-possessive warmth and genuineness.
10. **Catharsis** – the release of pent-up emotional energies.

As to how you enact the above, it is hoped after reading this chapter that they are no longer strangers to you and that you have sufficient insight to begin to enact them in your own therapeutic relationships.

Intuitively, I feel the cycle of this chapter is nearing completion and that it is time I moved to something else.

The way I make sense of the therapeutic relationship and those influences I blend into it might not be for you. Possibly you feel I have made too much use of psychotherapeutic and experiential material. I do not apologise for this; therapeutic relations are intensely personal things prone to the idiosyncracies of each carer. My way of relating is unique to me – a synthesis of sociological and psychotherapeutic biases, partly forged by my client experience. It works for me. You must now find one which works for you.

References

Alexander, F. M. 1976 *The resurrection of the body*. New York: Dell.

Barber, P. 1986 A process approach to education. *Nurse Educator* **11**, 40.

Barber, P. 1988 Learning to grow: the necessity for education processing in therapeutic community practice. *International Journal of Therapeutic Communities* **9**, 101–8.

Barber, P. 1993 Developing the 'person' of the professional carer. In Hinchliff, S. M., Norman, S. E. and Schober, J. E. (eds), *Nursing practice and health care*, 2nd edn. London: Edward Arnold, 344–73.

Barber, P. 1996 Social symbolism of health: the notion of the soul in professional care. In Perry, A. (ed.), *Sociology: insights in health care*. London: Edward Arnold, 54–82.

Barber, P. and Norman, I. 1987 An eclectic model of staff development: supervision techniques to prepare nurses for a process approach – a social perspective. In Barber, P. (ed.), *Mental handicap: facilitating holistic care*. London: Hodder and Stoughton, 80–90.

Berne, E. 1964 *Games people play*. Harmondsworth: Penguin.

Blumer, H. 1969 *Symbolic interactionism: perspective and method*. Englewood Cliffs: Prentice Hall.

Carter, F. M. 1981 *Psychosocial nursing*. New York: Macmillan.

Clarkson, P. 1989 *Gestalt counselling in action*. London: Sage.

Erikson, E. 1965 *Childhood and society*. Harmondsworth: Penguin.

Glasser, W. 1965 *Reality therapy*. New York: Harper and Row.

Gunner, A. 1987 Putting community care together: a rationale for nursing interventions using Henderson's model – a community perspective. In Barber, P. (ed.), *Mental handicap: facilitating holistic care*. London: Hodder and Stoughton, 12–24.

Harris, T. 1973 *I'm OK – you're OK*. London: Pan.

Henderson, V. 1969 *Basic principles of nursing care*, revised edn. Basel: Karger.

Heron, J. 1977 *Behaviour analysis in education and training*. London: British Postgraduate Medical Foundation and University of Surrey.

Kilty, J. 1982 *Experiential learning*. Guildford: Human Potential Research Project, University of Surrey.

Kilty, J. 1989 Personal communication.

Kroeber, T. C. 1963 The coping functions of the ego mechanisms. In White, R. (ed.), *The study of lives*. New York: Atherton, 178–98.

Lowen, A. 1967 *The betrayal of the body*. New York: Macmillan.

Lowen, A. 1972 *Depression and the body*. Baltimore, MD: Penguin.

Maslow, A. 1970 *Motivation and personality*, 2nd edn. New York: Harper and Row.

Menzies, I. 1960 *The functioning of social systems as a defence against anxiety*. London: Tavistock.

Nirje, B. 1976 The normalisation principle. In Kugel, R. and Shearer, A. (eds), *Changing patterns of residential services for the mentally retarded*. Washington: President's Committee for the Mentally Retarded.

Oakes, A. R. 1981 Near-death events and critical care nursing. *Topics in Clinical Nursing* **3**, 61–78.

Orem, D. 1995 *Nursing: concepts of practice*, 5th edn. New York: McGraw-Hill.

Orne, R. M. 1986 Nurses' views of nursing directors of education (NDEs). *American Journal of Nursing* **86**, 419–20.

Peplau, H. E. 1988 *Interpersonal relations in nursing: a conceptual frame of reference for psychodynamic nursing*. Basingstoke: Macmillan (first published in 1952 by Putman, New York).

Perls, F. 1969 *Ego, hunger and aggression*. New York: Vintage Books.

Polster, I. and Polster, M. 1974 *Gestalt therapy integrated*. New York: Vintage.

Reason, P. and Rowan, J. (eds) 1981 *Human inquiry: a sourcebook of new paradigm research*. Chichester: Wiley.

Rogers C. 1983 *Freedom to learn for the 80s*. Columbus: Merrill.

Rogers, M. 1970 *An introduction to the theoretical basis of nursing*. Philadelphia: Davis.

Rolf, I. 1977 *Rolfing: the structural integration of the human structure*. Boulder: Rolf Institute.

Roper, N., Logan, W. W. and Tierney, A. J. 1980 *The elements of nursing*. Edinburgh: Churchill Livingstone.

Rowan, J. 1983 *The reality game*. London: Routledge and Kegan Paul.

Roy, C. 1979 Relating nursing theory to education: a new era. *Nurse Educator* **4**, 16–21.

Rycroft, C. 1968 *A critical dictionary of psychoanalysis*. Harmondsworth: Penguin.

Trevelyan, J. 1989 Near-death experiences. *Nursing Times and Nursing Mirror* **85**, 39–41.

Tyne, A. 1978 *Looking at life – in hospitals, hostels, homes and units for adults who are mentally handicapped*. London: Campaign for the Mentally Handicapped.

Wilson H. S. and Kneisl, C. R. 1979 *Psychiatric nursing*. Menlo Park: Addison Wesley.

Wilson, H. S. and Kneisl, C. R. 1983 *Psychiatric nursing*, 2nd edn. Menlo Park: Addison Wesley.

Wright, D. 1974 *On the basis of social order*. Annual Meeting of the American Sociological Association. New York: American Sociological Association.

Yalom, I. 1970 *The theory and practice of group psychotherapy*. London: Basic Books.

Zinker, J. 1977 *Creative process in gestalt therapy*. New York: Vintage Books.

7 Sociology – its contributions and critiques

Abigayl Perry

Why sociology?

How can sociology promote understanding of nurses and their practices? What insights into nursing problems does it offer that are not already available in nursing theories? The purpose of this chapter is to provide an overview of the ways in which nursing dilemmas become issues in mainstream sociological theory. In other words, the organisation of modern nursing is not an isolated 'thing in itself' of concern only to nurses. Instead, its history, management and culture in the UK example are linked to the tasks of the health and welfare industry.

Sociology is only one of a number of disciplines which make up the specialism of health care. As a social science, it reflects the view that the health of the nation is likely to be decided around the Cabinet table rather than the operating table. The National Health Service (NHS) is, after all, heavily funded and controlled by the national government. Government policies are overt determinants of levels of health and service provision, expectations and definitions of health and health practices. Medicine is not, therefore, the only authority in society concerned with the formulation of health and illness concepts and the control of ill health as a social problem. Furthermore, an entire health industry, whether in a predominantly private or public system, intervenes in the doctor–patient relationship and the delivery of health care, e.g. multinational chemical and insurance companies, medical suppliers, the computer industry or the 'new technology', and a host of analytical chemists, paramedical and humbler groups which are needed to effect medical health practices.

Although nurses identify the dominance of the medical profession as the main constraint on their aspirations, this is seen by sociologists to be a secondary consideration (Witz, 1994, p.23). Through the sociological lens, nursing is an occupation whose social function is, and has been, constituted as a set of manual tasks within the agendas of the hospital medical establishment. The attainment of a semi-professional status by nurses has more to do with a unity administered through the 'welfare state' than with recent efforts on the part of nurse 'professionalisers'. Professional accreditation is always conferred from above via academic institutions, but it is earned from below in relevant organisational experiences. The rise of an elevated medical structure as the model of professional (career) development is not something which doctors achieved alone: it required institutional support. Medicine, like nursing, has been influenced by state-directed health policies and the structuring of work across industrial societies (Walby et al., 1994).

People are not only individuals; they are members of social groups and are treated as such in health organisations, whether they be practitioners or patients. There is nothing intrinsically wrong with a system that manufactures health care in relation to measurements of social rather than self-defined needs. For instance, a mass of research reveals that illness, disease and life expectancy occur in social patterns (Baggott, 1994), and that health needs are closely linked to social stratification (Townsend et al., 1990) and specific forms of oppression such as patriarchy or racism which predate the modern era (Doyal, 1995; Jones, 1994, Chapter 8). However, if treating the sick is highly stratified, diverse and a site for the deployment of contemporary power relations, then so too is nursing care. The structure of modern nursing is not an entity changing purely in relation to its own internal composition, but a dynamic part of an overall changing social situation. As such it is studied sociologically (Carpenter, 1993; Perry, 1993; Witz, 1992).

What is of particular concern to sociologists is the ideology or system of evaluation which defines and prioritises body parts, patients and health workers mainly in terms of a manifest utility to organisational powers in health and the wider society. The aim here is to review the practices of nurses as functions of the ideology behind health concepts, health professionalism and nursing theories. An ideology is not a system of benign beliefs. It embodies a political selection of the truth – the means by which dominant representations of reality are perpetuated without the necessity of providing proof. Thus, sociologists will argue that a professional ideology is a method whereby professionals sustain their untested proposition that more professionalisation causes better patient care, rather than increased patient control (Richman, 1987, p.131).

Nurses do not have to be professional social scientists. They do need sociological analysis to examine their changing roles in the distribution of power in health. When nurses were classified as mere generalists in a service dominated by medical specialists, not many people, except perhaps the patients, were particularly interested in nursing. Health care is now definitely an industry with commercial interests and a language of expediency: it is a social hierarchy. Given all of the economic calculus and political rationale, nurses have become careerists with a price on their work as a matter of survival. They come into competition, therefore, with other occupational groups over statuses at work. The source of these conflicts over *credentialism* lies in the wider society. Health workers are members of different social classes and identity groups, who are affected by status distinctions at work.

Readers who have been introduced to sociology will be aware that it incorporates various approaches. Its reports on knowledge show that there is not one way of thinking in society which can explain and predict everything that happens or is likely to occur. If this were so, we would be living under a dictatorship, and sociologists, if allowed to exist, would be reduced to commentating on the status quo. Instead, a number of perspectives enable theorists to question who makes the rules governing interpersonal action (interpretive or 'insider' sociology), and also to question the purpose of large-scale institutions which practise upon whole populations. This latter group includes structuralist theories such as functionalism, Weberian interactionism, Marxism and feminism.

Where does all of this sociological mentality and vocabulary lead us? Like other professional groups, sociologists bring their principles to bear on worlds which squeamish people would choose not to know, e.g. mental illness (Goffman, 1961; Prior, 1993), infertility and reproductive technologies (Pfeffer, 1993; Stanworth, 1987) or chronic illness and debility (de Wolfe, 1996). In the selection of topics which follows, more will be said about these different methods and vocations.

Nursing dilemmas

In nursing theory, professionalism is taken to be the only acceptable explanation of practice. Traditional debates concerning questions of 'Who should be allowed to nurse?' and 'How should they do it?', in response to 'Whose needs?' and 'What definition of health?' are discussed as either progressive or retrograde steps in the movement towards a higher occupational status. As an ideology, this approach exacerbates the insularity of nursing's leadership from everyone in health care (including the patient) which, in a way, it set out to solve. For it perpetuates, at the level of theory, the essentialist[7.1] position of the 'special case' or 'hostage' mentality – a superiority associated with unworldly virtue. It spreads a protective veil of innocence over the huge problem of powerlessness in nursing, occupational arrangements and patienthood. We never reach the comparative (real) world where the experiences of nurses are compared with those of others in similar status and class locations. Vying for a subordinate status or society-wide sympathy for the nursing service, these theorists avoid having to confront the objective conditions (i.e. tough standards and competition, deferred gratification and responsibilities) which signify everyday life in the professional middle class. The social reality of nursing, and of professionalism, is reduced to a state of mind (feelings and personal grievances), or at most a moral activism (humanism).

We do not learn that sympathy is the last resort of the true professional – an indication of a failure to problem-solve. We do not know how, despite the change to higher education, nurses continue to have a low status in the academy and in health. Furthermore, we do not know why caring and the carers who authenticate this objective continue to be undervalued in society anyway (Seabrook, 1985). The study of nursing theories requires investigation of social theories, including professional ideologies. I am, therefore, voicing a more controversial pedagogy in which the concerns of practitioners are open to debates within the larger academic and cosmopolitan, professional community.

> The lack of criticism or comment, in a field which is claiming to have arrived in the scientific world, but which is not yet established, may be damning evidence to the true state of nursing as a profession.
>
> (Hardy, 1986, p.103)

Nurses are not employed in the health service to express themselves as independent professionals or personalised carers, but to manufacture a system of help, and it needs to be stated that 'help', in most people's estimation, is a step up from 'care', which is taken to be 'the last resort'. The work that nurses do is largely in response to models implemented by their employers in which 'market forces' play a significant part. Subsequently, 'the majority of practitioners may be mystified by the version of nursing emanating from their professional associations and teachers' (Perry, 1993, p.48). Nurse theorists who exhort the benign theory of personalised caring (the 'stay as sweet as you are' syndrome) would be surprised to learn how similar this is to the model of vocationalism proposed by management in consumer (commercial) services (Hoggart, 1995, p.59).

Philosophical detachment is a source of spiritual strength in professional life. However, the more one is adrift from one's origins, the greater is the need for research, that is engagement with social issues. We know that professional caring philosophy is uplifting and effusive on the subject of professed values, but without a rigorous methodology how do we reach the nursing realities? For instance, nursing supervisors are busy with their paperwork and budgets, quality assurance staff are trying to cope with yet another rationing policy (skill mix in relation to predetermined levels of provision), with little time to be bothered with patients' complaints, nurse teachers are concerned, above all else, to preserve a sense of order in nursing even though the health service may be in complete disarray, community nurses have to deal with the increasing health risks in their clients' lives due to more cuts in social welfare provision, and frontline workers in the hospital or community receive the full reactions of the clients without the authority to bring about change. This latter group, which is the largest in nursing organisation and has the lowest status, consists of the nurses who are most likely to be 'client-orientated' but least able to do anything about it.

Sociologically speaking, this diversity in nursing practices suggests that nurses hold different orientations to their work. I have classified these in terms of three main categories: client orientation, management orientation and technical/scientific orientation (see Table 7.1).

Consequently, professionalisation is not the only occupational strategy in nursing. Nurses and other health practitioners seek to protect their work using credentialist strategies: educational, industrial and managerial (Mackay, 1989). Nursing is a multi-layered occupational structure, while patients are grouped according to clinical categories in order to be treated (Pearson and Vaughan, 1986).

Despite the 'whole person' approach in nursing, and official rhetoric that primary care is the answer, historic divisions between cure–care,

Table. 7.1　Different orientations in nursing work (from low to higher status in health structures)

1. **Client orientation:**
   Frontline nurses who work in the community or hospital at the lowest levels of the nursing hierarchy. Identify with the hardships in their clients' lives: pressures on their own standard of living may be linked to the situation of clients in their care. Emphasise the arduous nature of their tasks in the face of imposed definitions from 'above' of 'routine' work.

2. **Management orientation:**
   Nurse supervisors, managers and educators. Concerned with quality assurance in terms of maintaining control of skill definitions, and control over unqualified (unsafe) practitioners. Emphasise the work ethic as a moral imperative; first duty of nurses is loyalty to the nursing service to preserve a sense of order (at all costs).

3. **Technical/scientific orientation:**
   Specialist practitioners such as those working in intensive care, operating theatres, research units and midwifery staff. Emphasise the complementary nature of their roles to higher status groups and their superiority over lay management, nurse supervisors and teachers. Confident that the manner of their work expresses a direct link with scientific knowledge, and thereby with a professional status.

surgical–medical wards and hospital–community services continue to exert power in the health hierarchy. These processes contribute to status distinctions within medicine itself and between different areas of nursing. As previously mentioned, the bulk of nursing care is still carried out by those nurses with the lowest status. Sociologically, this may be analysed in terms of ethnic and class divisions:

> Women from ethnic minorities are concentrated in the auxiliary and state enrolled grades and white middle-class women in the registered grade in the prestigious teaching hospitals.
>
> (Abbott and Wallace, 1990, p.24)

In the absence of accessible knowledge based upon what nursing is when it is happening, nurses have used bureaucratic definitions to describe the working order, i.e. the accomplishment of tasks. In the absence of forums to develop understanding of their social roles on the wards or in the community, many problems arising out of service provision have been perceived as being due to personal inadequacy. For many nurses, especially those at the lower organisational levels, idealised versions of their roles do not explain everyday practice. These practitioners have to make conceptual leaps from their subordinate position on duty to the elevated codes of conduct governing the behaviour of doctors, the top professionals in health. However, this is not the whole story.

When overwhelmed by the lack of beds, porters or trolleys to accommodate patients, nurses and doctors may need to think heroically in order to carry on acting as decent human beings (Perry, 1996, p.3). Symbolic and sacred beliefs have an important place in health care, ensuring integrity in the face of another person's life/death struggle. As theories which explain the inadequacies of the social arrangements surrounding care, they are not very efficient. For many nurses, problems arising from objective conditions tend to be relegated to the complaints department, thus maintaining compliance at work (Turner, 1987, p.151).

Since the Second World War, academic education has become a route for many vocational groups seeking a professional status. Much has been said about the tense relationship between theory and reality, between the authority of the theory and the lack of authority in the workplace. It may be difficult for many nursing students to grasp that academic professional knowledge is supposed to maintain a gap between what is learnt and what is practised, so that practitioners may respond imaginatively to a client's individual needs. Professionals are meant to intervene and effect real differences in people's lives; to do this they need to be well placed in organisational and social structures. However, if nursing theorists continue to analyse professional nursing as a value largely independent of institutional arrangements, we shall never find out what prevents it from being.

Interestingly, research in the socialisation of nurses states that nurse managers use exhortations to professional behaviour as 'the mainstay of discipline within the nursing service' (Melia, 1987, p.167). This disciplinary approach also applies to nurse teachers. Both nurse managers and nurse educators apply behavioural techniques (the basis of educational/management theory) to staff and students with a lower status. Nursing education and practice are informed more by managerialism than by professionalism (as indicated in Table 7.1). An overarching middle-management ideology is the outcome of nursing's location in the occupational and class structure. It is an intermediary or manual occupation with aspirations of middle-class gentility (professional etiquette). In other words, a lower middle-class job performed largely by women along with certain levels of schoolteaching, social work and administrative work. Nurses' socialisation, whether in education or work, remains embedded in the values, experiences and frustrations of society's lower middle class[7.2]. An anti-intellectualism (a type of empiricist mentality) which exists at all levels of nursing is the effect, not the cause, of its social location.

Social differences between activities labelled as intellectual or manual work closely follow class, gender and wealth/hardship divisions. Middle-class jobs are characterised by mental capabilities, ethical responsibilities and educational and friendship networks. Working-class employment is marked by skill divisions. Craft skills, where judgement is not totally separated from the creator, by transfer to a machine or management function, lie somewhere between these two extremes. In the present occupational and prestige hierarchy, manual work, reduced to definitions of 'mindless' physical labour or 'bodies', does not command high status and rewards in the market-place, no matter how socially useful it may be.

New technology gives rise to new ways of working, and the status of professional groups may or may not be radically altered. If the public service ethos in medicine declines, doctors can pursue financial status, as dentists do. In consumer society this assures them of the rewards necessary to maintain a privileged position. Surgeons, who were once upon a time associates of the Barbers' Guild, have now overtaken the élite status of physicians. When Florence Nightingale's nurses were tending savage wounds on the battlefield, there were elements in the military and medical establishment who attempted to degrade the status of these women to that of Army camp followers. The social distance that nurses have travelled since the mid-nineteenth century, measured in terms of class, status and power, need not be underestimated.

Health and social care

Nurses have based their claims for a higher status on their central role in patient care, specialists and technical experts having a more 'remote-control' or intermittent presence at the patient's bedside. However, nurses have paradoxical roles in health organisation. Although nursing care has been central to medical hospital practices at the point of service delivery, it is marginal to medical and scientific education at the executive level of service provision. While nursing goals emphasise caring as a personal relationship, bureaucratic objectives encourage impersonality and standardised proce-dures in order to get the work done quickly. The actual healing of the sick demands time and involvement on the part of health practitioners, not of management. In the current context, caring has been largely removed from the control of professional groups and transferred to a management function. This is the case in school teaching as well as in nursing and social work.

Decisions concerning the number of doctors, nurses and patients, and funding matters, arise out of political processes in society (see Chapter 8). In the current context of the NHS, medical professionalism has been curtailed by a government-led strategy of 'market forces'. Where does this leave nurses? Caring work can very easily be viewed as something that people, especially women, do naturally. Does this mean that caring has been further devalued? Current conflicts between social carers and their employers, namely government departments, would indicate that this is so.

In a private system, health problems become the responsibility of individuals and not the state. In terms of hospital economics, the more operations it undertakes the more the hospital keeps going – the technological intensity of the system magnifies at the expense of labour-intensive care. In the USA, where health care is mainly a fee for service hospital business, it is frequently not physicians but the insurance companies who decide what treatments patients receive. Criticisms of overtreatment in the insured groups are paral-leled by concerns about undertreatment for those in underinsured and unin-sured groups. Furthermore, we learn that:

> Thirty-two per cent of all health care workers in the United States do not have health insurance. They are part of the 38 million Americans who face the same plight.
>
> (Navarro, 1993, p.10)

While health may be an unobtainable ideal for many people, research shows that illness is a common experience (Fitzpatrick *et al.*, 1984). The poor-est groups in society are the sickest; heart attacks and respiratory diseases are highest in the lowest social groups. Meanwhile, cuts in general welfare services, e.g. unemployment benefit, increase the need for general health care at the same time as cuts in the health service (due to administrative policies and length-of-stay procedures) decrease its availability in the population generally. Is community care the answer? At the moment, this area is seriously underfunded, yet staff and informal carers have to cope with the 'hopeless cases' – those who are unlikely to get better.

In an industrialised health system, with its throughput goals, nurses have expressed a decline in intrinsic rewards (job satisfaction). This has led to an increase in demands for better pay and working conditions. Technological changes in the modern hospital have affected nursing roles as well as medi-cine. The traditional model of nurse education has changed mainly because it is no longer appropriate to contemporary requirements. Nurses are now being educated for more differentiated roles as a result of more vertically structured administrative and management grades.

The redefinition of nursing practices stems from a combination of political, economic and social factors: first, a response to the reluctance of governments to finance full hospital and medical care for the poor; secondly, the growth of highly specialised health disciplines or paramedical occupations, from radiographers and physiotherapists to cytologists and haematologists; thirdly, the limited power of traditional health professionals in the political arena and in the market-place, e.g. we can no longer say that modern governments support a medical monopoly on decision-making in the health service; fourthly, technological and educational changes have altered nurses' social image. Instead of the 'lady nurse' with a vocational calling, we are presented with an image of a technically competent professional. The reality is heterogeneous groups of increasingly part-time hospital and community carers (Freidson, 1970; Salvage, 1985; Towers, 1996). Only a small proportion of nursing realities correspond to the ideal.

Sociology of nursing

The historical and current situation of nurses in health care is related to social issues which concern us all. For instance, it is difficult to discuss nurses' work without reference to the position of women in society and the lower status associated with women's employment (see Chapter 8). Potential conflicts between nurses and doctors, and between doctors and patients, are linked to gender- and class-based inequalities in society. A recent newspaper reported: 'Hysterectomies are on the increase, and class related: women without any further education are 14 times more likely to have one' (Ellman, 1996, p.14).

The recruitment of nurses is mainly from the 'buffer zone' (social class three on the Registrar General's scale), and from overseas. We all know that doctors' prestigious position has much to do with their 'gentlemen' status (knowledge and wealth), whatever their country of origin. Doctors are still mainly men from the upper middle class, while the majority of nurses and patients are women from lower social class backgrounds. What bothers sociologists is that 'personal judgements may colour supposedly professional and objective judgements' (Jones, 1994, p.285). This has serious implications for the way in which women patients are assessed and treated. For example, research reports in the *British Medical Journal* suggest that women may be discriminated against in the treatment and investigation of cardiac disease (Khaw, 1993; Petticrew et al., 1993). It emerges that when women visit their GPs with complaints of chest pain, they are likely to come away with a diagnosis of stress. If men present with chest pain, it conveys the serious implications of angina symptoms. At certain stages of life, men are more likely to die of coronary heart disease than women (Waldron, 1976), but this gender bias is not applicable throughout the life cycle.

In medicine, gynaecology is a high-status, surgical specialism (with a low proportion of women consultants). Gynaecological nursing has a fairly low status and this, I suggest, is partly caused by the hospital as well as the medical structure. Nurses as generalists may complain that the focus on a single body system is too narrow and that the tasks are repetitive. For whatever reasons, a female nurse does not automatically ally herself with the female patient. 'In fact, the more she falls in behind the medical model, with its support for male medical control, the less this is likely to occur' (Carpenter, 1993, p.112).

Nurses have been instrumental intermediaries between doctors and patients – prescription and cure. They have been medical and organisational *verifiers* (sometimes called interface workers). This means that they are at the bottom of the hierarchy of professional accountability in an organisation, but in the front line of the action. They have an intense but derived responsibility to keep the patient alive. Nurses may have some authority nowadays to deal with routine medical matters, but not to act upon a situation as it arises in the way that social workers do. If a patient is not progressing as the doctor ordered, the vigilant nurse does not vary the treatment, but calls the doctor. The pharmacist, who is not a doctor, has the authority to suggest remedies, but he or she is not regarded as directly responsible. Thus the nature of health professionalism varies in terms of control of work content and practices. In the sociology of the professions (Torstendahl and Burrage, 1990) this fundamental ambivalence in professional roles is an essential aspect of their autonomy and virtuosity – the power to act on their own (Burrage and Torstendahl, 1990; Jamous and Peloille, 1970).

All professional occupations are hierarchical in structure, but some individual practitioners, usually those at the top, have greater autonomy than others (Johnson, 1972). The history of nursing is located in the care of the poor (to which it is returning), the diseases of poverty and custodial care of the insane and the dispossessed. The history of medicine is associated with the physician's consultative role to the wealthy. Thus the status of these occupations is also linked to the status of the 'objects of care', conferring humility or nobility on those who do the caring.

Nurses have not been theoretically uninformed practitioners. Instead, assessment of the work that they do and the required standards of performance has been imposed by higher class and status groups. Nurses have gained knowledge from their observations of the varied nature of illnesses and treatments from the viewpoint of the sufferers. Generally speaking, health professionals have, in the past, relied upon the continuous flow of patient information relayed to them by nursing staff (an aspect of the doctor–nurse game cited below). However, the working conditions and mental horizons of nurses have been defined and overwhelmed by significant others. That nurses have been treated in undignified ways is apparent in the enacted drama of the doctor–nurse game (Stein, 1967; Stein *et al.*, 1990). 'It continues because the work culture and power relationships – including sexual politics – reinforce it' (Jones, 1994, p.486).

At the same time, nursing has long been accepted as socially useful work. Many new professional groups are not accorded this status attribute. For example, accountancy or advertising might be professions upon which the commercial world depends, but this involves more suspicion than trust. In nursing, the symbol of altruism can be seen as a compensation for the lack of economic rewards. Nurses as low-paid carers are highly thought of, but as careerists they may face the considerable criticism that social workers and teachers have received in recent years. They may be blamed for generating the very problems that they are supposed to contain, i.e. dependency in chosen populations.

An unstated bias, that nursing only has a history as middle-class respectability, is buried deep in the 'nursing service' culture. The sublimation of nursing's lowly class origins has been to the detriment of supportive networks and unified strategies for change. Ideas of middle-class gentility have masked class, gender and age distinctions between doctors and nurses and between general and psychiatric nurses (with their history as the keepers in custodial institutions). In addition, the drudgery of a harsh training suffered by young women (recruited from the working class and immigrant groups) has been almost totally over-looked. External controls over these nurses, used as a source of cheap labour, have been maintained by rigid hierarchies and the 'iron rule of obedience'. These many divisions continue to be a source of internal conflicts in nursing.

During its inception in the mid-twentieth century, the 'welfare state' was based upon professionalism and the *less eligibility principle* whereby certain groups of people were regarded as less deserving of resources than others. This process of stereotyping patients is expressed in the health sector in confused attitudes to cases of self-inflicted injury, e.g. drug abuse, attempted suicide, alcoholism and obesity to a lesser extent, psychosomatic illnesses such as anorexia, and sexually transmitted diseases.

Treatments available on the NHS are tax funded but mainly free from payment at the point of delivery. This does not mean that access to professional help is unrestricted. For instance, in the present system, to be defined as sick implies a medical category that is amenable to chemotherapy, surgery or psychiatric help. There is a crescendo of critical opinion which argues that professionals exercise considerable power in the control of who should or should not be treated (Hugman, 1991, p.113).

Individuals may be accused of escaping into illness because they are work-shy, malingerers or unable to accept adult responsibilities. Illness is perceived as a deviation from assumptions of normal social functioning: living up to one's responsibilities is defined as health (see Chapter 3). Talcott Parsons (1964), an American sociologist, was the first to show that illness is feared as a threat to social cohesion/social order. Behaviour that is considered to be inappropriate is too easily equated with deviance and antisocial activity. A patient who does not conform to medical prescription, for whatever reason, may be labelled as disruptive, i.e. unwilling to fulfil their *sick role* obligations (Carpenter, 1993, p.99).

This is a serious problem for those who are sick. These views also affect 'well patients', such as pregnant women. In the medical model, obstetrics is directly linked to gynaecology or disease pathology rather than to paediatrics or child health. The example below, taken from research on medicalised maternity services, illustrates the doctors' equation of normal as unusual.

> Consultant: Interesting, very interesting, most unusual.
> Registrar: You mean it was a normal delivery?
> Consultant: Yes – pushed the baby out herself!
>
> (Oakley, 1980, p.22)

Medical ideology equates health with medical intervention, and patient compliance with safety, especially in the case of antenatal care (Miller, 1996), hence the justification for its role in every pregnancy and health behaviours in general. This therapeutic strategy is known as *medicalisation*, which Illich (1975) viewed as the outcome of a medical imperialism – more areas of life become subject to medical definition and jurisdiction.

Illich's medicalisation thesis has been criticised (Cornwell, 1984; Strong, 1979), but it does draw attention to the power struggle in society over who is going to control, and profit from, health. For instance, medicine's monopoly has come up against the considerable 'market forces' of consumer industries and the accompanying dissemination of a new health consciousness, known as *healthism*, throughout society. Healthism, as the personalised consumption of health products and lifestyles, is embedded in holistic health and self-care movements, particularly in the USA. Like medicine, healthism locates the problem of and solution for health and disease at the individual level (see Chapter 3). 'Whereas medicine individualizes "disease", healthism individualizes "dis-ease"' (Crawford, 1980, p.381).

Crawford (1980) found that the national preoccupation with health in the USA is really overwhelmingly middle-class and supportive of wholly private solutions.

> In the healthists' world, the pursuit of health substitutes for, or may become defined as, doing politics. Where blue-collar workers are likely to talk of speed-ups or long hours, middle-class healthists are more prone to discuss their internal balance, stress, or adaptive mechanisms. Stress in you; exploitation in others.
>
> (Crawford, 1980, p.381)

People do not act – they have therapy. In the 'culture of complaint' (Hughes, 1993) which typifies popular culture in the USA, and increasingly in the UK, an all-pervasive 'victimhood' signifies a retreat from public and personal responsibility (i.e. the consequences of one's behaviour for others). The meaning of health, divorced from society and discussed in individualistic terms, is now promoted by health professionals. It leads not to social reforms, but to a consolidation of professional power and a subjectification of the patient. The new vocabulary of the healthists has become, according to May (1992a, 1992b), thoroughly accommodated within health professions in the UK and the new nursing. How can nurses therefore promote self-esteem and independence in patients? Professional nursing models propose contradictory tasks. On the one hand, they encourage patient advocacy as an individual's right to self-determine need; on the other, they insist on professionalism which presupposes patient dependency (Perry, 1993, p.73).

At the same time, there is little criticism of the present centralisation of caring as an executive management function. The pretensions of medicine may be criticised, but this does not mean that the old order in the NHS, medically prescribed though it was, should be seen to be decadent and its tools (knowledge and experience) pronounced obsolete. The NHS which we took for granted no longer seems to exist. In order to reform it, successive Tory governments have deformed it for purely political reasons (i.e. those who wish to benefit from medical expertise can pay for it). Therefore, the formally defined objectives of health care, or those who authenticated them, such as the doctors, have been questioned. What are the implications for nurses seeking careers in the current health service? Nursing's leadership wants professionalism, but the government would like to use nurses, as they have always been used, as interchangeable (cheap) labour – in this case, as a cheaper alternative to doctors where possible. Meanwhile, professionals everywhere notice a real decline in their expert status, career structure, working conditions and pay. Most public-spirited professionals nowadays are part of the salariat, the employed or even the economically insecure.

The key to sociological understanding of nurses as health practitioners, as we have seen, lies in the occupational role. It leads to the organisational framework in which the structure and ideology of nursing can be examined critically. Sociologists analysing changes in nursing refer to stratifying factors in society to explain the following:

- the distribution of authority between medicine and nursing, nurses and other health workers;
- the containment of health needs;
- the quality of existing provision; and
- the passivity of patients within various institutional settings.

Nurses' occupational roles are dependent upon the structure of industrial society, i.e. the health industry, rather than upon any conception of health. In the cure–care divide, and contestations over 'therapeutics', nurses have had little choice but to cling to a social model for maintenance and development. Unfortunately, the emphasis on caring models in 'health' often expresses an uncritical optimism about the extent to which professionals have the power to influence the health status of individuals and whole communities. Meanwhile, reported rates of illness continue to rise in the light of increased pressures and insecurities in people's lives throughout all levels of society.

Bureaucracy: its hidden agendas

The NHS in the UK is the largest employer in western Europe; 50 per cent of its work-force is female, in line with national trends, and it is also a growth industry. It is of importance to the economy, and to the pay and conditions of the work-force and of women workers in particular (Perry, 1996, pp.1–2).

Large-scale bureaucracy is a major institutional form in modern societies, and the NHS is clearly no exception. How can the subservience of nurses in health bureaucracy be understood without reference to the exercise of power by individuals or groups in positions of authority?

It is sociologists who put forward the shocking idea that authorities create deviance by 'establishing a social norm in which it is acceptable to cheat, steal and lie' (Schaef and Fassel, 1988, p.67), thus separating us from our public-spirited awareness. In the present corporate structures, careerist individuals have a tendency to set up their own systems of patronage so that they may gather like-minded minions around them. This is an aspect of the hidden agenda in nursing (Perry, 1993). For example, a positive ward report may depend more on the personal preference of the ward sister or charge nurse than on the competence of subordinate members of staff. The rewarding of certain individuals over others is not always based on openly professed goals or merit. This is creative use of the rules and inconsistency in valuing the work of different individuals.

Marxists analyse power in terms of the dominance of middle-class values in all capitalist institutions – respectability as ideology. Weber, the founder of interactionism, drew attention to the way in which individuals invested with authority may not always use it rationally. Institutions do not, therefore, function only at the level of appearance. Using Goffman's (1959) *dramaturgical model*, the ways in which some people devote their energy, and that of underlings, to promoting themselves symbolically as indispensable at work can be analysed. These people are the biggest time-wasters in any organisation (Jacobs, 1969), yet they are often rewarded with more power by management in the mistaken belief that the work only gets done because they act as the coercive arm of management. So long as management goals appear to be served, the quality of the product and personal interaction between staff is not seriously questioned.

The promotion of these competitive values, expressed in authoritarian leadership styles and closed communication systems, may be particularly offensive and distressing to those who have chosen to be carers (see Chapter 6). This may be one of the reasons for the high turnover of staff in the caring fields of nursing and social work.

Michels' (1949) rule of power states that those who rise to positions of authority tend to become corrupted (Haralambos with Heald 1980, p.288). Thus, high places in an organisation always constitute an élite. While some individuals benefit from this, others are set up to fail. Living up to high standards of care may render an employee deviant within an organisation in which corporate values hold sway in service delivery. If organisational theory is to be useful to nurses in understanding modern health bureaucracies, then it needs to be interpreted critically (Schaef and Fassel, 1988). Otherwise, one would have to accept that all those who hold positions over us are the most talented and best suited for the posts (Davis and Moore, 1967), and also that individual complaints are personal grievances and not the result of problems in the organisation. Furthermore, it would need to be agreed that competitive ways of working naturally take precedence over democratic or more co-operative methods (Strong and Robinson, 1988).

Sociological research on gender and race inequalities in employment has shown how informal patronage in organisations operates as a mode of discrimination in selection procedures (Jewson and Mason, 1986) and barriers to career opportunities (Crompton and Sanderson, 1986). Individuals are selected and judged on an unfair basis of ascription rather than achievement in education and work. This process is known as occupational segregation by ascribed characteristics, such as gender, race and age (Blaxall and Reagan, 1976). Looking across the economy, it can be seen that those with minority group status continue to occupy the lower levels within all occupations.

Nursing and patient care

Sociologists believe that concepts of health and the roles of health carers and patients are socially defined. How nursing is organised is an important aspect of the way in which a society constructs gender roles through political processes. In the former Soviet Union, for instance, medicine was an overwhelmingly female occupation, 90 per cent of primary care physicians being women. At this level, medicine was regarded as women's work, men taking up better career options in hospital administration, industry, the armed forces or Party officialdom. The relatively lower status of primary medicine was not due to the fact that women did this work, but rather women did it because it was regarded socially as a lower status profession than, say, engineering (Navarro, 1977). Comparative and cross-cultural studies clearly show that men or women are not naturally best suited to be doctors or nurses.

Nurses are not only employed in the health service to do the patient's housework, nor are they technicians whose work is amenable to management ideals concerning the timing and sequencing of appropriate acts. For instance, giving an injection can be broken down into detailed tasks, and reduced to a skill rather than an action involving judgement, i.e. adjustment to the needs of particular patients. Apart from the administrative and legal procedures informing drug use, nurses decide where is the best place to give the injection and the way in which to carry out the procedure gently and safely. The nurse takes into account skin and muscle tone, age and condition, and how best to reassure and reduce the patient's apprehension or fear. The practice of nurses, like that of doctors, does not take place in a vacuum, but is governed by abstract professional principles and concrete organisational rules.

Nurses have a social purpose to ensure that individuals are integrated into the sick role so that the doctor–patient relationship can be effective (Jones, 1994, p.402). At the same time, their presence at the bedside requires that they respond to the patient's personal needs. If a surgeon removes a kidney instead of repairing a hiatus hernia, what does the nurse tell the patient and the relatives? This is not, by the way, a fictitious example. Medical sociologists are inclined to take a conflict rather than a consensus perspective on the doctor–patient relationship (Annandale, 1989; Mechanic, 1995).

Studying nursing in its social/occupational context helps to rescue carers in general from social oblivion. It also provides insights into the problems that women face in having this type of work taken seriously, either in employment or in the home. While nursing was regarded as purely women's work it was not seen as a proper job, but as an interim occupation before women got down to the serious business of marriage and nurturing within their own families. Demographic change, especially the reduction in the number of school-leavers, means that there is no longer a ready supply of young recruits to nursing. Nursing is seeking new labour markets, i.e. mature entry and part-time work, and ways of retaining staff through improved systems of training and communication. Nurses work in situations of high turnover for staff and patients, and may not be able to rely upon a long-term building up of team relationships.

Curative science, anatomical pathology, pharmacology and other important disciplines (see Chapter 4) have acted as a collective underpinning to a medical ethos which has perhaps marginalised people's own experiences of illness. It is social scientists who have begun to explore the importance of cultural beliefs in diagnosis, treatment and prescribed outcomes. Furthermore, the majority of ill people suffer from chronic illnesses which require long-term care and support. Although people appeal to medicine for help, their conditions cannot be cured or contained in the consulting room – they have to manage at home as best they can (de Wolfe, 1996).

The change from hospital to community care implies that the careers of nurses and doctors are no longer solely based upon curative techniques. It also assumes that all patients have clean, comfortable homes and stable family settings in which to recover. This has led sociologists to question the meaning of community care.

> For everyone in health care, 'community' is an exceedingly familiar adjective. Community care, community nursing and community medicine are terms used routinely. Patients are admitted and discharged to 'the community', so describing the influence of community would seem to be a straightforward project.
>
> (Greenwell, 1996, p.133)

The researcher discovered that this was far from being the case.

> The hospital is positioned as the central institution and 'the community' is the amorphous locality that surrounds the hospital.
>
> (Greenwell, 1996, p.133)

It seems that 'community' is defined negatively as 'non-hospital', meaning that it is defined by what it is not. While this term has become increasingly popular in the vocabulary of the new professionals (politicians, media personnel, shopkeepers/retailers and anyone working in a service industry nowadays), it tends to be regarded as a fairly meaningless concept in sociological theory. A question which concerns sociologists is whether the modern family, limited to two generations, is capable of shouldering the informal burden of 'community care', especially in the case of families with fragile resources.

With the decline in family size, increased distances between ageing parents and their grown-up children, and the large numbers of married women in employment, the resources of women as family carers are limited.

High-risk society

To sociologists, the 'main killers' are not invisible germs but obvious things such as bad housing, poverty, inherited nutritional disadvantage and industrial health hazards. The British epidemiologists Doll and Peto (Open University, 1985) estimate that over 75 per cent of cancer deaths in industrial societies are preventable, i.e. they could be avoided. They argue that the majority of cancers are caused by adulterated food (additives), cigarette smoking, alcohol and deregulated industries resulting in unhealthy working and living environments (see Chapter 5). It appears that the pathogenic quality of modern life makes us ill.

> In the past, the hazards could be traced back to an undersupply of hygienic technology. Today they have their basis in industrial over-production.
>
> (Beck, 1992, p.21)

Sociological research demonstrates that theories of health and illness arise out of particular social conditions and cultures (Armstrong, 1983). The literature on health beliefs shows that people's attitudes are influenced by official definitions, of which there are several in currency (Jones, 1994, p.368), with biomedicine leading the field of enquiry.

> Most patients ... have been conditioned to believe that the doctor alone knows what makes them sick and that technological intervention is the only thing that will get them better.
>
> (Capra, 1982, p.163).

Capra (1982) concludes that overcoming this medical dogma would require nothing short of a cultural revolution. So where does this leave nurses? As non-technological, palliative carers they are unlikely to have a high status in Beck's (1992) *Risk Society*. Some midwives make claims to be 'experts' in low-risk births, but this may threaten their credibility as a professional group because 'Prestige and power are given to those who manage high-risk situations, not to those who attend low-risk births' (DeVries, 1993, p.144).

This may not make sense to nurses or midwives, but it is industrial logic, not the fault of doctors. In western technological societies, the natural sciences create knowledge but modern states transform it into power. Social progress is reduced to notions of the profits that modern economics bring, e.g. how many car owners there are in the population. Subsequently, a patient's progress is measured in terms of responses to technological treatments such as surgery or chemotherapy, and not in terms of his or her quality of life. Progress is thus equated with consumption patterns.

Patients may be discharged back into the situations which gave rise to their health difficulties in the first place (Chapman, 1984). The patient's recovery post-surgery is confined to ensuring that he or she is still alive afterwards. Community nurses have to contend with post-operative problems such as infected suture lines which require stringent hygiene and take time to heal. Chemical treatments often have appalling consequences, such as long-term disability in the practolol syndrome and deformities in the case of thalidomide (Melville and Johnson, 1982). Medicine has been used to shape the whole of contemporary health knowledge, so patients demand prescription drugs and look to doctors for answers to many social as well as health problems.

Human societies are unequal societies. The ideas or theories available to explain 'how people should lead their lives' closely resemble the assumptions of those powerful enough to impose their views on others. These powerful meaning systems are called ideologies – the means whereby individuals interpret the way they feel, reason and act, and judge the performance of others.

The way one acts may be largely constrained by others, as in the case of nursing. Many people struggle against the unfairness of these forces in their lives. If sceptical sociologists have anything to offer, it is that institutional practices may be harmful to spiritual or physical health. This perspective is shared by some health users who form themselves into pressure groups to effect more humane methods of treatment and care. Another example is medical fashion, which may be unrelated to better health practice. This was the case with the dramatic decline in breast-feeding in the USA. Although this proved detrimental to infant health, it lasted until the scandal over Nestlé's milk powder and pressure from mothers reversed the medical trend (Francome, 1986). Professionals need to reflect upon the implications of their own truths before advising clients. Disease or health models may pose problems in terms of biology/individual need, but the solutions tend to be social or collective.

Altered states of mind and matter

Social scientists believe that all significant human behaviour is learned. In primary socialisation in the family, children learn to become members of the human group. Subsequent socialisation in school, peer group and work illustrates the changes and conflicts encountered as individuals come into contact with new people and situations. Individuals not only learn to adapt to conventional ways in society, they also acquire the mental capabilities to allow them to communicate meaningfully with other human beings. Of course this potential is not always expressed, depending as it does on opportunities for emotional and social security. These ideas are raised and discussed in introductory sociology textbooks, but also in nursing models concerned with personal growth and development, such as those of King (1981) and Peplau (1952; see Chapters 1, 5, 6 and 10).

Occupational groups undergo intellectual or symbolic changes in preparation for their roles and status positions. This represents part of the formal socialisation of educated groups, but is largely informal in manual occupations, i.e. learning one's place on the job. For future professionals, the process forces students to discard lay imagery and to internalise the correct moral principles and 'power of thought' (academic know-how). This personal conversion forms an introduction to the knowledge base relating to the claims of the occupational group. In the case of medical students, it has been observed that the learning of the medical role consists of an alienation of the student from the lay medical world (Hughes, 1958).

A consequence of the esoteric learning is the justification of jargon which only the initiated understand. Through the use of their *jargon of authenticity* (Adorno, 1973), professionals put themselves forward as sharers in a higher culture – individuals with an essence of their own that is distinct from the common herd (Adorno, 1973, p.18). This perpetuates the alienation of patients from what is happening to them. Encounters with the scientific mentality of medicine usually render patients' bodies inert and their minds irrelevant. Supported by the impersonality of the hospital bureaucracy, emotions and other messy human affairs are excluded from the clinical environment.

Social approaches in health care attempt to overcome distinctions between physical, mental and psychosomatic illness. In psychoanalytical theory all illness is considered to be self-motivated, although not in a self-conscious way. This means that it is necessary to a certain extent in the maintenance of a stable personality. In popular usage, psychosomatic has come to mean 'not really ill'. This assumption overlooks the widespread nature of illness, the devastation it causes in people's lives, and the significance of stress in producing vulnerability to a range of diseases, from the common cold to heart attacks (Fitzpatrick, 1986; see Chapter 5).

It seems that some people react to stressors in their lives by having nervous breakdowns, while others fall ill with an unexplained physical 'disease'. Whatever the trigger factor and the effects, these people are not imagining an illness which is not there. However, in order to understand the altered states brought about by illness – the solitude and heightened introspection (see Chapter 6) – it is helpful to turn to literature rather than to scientific texts (Green, 1964; Solzhenitsyn, 1971). Little has been written from the viewpoint of medical learning. One learns about the experience of illnesses which have defied medical interpretation from self-help groups organised around specific symptoms, such as the Myalgic Encephalomyelitis (ME) Association. Health and illness always involve psychological and physical causes and effects.

According to Goffman (1961), doctors maintain their impersonality in treating patients by two main methods. First, they can anaesthetise the patient. By the time the powerful suppressing effects of the anaesthetic have worn off, the patient has been turned over to the nursing staff. They are no longer medical problems but nursing problems. Secondly, doctors can treat the patient as a non-person by ignoring the fact that a person has to accompany their body to the medical workshop. Apart from greeting the patient 'with what passes as civility, and said farewell to in the same fashion, everything in between goes on as if the patient weren't there at all, but only as a possession someone has left behind' (Goffman, 1961, p.298).

Doctors as scientific workers receive job satisfaction from the use of individualised technology which maintains the distance between élite professionals and patients. This is often contrasted with nurses, whose personal interaction with patients is essential to their stated satisfaction with their work (Chapman, 1976). However, because doctors are professionals cast in the scientific (perfectionist) mould, they are more likely to give people time to recover in hospital after treatments than managers. This surely has implications for many nurses whose careers are tied to the NHS management structure, especially in matters of 'quality assurance' (health care rationing).

The impersonal approach of medicine can also serve humane purposes. Doctors accept the burden of the disease, as most healers do, and responsibility for the patient's recovery. In other cultures, healers are more concerned with the misfortunes illness brings, and not its causes; they do not usually accept responsibility to produce a cure. Medical authority may alleviate the aura of personal inadequacy emanating from the sick person, as all illness is associated with a certain deviance, ranging from carelessness, such as 'catching cold', to divine retribution, as with some sexually transmitted diseases (Carter and Watney, 1989). To be ill means there has been a deviation from the norm of being healthy, and ill people are often judged by those around them to be at fault. In the meantime, research shows that while illness is a common experience, to many people health may be an unobtainable ideal (Perry, 1996, p.6).

The problem of defining health

Many nurses think that personalised caring and emotion work (Smith, 1992) literally mean catering to the patient's every need. This would be an impossible task even if there was one nurse for each patient. Health and nursing care are matters of individual behaviour but also involve social responsibility, such as public health. Instruction given by nurses to people on how to take care of themselves in unhealthy, damp housing is not, on its own, likely to be effective. Being healthy is not totally dependent upon the isolated activity of individuals, be they professionals or patients – it has wider consequences.

Some people think that health, like human nature, is a timeless truth. However, it is a social judgement located in culture which varies between and within societies and groups over time. Health as a social, relative concept is a variable – a factor which changes according to circumstances. Health and illness can be measured objectively in terms of frequency of conditions observed over time, and subjectively by investigation of cultural attitudes and individual and group beliefs. Health practitioners will be familiar with a variety of definitions ranging from health as medical treatment, a state of mind, to the all-encompassing construct of the World Health Organisation (see Chapter 3).

Generally speaking, health is understood in functional terms as the absence of disease or disability and the ability to continue to carry out one's social activities. There are three main criteria for judging wellness:

- the subjective feeling of well-being;
- the absence of symptoms; and
- the ability to perform activities which those in good health can perform.

The criteria for judging illness are derivative, i.e. the degree to which it interferes with ordinary activities and the originality or novelty of the experience – when it has just happened and has not happened that way before (Pearson and Vaughan, 1986, p.43).

Social research on lay beliefs shows that these vary, but are class-related (Blaxter and Paterson, 1982; Cornwell, 1984). Among working-class people, health is generally regarded as being able to cope with one's job/ housework/looking after children, and with misfortune. Middle-class people, having relatively more security, are likely to describe it in terms of positive well-being, but

> Whatever meaning is given to health by lay people, ill health represents a breakdown in the normal, expected state of health ... a situation where things go wrong, a deviation from how things should be, and usually are.
>
> (Miles, 1991, p.42)

In the functionalist model, health is described as 'the state of optimum capacity of an individual for the effective performance of roles and tasks for which he has been socialized' (Parsons, 1979, p.132). Healthy individuals are essential for the smooth running of their own lives and that of the social system. Illness is an undesirable disruption. Systems theories and adaptation models in nursing illustrate this approach, for example Neuman (1980), Orem (1980) and Roy (1976).

Problems arise for functionalist theorists if health or the 'flight into illness' are too highly valued. The sick role is a conditional one, and the purpose of doctors, the gatekeepers, is to ensure that illness is under control like acute disease episodes, i.e. of short duration. Problems arise because the majority of sick people have chronic conditions, incurable mental illnesses or diseases of old age. Thus the treatment that they receive may be medical, but it may not be appropriate to their needs. The patient role is not completely accommodating, because it is assumed that people may find it more desirable than the continued struggle with their everyday lives. On the other hand, too low a level of health would represent a poor return on society's investment in its members. If health expectations continue to rise due to the rising standard of living, then the demand for medical services may exceed supply. This implies that it is in society's interest to exclude certain people from the general prosperity in order to keep health costs down. This approach is frequently criticised by other sociologists as a justification for the status quo – the continued dependence of patients on the exclusive knowledge of the experts (Hart, 1985; Morgan *et al.*, 1985).

Sociologists question self-evident 'truths' about how normality is socially constructed. It is by no means true of all societies that mad people came to be regarded as mentally ill and institutionalised, unmarried mothers criminalised and cast in chains, or that the causes of illness in the living were to be sought in the dissection of the dead. The relativity of these truths, as specific social and cultural judgements, usually only becomes obvious when viewed historically. The social order that exists may not exist because of need but power; the activities of men in controlling the behaviour of others. This is the basic assumption underlying Foucault's path-breaking analyses:

1. *Madness and civilisation – a history of insanity in the age of reason;*
2. *The birth of the clinic – an archaeology of medical perception;* and
3. *Discipline and punish – the birth of the prison.*

(Foucault, 1973a, 1973b, 1977)

Class, role and health status

Sociologists have shown that social class is a significant factor in the distribution of mental illness. In the USA it is almost fashionable among white middle-class professionals to seek support from an analyst for neurotic symptoms such as anxiety and depression. For these wealthy Americans, illness is to a certain extent a necessary part of their mental health. In order to cope with the pressures of middle-class role expectations, the well-off can afford to pay for the personal services of a range of therapists. This is not the case for others, especially young mothers with limited means. Brown and Harris' (1978) study of 600 women in London found that a far higher proportion of working-class mothers were vulnerable to depression and an inability to cope with crises than middle-class mothers or working-class women without children. Isolation in the home with three or more small children and little emotional support from partners led to a lower level of self-esteem among these working-class mothers. The solution probably has as much to do with the availability of pre-school nursery places as with psychiatric help.

Until the confirming evidence of the Black Report (Townsend and Davidson, 1982), illness and premature death were not widely accepted by health educators as the products of class inequalities, but rather as the result of individual mismanagement. This report showed that the distribution of health probabilities closely followed the distribution of income and wealth. Morbidity and mortality rates remain connected, as they always have done, to hardship and poverty. The researchers observed marked class distinctions for most causes of death, particularly respiratory diseases and accidents. These conditions were related to health risks in the social environment. The findings revealed that the middle classes benefited more from the health service than the working classes. It is true to say that, as the need increases, so the number and quality of the services available decreases. This phenomenon is known as the *inverse care law* (Tudor Hart, 1975, p.205).

It is commonly assumed that divisions between individuals and groups are natural. Sex-based inequalities at work and in the family have been interpreted as extensions of a biological destiny, as if men and women were immutable opposites. Although one might not expect to find women in top positions in male-intensive occupations, it is surprising to find that they have not 'made it' even within occupations in which they predominate. Nursing as a female-intensive occupation illustrates these trends. While the nursing profession is made up of over 90 per cent women, men are over-represented in educational, managerial and supervisory posts. Despite the equality legislation of the 1970s, the accomplishments of men in work tend to be more rewarded than those of women employees. Male nurses are seen primarily as men and managers, and secondarily as nurses (Gaze, 1987). The employment of more men in nursing does not lead to improved conditions, but to greater competition for career posts. Furthermore, it needs to be stated that women do not work because they want to be like men. They want to be independent and need to be providers on a regular rather than a casual basis. Generally speaking, the situation of women in the health service, as nurses, doctors or administrators, reflects a female status in the wider society.

> In 1970, 26 per cent of students entering medical schools in Great Britain were women. In 1980, the equivalent figure was 38 per cent and in 1989, 49 per cent.
>
> (Elston, 1993, p.27)

Despite the rise in female intake in medical schools, a trend which is continuing, these women, once they have qualified, experience difficulty in obtaining posts in high-status specialisms such as surgery and obstetrics. The majority of women doctors are general practitioners, and this is not necessarily the result of personal choice (Elston, 1993, p.56).

All societies have systems of organising activities and assigning differential prestige, usually along the lines of gender and age stratification. In complex industrial societies there are further dimensions, such as class power/powerlessness, ethnicity, sexual orientation and lifestyle identity. The assumption that all societies have rules for regulating and rewarding the behaviour of individuals and social groups may not be acceptable to individuals who believe in 'freedom of choice'.

Sociologists investigate health care

Methods of investigation

Sociologists of health question the following:

- purely biological definitions of health and illness;
- a medical monopoly in health care;

- understandings of patterns in illness and health as random or natural events; and
- rationing procedures in health care systems.

In order to carry out research, sociologists use a variety of methods and techniques.

Despite the popularity of the laboratory experiment in the natural sciences and in psychological studies on compliance, it is almost never used in sociology. The reasons for this are both practical and ethical. In practical terms, sociologists often study large groups of people and they go out into the 'field' because in a clinical situation people would not act as they usually do (O'Donnell, 1981, p.24). For example, Goffman's (1961) participant observation sprang from his fieldwork in an American psychiatric hospital as a member of staff.

In clinical trials, patients are divided into experimental and control groups. This means that one group of patients will receive a new drug treatment, while others will be given placebos or nothing at all. Patients who receive placebos cannot be informed of the true nature of the research, otherwise it would be 'biased' (Hibbert, 1996). This type of manipulation of people is considered to be morally dubious in sociology, which instead offers other comparative methods, such as surveys and content analysis, to nurse and health services researchers.

The most popular method for obtaining information about health beliefs and behaviour is the social survey. Most nurses are probably familiar with the techniques of questionnaires and interviews associated with opinion polls and attitude testing of whole populations or smaller representative samples. Surveys provide a mass of data about the characteristics of the population, ranging from age and income distribution to causes of death and disease. Survey analysis at its most productive involves the coding and identification of significant features and trends. This is a recognised method for assessing the following:

- people's health needs;
- the quality of service provision;
- the benefits of clinical treatments;
- accidents at work, in the home and surrounding environment; and
- the use of technology in medical practice.

Theories

There are three main theoretical approaches in sociology, namely functionalism, interactionism and Marxism. These traditions were founded by Durkheim, Weber and Marx in the nineteenth century, when the study of explanations of human behaviour (social theories) devolved from metaphysics (philosophy and theology) into social science. In other words, knowledge became firmly associated with particular forms of secular society. These three perspectives are represented in sub-specialisms such as the sociology of the professions and the sociology of health care.

Functionalists as consensus theorists view unequal relationships between doctors and patients as largely benign (Parsons, 1964). They accept that the professional authority of physicians over the laity is a necessary part of the acceptance of treatment. The medical encounter is considered to be an essentially cooperative enterprise which prevents sick people from being isolated or derided as deviants (scroungers). Illness as potentially disruptive behaviour is integrated and controlled via institutionalised medicine. Critiques of this approach are many, but Carpenter's (1993, p.98) account includes an analysis of nurses' roles.

Interactionists and Marxists analyse the organisation of health care, professional roles and patienthood in terms of different interest groups. In the interactionist framework, the nurse's role is conflictual – it embodies fundamentally different views (Melia, 1987). These theorists may ask: 'Is the primary obligation of the nurse to the doctor, the organisation or the patient?' Symbolic interactionists or 'insider' sociologists have studied the socialisation of carers in personal service occupations (the American term), such as medical students (Becker *et al.*, 1961) and student nurses (Davis, 1975). In both of these studies, understanding of clients' needs was found to be a secondary consideration. The primary concern was promotion of a professional identity.

Important contributions are made in other disciplinary areas. In the sociology of the family, feminists and psychotherapists have provided radical critiques of the role of the modern family in the production of healthy individuals. Using data on mental illness, such as rates of depressive neurosis and case studies on schizophrenia, they suggest that normal family life may produce passive and neurotic rather than creative and emotionally stable individuals (Morgan *et al.*, 1985; Oakley, 1976).

Specific contributions

Sociologists have for some time been concerned with the influence of social isolation on health. In 1897, Emile Durkheim published his study *Le Suicide* (republished in 1952), in which suicide was defined as the ultimate retreat from the performance of social roles. (This sociologist must have had a sense of humour!) Durkheim argued that suicide, like crime or divorce, was a symptom of problems in society rather than a weakness in an individual's personality. He believed that a person's health resulted from involvement in social roles and relationships – a lack of these would lead to a sense of failure, loneliness and suicide. In particular, Durkheim was concerned with the negative effects of rapid social change (industrialisation) and the break-up of traditional communities (urbanisation). The study concluded that suicide rates were the consequence of the degree of a person's integration within social groups. Changes in suicide, crime or divorce rates could be analysed as the effects of changing social values and conditions, i.e. breakdown in family or working life, in communities or whole societies.

The patterns that Durkheim identified are still prevalent today. The rates of suicide, morbidity and mortality are generally higher among single and divorced people than among married couples. More men commit suicide than women (although the rate of treated depression is higher in women than in men), and the rate rises with advancing age, due to increasing isolation and poverty. This approach provides insight into those who are 'at risk', the parasuicide rate being much higher.

In the 1950s, American sociologists developed the study of illness and the social institution of medicine in the context of deviance and social control. The work of Parsons (1964), following on from that of Durkheim, signifies the move to a view of illness as social disruption, not spiritual inadequacy. Parsons (1964) sees overcoming of the sick role in the patient's acceptance of medical prescriptions. Patients are relegated to a subservient role which Parsons argues is essential to avoid the sick forming themselves into a group of 'non-productive' people. This social sickness model echoes concerns of a curative medicine. Both have difficulty in accommodating illness that is not of a short-term nature.

Symbolic interactionists have contributed understandings of the problems which arise out of the impersonal values of modern, large-scale organisations. Using the concept of the *total institution*, Goffman (1961) analysed the process of becoming an inmate – a mental patient – as a degrading experience. Through a complicated system of punishments and rewards, the inmate is induced to conform to the house rules. It is hardly surprising that release, rather than rehabilitation, became the ultimate goal. This is institutional rationality taken to its logical extreme: the system designed to run the place is more insane than the patients. This does not, Goffman reassures us, render all staff and patients totally functional to the 'machinery', i.e. the continued production of mentally ill people. He provides examples of resistance by staff and patients to the imposition of the system's values on personal identity. This critical study of *negotiated order* within mental institutions has implications for all those working in organisations geared to their own goals (corporatism).

Further critiques of institutionalised care have been provided by Marxists and feminists. These writers have discussed the role of women as the main producers and consumers of health care in male-dominated societies (Doyal, 1985; Ehrenreich and English, 1976). They see the position of women in the family and employment as the result of a repressive system – not purely a matter of individual choice. Women in families have responsibilities to maintain emotional stability and mental health, a hygienic and safe environment and care of the sick and dependent. The study of the family requires an understanding of its relationship to concepts of health and to women's roles as formal and informal carers (Graham, 1984). Instead of the family being a place of stability and refuge from the competitive 'outside' world of work and politics, feminists reveal the numerous conflicts and abuses of power in relationships between husband and wife, parents and children, and young and old (Dingwall, 1987; O'Bryne, 1988; Pizzey, 1974).

Sociologists are concerned that many families do not have the resources to cope with the social pressures that arise from increasing divorce, unemployment, poverty and long-term sickness, as well as class and racial inequalities and the cuts in social and health provision. Illness in the family can be devastating, as providers cannot work and carers cannot look after the children. Social researchers use statistics from various government publications in the investigation of families, households and health. They take into account a host of demographic variables, such as the distribution of age, mortality, fertility, occupations, immigration, income and poverty. This mass of material is obtained notably from the General Household Survey, Social Trends and the Office of Population Censuses and Surveys (OPCS).

Feminist sociologists and historians have also addressed the situation of nurses in medicine and health (Davies, 1976; Gamarnikow, 1978). They see the position of women in the family and the public health domain as the product of social divisions. Consequently, they reject the essentialist view of some early nurse reformers and contemporary nurse theorists, that women are naturally suited to make a specific contribution to health care. Women are basically cheaper workers and historically their work has been undervalued by employers for this obvious reason. Occupations that have been successful in their claim to a professional status have been male-intensive with upper-class connections, as we have seen. Those which have not succeeded have been female occupations which rely upon open recruitment and immigrant labour (Stacey, 1988; White, 1986).

Marxists as political economists have drawn attention to a fundamental tension in health care. This is the problem of trying to operate as a public service and at the same time as an industry, subject like any other to free 'market forces'. On the one hand, the public service ethos attempts to induce members of its labour force to be spread equitably between the different branches of the service so that all of the work, even the least desirable, is accomplished. On the other hand, as an industry, competition from the market results in high labour shortages in low-wage, low-prestige sectors of the service.

In a capitalist economy, the health industry with its market-driven strategy has to realise profit; all health institutions are committed to the consumption of health goods and services. For example, expensive foetal monitors are introduced into routine obstetric care. Huge profits are made by the pharmaceutical industry, which relies for its existence on the continued emphasis on symptom relief (it makes a fortune from over-the-counter remedies for indigestion). Routine medical care, i.e. general practice, has become increasingly dependent upon prescription drugs and patient details displayed on a computer screen. Doctors do not have to recommend self-medication – the whole population is already addicted (Inglis, 1983). In modern societies, where no one is allowed to rest, we are busy consuming products even when we are sick or immobilised in front of a television set.

Sociologists of health have a strong, if critical, belief in preventive measures. This is in contrast to biomedical health, in which resources are concentrated towards coping with illness after it has occurred. People swallow pills in an effort to relieve the symptoms, because the causes remain a mystery. Illich (1975) sees this *clinical iatrogenesis* as an inevitable consequence of dependency on medical dogma in western industrialised societies. Arguing against 'the establishment', he concludes that the dynamic of human behaviour, including health, is less biological than social.

Changing patterns of ill health

With the development of industrialism in British society, all manner of relationships between people changed. To some sociologists the most relevant of these changes were:

- the separation of the family from the working environment, resulting in specific problems of combining childcare and work for working-class families;
- the coming together of different classes of people in the industrial towns, giving rise to public health and social problems associated with widespread poverty.

The establishment of sociology as an academic discipline arises out of an analysis of these nineteenth-century conditions and social upheavals. Its humanitarian concerns are reflected in classic texts such as *Capital* (first published in 1867; Marx, 1974), *The Division of Labour in Society* (first published in 1886; Durkheim, 1933) and *The Protestant Ethic and the Spirit of Capitalism* (first published in 1904; Weber, 1958).

> In 1917 it was safer to be a soldier on the Western Front than to be born in England. For every nine soldiers killed in France, twelve babies died within their first year of life, in Britain. The infant casualty rate was 1000 per week.
>
> (Iliffe, 1983, p.11)

The Registrar General's social class scale (Blane, 1991, p.116) was introduced in 1911 to aid analysis of variations in infant mortality statistics in particular and demographic statistics in general. The greatest discrepancies between the death rates of the upper classes and those of the rest of the population occurred predominantly in infancy and childhood (Leete and Fox, 1977). Historically, western disease patterns have changed from infectious epidemics to degenerative conditions associated with an increasing lifespan and chronicity.

> In 1901, average life expectancy in the United Kingdom, at birth, was only 45.5 years for men and 49 years for women. In 1991 a newborn male could expect to live 73.2 years on average, a newborn female, 78.8 years.
>
> (Baggott, 1994, p.4)

Control of contagious epidemics during the first part of the twentieth century is often attributed solely to developments in medical science and technology. Examples cited include the safer techniques of modern surgery and the use of anaesthetics, the discovery of antibiotics and improved diagnostic testing. However, the many doubts which exist about medicine's effectiveness make it difficult to accept this view uncritically (Weindling, 1992). After all, one of the major effects of the increasing scale of medical organisation has been the rise in the numbers of people diagnosed as sick (Gomm, 1979).

Sociologists and some medical historians believe that social change has had a greater impact on patterns of health than changes in medical theory. Improved diet and working conditions have enabled people to build up resistance to infectious diseases. Furthermore, the decline in malnutrition, together with a reduction in family size, have had a significant effect on the rates of maternal and infant mortality. Medical intervention is but one aspect of social health promotion (Hart, 1985).

Despite a significant shift in disease burdens, patterns of inequality between different classes persist over generations. In nearly all disease categories, the poorest occupational classes are more affected than the rich.

> This applies equally well to coronary heart disease, stroke and peptic ulcers, which are still sometimes mistakenly referred to as 'diseases of affluence' or 'executive diseases' when in fact they are more common in the manual classes.
>
> (Whitehead, 1990, p.394)

While there has been a rise in general standards of health since the establishment of the National Health Service, marked class gradients are evident at every stage of life. It seems that poverty remains as significant a 'killer' nationally as it is worldwide.

Conclusion

In this chapter I have argued that nursing and health care arise out of institutional arrangements. If health problems are located in individual behaviour rather than in social conditions, then attention is diverted away from the social factors which cause ill health and, in turn, the social reforms necessary for its improvement. At first glance, the self-care concept prevalent in nursing models appears to be a considerable improvement on the 'helpless' patient confined to bed. However, critics of this approach see it as a way of pushing the responsibility back on to individuals in an attempt to justify the reduction in social provision (Crawford, 1977; Pearson and Vaughan, 1986).

Under the influence of the Conservative government's privatisation strategies, hospitals have become technological treatment centres and not the places of care we have relied upon previously. In other words, they have only recently been reduced to their long-professed specialist functions. Patients needing longer-term care have been 'de-housed' back into the environments which gave rise to their problems in the first place. This system does not require caring nurses and other such helpers – it needs relatively fewer technical specialists.

The proposed modular or privatised system of health care is divided up into economic units – everything and everyone becomes a unit of cost. As a consumer or 'Sainsbury's' model of provision, it is based on a self-service, not a self-care, society. For instance, looking across social institutions we can see that this is the model which informs the various modular courses operating in further and higher education, including the nursing curriculum. I tend to view these developments negatively,[7.3] as opportunism (not educational opportunity) and popularism (not pluralism/multiculturalism).

The economistic perspective expounded by the previous government, postulates the existence of 'rational man' – he who is able to make informed choices from a range of market options. In order to participate in the health market, consumers have to be reasonably wealthy, or at least heavily insured, highly knowledgeable and well informed, and hopefully strong enough to travel widely to seek the best quality service. This is a form of health tourism which may not suit the majority of sick, injured and vulnerable people.

Despite modern governmments' presumption that community care is the answer, they are still heavily funding highly techological hospital treatments. Community care remains as always the poor relation. Closing the asylum doors has not meant that mental illness has gone away. Many of these people, out on the streets, have ended up in the criminal justice system.

Sociological analysis is essential to an understanding of current changes and developments in nursing and health systems. I have demonstrated above sociology's contributions and critiques – analysis which is not available in nursing theories. It may appear to many readers as a 'worst-case' scenario, but it is the job of the sociologist to acknowledge major social trends, and to do so with candour. Nurses may want just to be kind and caring nurses – they may wish to keep the theory and politics out of nursing. In contemporary society, however, we have to 'see' through contemporary lenses because change, by definition, does not come upon us in old, familiar ways.

Learning activities

Social science disciplines require students to be imaginative – to 'put themselves in another person's shoes'. Students learn ways of transforming themselves, through ideas, into the world of others. In psychology, we enter the world of individual feelings which underlie cultural traits. In sociology, we enter the systems of meaning which people use to interpret their everyday lives. The discussions outlined below will help students to develop their sociological imagination, to have empathy towards social experiences which may differ from their own.

Topic area 1 – the problem of defining health

Working in pairs, consider the questions below from a sociological perspective:

1. What is health/mental health?
2. Who are the sick/mentally ill?
3. Why are some people healthier than others?
4. What are the 'main killers' today?
5. What were the 'main killers' in the past?
6. What are society's attitudes to mental illness, the elderly, death and dying, drug abuse and HIV/AIDS?
7. What does it feel like to be a professional?
8. How do you think people's health could be improved?

FURTHER DISCUSSION

1. Interview your partner to identify his or her health needs with regard to medical, psychological and social aspects.
2. What does it feel like to be a patient?
3. How do you think your own health could be improved?

Topic area 2 – health and social stratification

Small group discussion – each group should select a note-taker and a speaker to present the group's findings to others in a forum discussion.

Within the social model of health, how would you account for the variations in health status between men and women or middle- and working-class groups or young and old people, or different ethnic/cultural groups, in relation to the following:

1. mortality and morbidity rates;
2. health and safety at work;
3. violence in the family;
4. greater life expectancy.

Endnotes

7.1 Essentialist thinking is a theory of difference ('them' and 'us' view) based upon a series of contradictory assumptions about nature and values. In contemporary culture it has become a form of fundamentalism – an ideology espoused by a leadership in many an interest group, whether it be an academic discipline, identity group or political party. It attempts to explain the special interests of a group as a type of ethical truth for all of us, and for all ages. At one level, moralising about the superiority of one's values appears to be the only certainty – a retreat from any confrontation with the unpleasantness of reality (the disruptions, disorders and humiliations). This may produce an aura of security, but without reference to social and political frames (causal factors) it is unlikely to be more than a nostalgia for a (mythical) future. At the level of political and social theory, this moralism is the means whereby the powerlessness of a group, based on class, race, sexuality or gender, is turned into a distinct 'specialness' which does not challenge conventional arrangements. In the nursing example, professional caring philosophy emphasises the 'uniqueness' of the care that nurses give, but as an adaptation rather than a challenge to the cure–care divide, and the subordinate place of nurses in health and the academy. Leaders speak 'on behalf of all nurses' because nursing is taken to be a unified, stable and professional structure although, paradoxically, science (biological or social) is regarded with great suspicion. While political philosophy is significantly absent from these accounts, moral philosophising, in its present form of relativism, runs riot. Well, not quite. All of this relativism does end somewhere, usually in a wilderness of individual meanings summed up in Mrs Thatcher's maxim: 'There is no such thing as society. There are individual men and women, and there are families' (quoted in Hoggart, 1995, Part One). The version of nursing that emanates from these theorists is too sentimental to be the 'old' professionalism, but is probably the 'new' vocationalism, i.e. individualism and a good-natured conformism. Of particular concern to sociologists are the following: first, the degree to which nursing's benign theory of personalised caring resembles the model of 'professionalism' in consumer services and retail trades (Hochschild, 1983); and, secondly, whether this model signifies future developments in public service professionalism. In terms of sociological measurement, these factors would indicate that the majority of nurses have moved only marginally over the 'class-divide' line, from social class 3 manual to social class 3 non-manual, rather than social class 2 (Registrar General's scale).

Essentialism is represented in numerous current debates in post-modernism and in feminist theory (the infantilising 'woman as victim' view). According to these feminists, men and women are seen to be mutually exclusive categories, i.e. unlike men, women are essentially 'good', nurturing and non-aggressive. These are issues of sexual politics and need to be argued. Thus, the essentialist view has been severely criticised by socialist feminists for failing to address significant social forces maintaining inequalities and subordination in the lives of women which are reduced to some timeless dominance of masculine values over feminine ones (Segal, 1987). Since medicine and nursing are, historically, 'gendered' occupations with differential class associations, it is hardly surprising that issues of sexual politics (see Chapter 8) and class cultures are relevant to analyses of health care policies and practices.

7.2 Nurses' social location in the lower-middle classes is shared by other public sector employees, but also by the majority of those in the work-force, electorate and population in general. In terms of numbers, one would expect people in these strata to have a considerable influence in work, politics and society. However, this is not the case. Even though the values of the majority are predominant in liberal democratic societies such as the UK, and expressed in the previous government's 'back to basics' rhetoric, the material and business interests of less obvious but more powerful groups tend to be uppermost (Hoggart, 1995; Zavarzadeh and Morton, 1991).

7.3. By way of contrast, an optimistic view of modularisation in the nursing curriculum is presented in Chapter 9 of this volume.

References

Abbott P and Wallace C. 1990 Social work and nursing: a history. In Abbott, P. and Wallace, C. (eds), *The sociology of the caring professions*. London: Falmer, 10–28.

Adorno, T. W. 1973 *The jargon of authenticity*. Evanston, IL: Northwestern University Press.

Annandale, E. C. 1989 The malpractice crisis and the doctor–patient relationship. *Sociology of Health and Illness* **11**, 1–23.

Armstrong, D. 1983 *An outline of sociology as applied to medicine,* 2nd edn. Bristol: Wright.

Baggott, R. 1994 *Health and health care in Britain.* Basingstoke: Macmillan.

Beck, U. 1992 *Risk society: towards a new modernity.* London: Sage (translated by M. Ritter).

Becker, H. S., Greer, E. C., Hughes, E.C. and Strauss, A. L. 1961 *Boys in white: student culture in medical school.* Chicago: University of Chicago Press.

Blane, D. 1991 Inequality and social class. In Scambler, G. (ed.), *Sociology as applied to medicine,* 3rd edn. London: Baillière Tindall, 109–28.

Blaxall, M. and Reagan, B. (eds) 1976 *Women and the workplace.* Chicago: University of Chicago Press.

Blaxter, M. and Paterson, E. 1982 *Mothers and daughters: a three-generational study of health attitudes and behaviour.* London: Heinemann Educational Books.

Brown, G. and Harris, T. 1978 *The social origins of depression.* London: Tavistock.

Burrage, M. and Torstendahl, R. (eds) 1990 *Professions in theory and history: rethinking the study of the professions.* London: Sage.

Capra, F. 1982 *The turning point: society and the rising culture.* London: Fontana.

Carpenter, M. 1993 The subordination of nurses in health care. In Riska, E. and Wegar, K. (eds), *Gender, work and medicine.* London: Sage, 95–130.

Carter, E. and Watney, S. (eds) 1989 *Taking liberties: AIDS and cultural politics.* London: Serpent's Tail.

Chapman, C. 1976 The use of sociological theories and models in nursing. *Journal of Advanced Nursing* **1**, 111–27.

Chapman, P. 1984 Specifics and generalities: a critical examination of two nursing models. *Nursing Education Today* **4**, 141–3.

Cornwell, J. 1984 *Hard-earned lives: accounts of health and illness from east London.* London: Tavistock.

Crawford, R. 1977 You are dangerous to your health: the ideology and politics of victim blaming. *International Journal of Health Services* **7**, 663–80.

Crawford, R. 1980 Healthism and the medicalization of everyday life. *International Journal of Health Services* **10**, 365–88.

Crompton, R. and Sanderson, K. 1986 Credentials and careers: some implications of the increase in professional qualifications among women. *Sociology* **20**, 25–42.

Davies, C. 1976 Experience of dependency and control in work: the case of nurses. *Journal of Advanced Nursing* **1**, 273–82.

Davis, F. 1975 Professional socialization as subjective experience: the process of doctrinal conversion among student nurses. In Cox, C. and Mead, A. (eds), *A sociology of medical practice.* London: Collier-Macmillan, 116–31.

Davis, K. and Moore, W. E. 1967 Some principles of stratification. In Bendix, R. and Lipset, S.M. (eds), *Class, status and power,* 2nd edn. London: Routledge and Kegan Paul, 47–53.

DeVries, R. G. 1993 A cross-national view of the status of midwives. In Riska, E. and Wegar, K. (eds), *Gender, work and medicine.* London: Sage, 131–46.

de Wolfe, P. 1996 A world without illness? The 'thinking away' of the chronically sick. In Perry, A. (ed.), *Sociology: insights in health care.* London: Edward Arnold, 107–32.

Dingwall, R. 1987 No need to panic. *Nursing Times and Nursing Mirror* **83**, 28–30.

Doyal, L. 1985 Women and the NHS. In Lewin, E. and Olesen, V. (eds), *Women, health and healing.* New York: Tavistock, 236–69.

Doyal, L. 1995 *What makes women sick: gender and the political economy of health.* Basingstoke: Macmillan.

Durkheim, E. 1933 *The division of labour in society.* New York: Free Press.

Durkheim, E. 1952 *Suicide.* London: Routledge and Kegan Paul.

Ehrenreich, B. and English, D. 1976 *Witches, midwives and nurses: a history of women healers.* London: Writers and Readers Publishing Co-operative.

Ellman, L. 1996 Sugar and spice and not very nice. *Independent on Sunday* (Supplement), 4 February, p.14.

Elston, M. A. 1993 Women doctors in a changing profession: the case of Britain. In Riska, E. and Wegar, K. (eds), *Gender, work and medicine.* London: Sage, 27–61.

Fitzpatrick, R. 1986 Social causes of disease. In Patrick, D. and Scambler, G. (eds), *Sociology as applied to medicine,* 2nd edn. London: Baillière Tindall, 30–40.

Fitzpatrick, R., Hinton, J., Newman, S., Scambler, G. and Thompson, J. 1984 *The experience of illness.* London: Tavistock.

Foucault, M. 1973a *Madness and civilization: a history of insanity in the age of reason.* New York: Vintage Books.

Foucault, M. 1973b *The birth of the clinic: an archaeology of medical perception.* London: Tavistock.

Foucault, M. 1977 *Discipline and punish: the birth of the prison.* Harmondsworth: Penguin.

Francome, C. 1986 The fashion for caesarians. *New Society* **75**, 100–101.

Freidson, E. 1970 *Professional dominance.* New York: Aldine Atherton.

Gamarnikow, E. 1978 Sexual division of labour: the case of nursing. In Kuhn, A. and Wolpe, A. (eds), *Feminism and materialism: women and modes of production.* London: Routledge and Kegan Paul, 96–123.

Gaze, H. 1987 Man appeal. *Nursing Times and Nursing Mirror* **83**, 24–7.

Goffman, E. 1959 *The presentation of self in everyday life.* New York: Anchor Books.

Goffman, E. 1961 *Asylums: essays on the social situations of mental patients and other inmates.* Harmondsworth: Penguin.

Gomm, R. 1979 Social science and medicine. In Meighan, R., Shelton, I. and Marks, T. (eds), *Perspectives on society.* Sunbury on Thames: Nelson, 240–60.

Graham, H. 1984 *Women, health and the family.* Brighton: Wheatsheaf.

Green, H. 1964 *I never promised you a rose garden.* London: Pan.

Greenwell, J. 1996 Sociology of the NHS: when does the community decide? In Perry, A. (ed.), *Sociology: insights in health care.* London: Edward Arnold, 133–61.

Haralambos, M. with Heald, R. M. 1980 *Sociology: themes and perspectives.* Slough: University Tutorial Press.

Hardy, L. 1986 Identifying the place of theoretical frameworks in an evolving discipline. *Journal of Advanced Nursing* **11**, 103–7.

Hart, N. 1985 *The sociology of health and medicine.* Ormskirk: Causeway.

Hibbert, C. 1996 Medical therapeutic research: ethical and legal issues in randomised control trials. In Perry, A. (ed.), *Sociology: insights in health care.* London: Edward Arnold, 186–210.

Hochschild, A. R. 1983 *The managed heart: commercialization of human feeling.* Berkeley: University of California Press.

Hoggart, R. 1995 *The way we live now.* London: Pimlico.

Hughes, E. 1958 *Men and their work.* Glencoe, IL: Free Press.

Hughes, R. 1993 *Culture of complaint: the fraying of America.* New York: Oxford University Press.

Hugman, R. 1991 *Power in caring professions.* Basingstoke: Macmillan.

Iliffe, S. 1983 *The NHS: a picture of health?* London: Lawrence and Wishart.

Illich, I. 1975 *Medical nemesis: the expropriation of health.* London: Calder and Boyars.

Inglis, B. 1983 *The diseases of civilization.* London: Granada.

Jacobs, J. 1969 Symbolic bureaucracy: a case of a social welfare agency. *Social Forces* **47**, 413–22.

Jamous, H. and Peloille, B. 1970 Professions or self-perpetuating systems? Changes in the French university hospital system. In Jackson, J. A. (ed.), *Professions and professionalization.* Cambridge: Cambridge University Press, 111–52.

Jewson, R. and Mason, D. 1986 Modes of discrimination in the recruitment process: formalisation, fairness and efficiency. *Sociology* **20**, 43–63.

Johnson, T. 1972 *Professions and power.* London: Macmillan.

Jones, L. J. 1994 *The social context of health and health work.* Basingstoke: Macmillan.

Khaw, K. T. 1993 Where are the women in studies of coronary heart disease? *British Medical Journal* **306**,1145–46.

King, I. M. 1981 *A theory for nursing.* New York: Wiley.

Leete, R. and Fox, J. 1977 Registrar General's social classes: origins and uses. *Population Trends* **8**, 1–7.

Mackay, L. 1989 *Nursing a problem.* Milton Keynes: Open University Press.

Marx, K. 1974 *Capital: a critical analysis of capitalist production. Vol. 1.* London: Lawrence and Wishart.

May. C. 1992a Individual care? Power and subjectivity in therapeutic relationships. *Sociology* **26**, 589–602.

May, C. 1992b Nursing work, nurses' knowledge, and the subjectification of the patient. *Sociology of Health and Illness* **14**, 472–487.

Mechanic, D. 1995 Sociological dimensions of illness behavior. *Social Science and Medicine* **41**, 1207–16.

Melia, K. 1987 *Learning and working: the occupational socialization of nurses.* London: Tavistock.

Melville, A. and Johnson, C. 1982 *Cured to death: the effects of prescription drugs.* London: Secker and Warburg.

Michels, R. 1949 *Political parties.* Glencoe, IL: Free Press.

Miles, A. 1991 *Women, health and medicine.* Milton Keynes: Open University Press.

Miller, T. 1996 Exploring the process of becoming a mother: narratives and narrative construction around childbearing. *Medical Sociology News* **21**, 24–32.

Morgan, M., Calnan, M. and Manning, N. 1985 *Sociological approaches to health and medicine.* London: Croom Helm.

Navarro, V. 1977 *Social security and medicine in the USSR.* Lexington: Heath.

Navarro, V. 1993 *Dangerous to your health: capitalism in health care.* New York: Monthly Review Press.

Neuman, B. 1980 The Betty Neuman health-care systems model: a total person approach to patient problems. In Riehl, J. and Roy, C. (eds), *Conceptual models for nursing practice*, 2nd edn. New York: Appleton-Century-Crofts, 119–34.

Oakley, A. 1976 The family, marriage, and its relationship to illness. In Tuckett, D. (ed.), *Introduction to medical sociology.* London: Tavistock, 74–109.

Oakley, A. 1980 *Women confined: towards a sociology of childbirth.* Oxford: Martin Robertson.

O'Bryne, J. 1988 High abuse figure indicates low status of old people. *Geriatric Nursing and Home Care* **8**, 6.

O'Donnell, M. 1981 *The new introduction to sociology.* London: Harrap.

Open University 1985 *Experiencing and explaining disease.* Course U205, Health and Disease, Book VI. Milton Keynes: Open University Press.

Orem, D. E. 1980 *Nursing: concepts of practice*, 3rd edn. New York: McGraw-Hill.

Parsons, T. 1964 *The social system*. New York: Free Press.

Parsons, T. 1979 Definitions of health and illness in the light of American values and social structure. In Jaco, E. G. (ed.), *Patients, physicians and illness*, 3rd edn. New York: Free Press, 120–44.

Pearson, A. and Vaughan, B. 1986 *Nursing models for practice*. London: Heinemann.

Peplau, H. E. 1952 *Interpersonal relations in nursing*. New York: Putnam.

Perry, A. 1993 A sociologist's view: the handmaiden's theory. In Jolley, M. and Brykczynska, G. (eds), *Nursing: its hidden agendas*. London: Edward Arnold, 43–79.

Perry, A. 1996 Introduction. In Perry, A. (ed.), *Sociology: insights in health care*. London: Edward Arnold, 1–10.

Petticrew, M., McGee, M. and Jones, J. 1993 Coronary artery surgery: are women discriminated against? *British Medical Journal* **306**,1164–66.

Pfeffer, N. 1993 *The stork and the syringe: a political history of reproductive medicine*. Cambridge: Polity Press.

Pizzey, E. 1974 *Scream quietly or the neighbours might hear*. Harmondsworth: Penguin.

Prior, L. 1993 *The social organization of mental illness*. London: Sage.

Richman, J. 1987 *Medicine and health*. London: Longman Group.

Roy, C. 1976 *Introduction to nursing: an adaptation model*. New Jersey: Prentice-Hall.

Salvage, J. 1985 *The politics of nursing*. London: Heinemann.

Schaef, A. W. and Fassel, D. 1988 *The addictive organization*. San Francisco: Harper and Row.

Seabrook, J. 1985 The fall of the caring classes. *New Society* **73**, 190–92.

Segal, L. 1987 *Is the future female? Troubled thoughts on contemporary feminism*. London: Virago.

Smith, P. 1992 *The emotional labour of nursing*. Basingstoke: Macmillan.

Solzhenitsyn, A. 1971 *Cancer ward*. Harmondsworth: Penguin.

Stacey, M. 1988 *The sociology of health and healing*. London: Unwin Hyman.

Stanworth, M. (ed.) 1987 *Reproductive technologies: gender, motherhood and medicine*. Cambridge: Polity Press.

Stein, L. 1967 The doctor–nurse game. *Archives of General Psychiatry* **16**, 699–703.

Stein, L., Watts, D. and Howell, T. 1990 The doctor–nurse game revisited. *The Lamp* **47**, 23–6.

Strong, P. 1979 Sociological imperialism and the profession of medicine: a critical examination of the thesis of medical imperialism. *Social Science and Medicine* **13A**, 199–215.

Strong, P. and Robinson, J. 1988 *New model management: Griffiths and the NHS*. Coventry: University of Warwick, Nursing Policy Studies Centre.

Torstendahl, R. and Burrage, M. (eds) 1990 *The formation of professions: knowledge, state and strategy*. London: Sage.

Towers, B. 1996 Health care and the new managerialism: policy, planning and organisations. In Perry, A. (ed.), *Sociology: insights in health care*. London: Edward Arnold, 30–53.

Townsend, P. and Davidson, N. 1982 *Inequalities in health: the Black Report*. Harmondsworth: Penguin.

Townsend, P., Davidson, N. and Whitehead, M. 1990 *Inequalities in health: the Black Report 1980 and the Health Divide*. London: Penguin.

Tudor Hart, J. 1975 The inverse care law. In Cox, C. and Mead, A. (eds), *A sociology of medical practice*. London: Collier–Macmillan, 189–206.

Turner, B. 1987 *Medical power and social knowledge*. London: Sage.

Walby, S., Greenwell, J., Mackay, L. and Soothill, K. 1994 *Medicine and nursing: professions in a changing health service*. London: Sage.

Waldron, I. 1976 Why do women live longer than men? *Social Science and Medicine* **10**, 349–62.

Weber, M. 1958 *The protestant ethic and the spirit of capitalism* (translated by T. Parsons). New York: Scriber.

Weindling, P. 1992 From infections to chronic illness: changing patterns of sickness in the nineteenth and twentieth centuries. In Wear, A. (ed.), *Medicine in society: historical essays*. Cambridge: Cambridge University Press, 303–16.

White, R. 1986 *The effects of the NHS on the nursing profession 1948–1961*. London: King Edward's Hospital Fund.

Whitehead, M. 1990 The health divide. In Townsend, P., Davidson, N. and Whitehead, M., *Inequalities in health: the Black Report 1980 and the Health Divide*. London: Penguin, 221–356.

Witz, A. 1992 *Professions and patriarchy*. London: Routledge.

Witz, A. 1994 The challenge of nursing. In Gabe, J., Kelleher, D. and Williams, G. (eds), *Challenging medicine*. London: Routledge, 23–45.

Zavarzadeh, M. and Morton, D. 1991 *Theory (post)modernity opposition*. Washington: Maisonneuve Press.

Power, politics and policy analysis in nursing

8

Jane Robinson

The word 'politics' is enlisted here when speaking of the sexes primarily because such a word is eminently useful in outlining the real nature of their relative status, historically and at the present. It is opportune, perhaps today even mandatory, that we develop a more relative psychology and philosophy of power relationships beyond the simple conceptual framework provided by our traditional formal politics. Indeed, it may be imperative that we give some attention to defining a theory of politics which treats power relationships on grounds less conventional than those to which we are accustomed. I have therefore found it pertinent to define them on grounds of personal contact and interaction between members of well-defined and coherent groups; races, castes, classes and sexes. For it is precisely because certain groups have no representation in a number of recognised political structures that their position tends to be stable, their oppression so continuous.

(Millett, 1977, p.24)

A personal note to begin

The approach to politics and policy analysis presented in this chapter represents an airing of some of the ideas which have been fermenting for most of the past 15 years. Entry in 1977 into the (part-time) world of academia to study for an MA by research began the slow and often painful process of consolidation of previously disjointed ideas and experiences. The process can be compared to peering down the tube of a kaleidoscope and seeing at first only a jumble of assorted shapes and colours. Shake the tube gently and suddenly a coherent pattern emerges; turn it again and the colours and images present in sharply different focus. The contents of the kaleidoscope are unchanged, but there is a constant stream of opportunities to see them in different profiles and orderings of significance. The process of conceptual clarification is always demanding higher levels of refinement. Hence the drive to clarify one's ideas is never complete, for they are being tested and re-tested continuously by various means (see Chapter 10). Publication is one vital stage in this testing process, and looking back over the years certain themes recur in my tentative attempts to express in public the issues which concerned me greatly. Questions of power and oppression are never far from the surface, especially in relation to women; women as either the recipients of health care services or women as part of the health care delivery system. And women in these situations are often divided on two sides of a fence, instead of pressing together for the recognition of their problems as valid policy issues in the public, political world of men. I wrote on these themes concerning women in Jolley and Allan's book *Current Issues in Nursing* (1989), with which this chapter could usefully be read in conjunction. Here I am beginning to locate the study of nursing political issues within a developing critical policy analysis tradition. It draws on many different sources of literature, and beginning to make sense of its jumble of origins takes us back to the unshaken kaleidoscope. Nevertheless it is a beginning, and in the first part of the chapter I set out some basic definitions, supported by certain key references. In the second, much longer part, I begin to construct an analysis of several of the most well-known published works on nursing politics. The re-working of other people's ideas is another important way of moving conceptual analysis further[8.1]. The reader is left to draw his or her own conclusions as to whether the product 'fits' the experience of his or her own 'life world'. Whether it does or not, readers are invited to participate themselves in taking up the challenge, and to refute or refine the ideas so presented. The creation of knowledge is not some elite form of occupation for the chosen few – it is something with which we should all be concerned and in which we should actively participate.

Introduction

The 1980s have seen an upsurge of interest in what may be termed 'the politics of nursing'. A succession of books, all with nursing and politics in their titles, have been published (Clay, 1987; Salvage, 1985; White, 1985, 1986a, 1988), and speakers urging nurses to become more political have become a familiar aspect of the Nursing Conference circuit. Yet, despite all the *talk* of politics and political consciousness in nursing, there has been little theoretical development derived from the now fairly substantial case-study literature on nurses' experiences of unequal power relationships and the welcome awakening of interest in a subject previously considered taboo by the professional nurse. We are able to describe but not yet to *explain* the phenomenon. This is not at all surprising – the discourse of public policy is the discourse of *men*. Feminist theorists (with whom nurse theorists share much in common but also some important differences; Robinson, 1989) have recognised and struggled with this problem. The quotation taken from Kate Millett's book *Sexual Politics*, with which this chapter began, illustrates how the very basis of 'taken for granted' assumptions about the nature of special relationships has to be questioned in order to begin to understand the *unquestioning* acceptance of oppression by certain social groups.

Part One: the development of a critical approach to politics and policy analysis in nursing

To begin to understand political issues in nursing in terms of unequal power relationships requires the study of a complex web of social interactions. They are complex because they involve nursing's relationship to both specific and general government policies on health and welfare, and also to its own internal policies. These are developed against the backdrop of the social and economic circumstances in which the activity of nursing is practised – so these too should inform the debates. This contextualisation of issues proved crucial in the 4-year study of the management of nursing following the implementation of general management in the National Health Service (Robinson and Strong, 1987; Robinson et al., 1989; Strong and Robinson, 1988, 1990), for without the analysis of the broad picture it would not have been possible to illuminate how relatively unimportant nursing is to government and to managers in comparison with medicine. This insight led us to conclude that nursing remains in the social equivalent of an astronomical Black Hole. It appeared from our empirical evidence that even when nurses themselves were trying actively to break free from the negative gravitational force of tradition, and not all of them were, others on the outside showed little interest in trying to harness, or even to understand, the frustrated energies locked deep within the occupation of nursing. And this was not, apparently, a temporary aberration in policy matters, for the process whereby many senior nurses were side-stepped and stripped of their power during the structural changes in the NHS following the Griffiths Report (NHS Management Inquiry Team, 1983) appears to be continuing unabated with the resignation of one of the most formidable Regional Nursing Officers in the country (*Nursing Times and Nursing Mirror*, 1989).

Perspectives on power, politics, policy and decision-making

Before going further with this particular line of critical policy analysis, it is important to stand back and to set it within more conventional definitions of politics and policy studies. Pollitt *et al.* (1979) and Ham and Hill (1986) argue that because the terms politics and policy[8.2] have evolved untidily, writers should avoid the intellectual imperialism of insisting upon tight, stipulative definitions. Indeed, as Millett (1977) argues, the unquestioning acceptance of imposed definitions can lock us into accepting the very assumptions we ought to be questioning. At first sight definitions *appear* nevertheless to be relatively straightforward. The Greek word *polis* is the root for both English words *policy* and *politics* which, according to the Shorter Oxford English Dictionary, refers to issues concerned with citizenship, government and the state. Hence political *theory* has been concerned traditionally with the science and art of government, and in particular with the form, organisation and administration of the whole, or some part, of the state. Things are less straightforward, however, when we return to the *applied* aspects of policy and politics. First, it is important to recognise that the terms policy analysis, policy studies and public administration have often been used interchangeably. Secondly, such studies are *multidisciplinary* and may draw on the insights of disciplines as varied as economics, psychology, sociology, history and anthropology. Thirdly, they consist of two main approaches, used either simply or in conjunction with one another:

- the description, evaluation and solution of practical problems;
- the analysis of the way in which societies go about these same tasks.

In other words, policy studies involve *both* the acquisition of knowledge and the development of theories about problems *and* an understanding of the political issues involved in solving them. These issues turn centrally on the question of *power* and how it is mediated in the policy process. Policy studies in nursing can help therefore not only to clarify some of the political issues involved in providing a nursing service within a health care system, but also to unravel some more general aspects of power in the policy-making process.

The substantive *area* of nursing is, of course, the subject matter of nursing policy studies. There may, however, be many different *topics* within it. For example, policy may be analysed in respect of clinical nursing, nurse education, nurses' pay or the management of nursing. The study of each of these policies involves, as mentioned above, *many different modes of thinking* – sociological, economic, historical, political theory, psychological, and so forth. Hence the claim that policy studies is a multidisciplinary activity. Thus collections such as *Readings in the Sociology of Nursing* (Dingwall and McIntosh, 1978), *Re-writing Nursing History* (Davies, 1980a) and *Understanding Nurses: the Social Psychology of Nursing* (Skevington, 1984) all help to illuminate in some way political issues in nursing.

The impossibility of merely *describing* events without seeking to draw policy lessons from them is also increasingly acknowledged. Hence the analysis *of* policy becomes almost invariably a case *for* policy. In this sense the activity can never be value-neutral. Rein (1976) challenges researchers to acknowledge this situation. However, as he notes, this does not mean abandoning scholarly values. Rein also urges the importance of a sceptical approach and the need to develop a value-critical stance to policy issues. This requires the analyst to question his or her own values as well as those he or she seeks to study. Nurses, in particular, need to take this lesson to heart or their writing on policy issues can become barely concealed polemic.

Policy studies implies then not just the gathering of facts about an issue, but also the analysis of how and why the issue becomes, or does not become, 'a problem' worthy of public attention and solution. It follows that one of the central topics of policy studies is how and why some issues get selected as a serious problem for public concern while others, potentially no less important, are neglected. The how and why crucially concern matters of power and influence. Nursing, with little of either, is rarely an issue in public policy. An important topic for research must therefore be when, and about what, nursing issues become matters for public concern.

Two important interrelated issues arise from the above discussion for nursing policy studies. First, where is nursing placed in relation to the location and exercise of power – power both external and internal to the profession? Secondly, where does nursing stand in relation to particular institutional frameworks for health and social welfare? In order to move forward on these issues it is important to investigate further the nature of power and decision-making.

Power and decision-making

There are many theoretical analyses of the nature of power and of its distribution within society. Ham and Hill (1986) group the major studies which examine the relationship of power to decision-making into three broad categories which theorists have developed over the past 15 years. First, there are those which study the power to make key, concrete policy decisions. These are generally focused on actual decision-making behaviour. They analyse whether the power to make decisions is concentrated within one or several élite groups or, alternatively, through a pluralistic system in which various regulatory mechanisms ensure that ultimately the majority view prevails. This approach embodies the notion of an ultimate rationality in decision-making and the power to ensure a consensus in policy terms in order to achieve that goal. It tends to focus, therefore, on studying those who already hold a considerable measure of power to shape events!

The second group of studies originates from the critiques of the nature of power portrayed in the first. They are concerned with analysing the power to keep key issues *off* the policy agenda – and involve the nature of non-decision-making. Bachrach and Baratz (1962) were among the first to develop an argument for this approach to policy studies, and their original article remains highly relevant. This perspective has, in turn, been criticised because of the empirical difficulty of demonstrating the nature of a non-decision. Nevertheless, writers such as Crenson (1971) have illustrated, for example, the indirect influence of the economic power of a major industrial monopoly in preventing the passage of clean air legislation.

The third dimension of power (as developed by Lukes, 1974) is the product of more than a decade of debate over the validity of the first two perspectives. Lukes' (1986) position, which is developed from and loosely related to the second, argues (despite the even greater problems of empirical validation) that power concerns the subtle and complex ways in which 'the sheer weight of institutions – political, industrial and education' (p.38) serve to shape people's cognitions, perceptions and preferences. As a result:

> they accept their role in the existing order of things, either because they can see or imagine no alternative to it, or because they see it as natural and unchangeable, or because they value it as divinely ordained and beneficial. To assume that the absence of grievance equals genuine consensus is simply to rule out the possibility of false or manipulated consensus by definitional fiat.
>
> (Lukes, 1986, p.24)

Other authors have explored similar ideas, and the study of policy in the field of health care provides rich examples of his view that power is sustained through the values of dominant belief systems. Alford (1975) argues that the politics of health care are governed by dominant, challenging and repressed structural interests. He sees the sustaining of the medical model of health and illness as being of fundamental importance to the maintenance of the dominant structural interests and therefore the power of the doctors. Certainly the events observed in the 4-year study of the management of nursing after the implementation of Griffiths, referred to above, could be explained as a fundamental struggle by the government, represented by general managers, to challenge the dominant power of medicine. The invisibility of nursing in this struggle merely confirms its status as a repressed policy interest (see Chapter 7).

Ideology, politics and health care

The position arrived at so far suggests that politics may be seen as the possession of power to ensure that:

- certain issues become defined as valid for policy concern and therefore receive a place on the public policy agenda; or
- certain issues are kept off the public policy agenda, whether deliberately or by default.

Women's issues, of which nursing may be seen as one subset, are rarely counted as matters of valid policy concern except in time of national emergency, such as war. Even then the issues tend to be defined in ways which ensure that they can be removed from the agenda as soon as the emergency is over. Child-care facilities, for instance, are seen as important in order to release women to contribute to the national work effort, rather than to enable them to pursue careers and fulfil their individual potential. Clearly, a third crucial aspect of power must then concern *the ability to define issues in such a way that they can meet certain chosen means and ends.* Means and ends imply values, and values involve an underlying ideology. Hence policy is never value-neutral, but is always founded on an implicit or explicit belief system (see Chapter 5). For example, if women's first obligation is to their home and children it follows, according to this particular value system, that child-care facilities are unnecessary unless a greater obligation (the national good) intervenes, when the first may take a lower priority than the second.

Describing issues in this way may sound emotive, and it is crucial to emphasise that the underlying system of ideas *is* neutral. It is only when the ideas are put into practice and, as a result, some people's interests suffer at the expense of others that feelings and emotions come into play. The Shorter Oxford English Dictionary defines ideology in two ways:

- the science of ideas; the study of the origin and nature of ideas;
- a system of ideas concerning phenomena, especially those of social life; the manner of thinking characteristic of a class or an individual.

It is the incorporation of ideas into a system which can command the power to define goods and services according to their *value* which translates ideology into a political belief system. Hence, in a detailed study of welfare work, Cousins (1987) sees contradictions in the values applied to caring work such as nursing. On the one hand, there is a 'factory-like logic' where welfare labour is subjected to wage pressure and de-skilling similar to that applied in the private sector reflecting Marx's ideas of an *exchange value* for labour. On the other hand, Cousins argues that welfare services are produced also in terms of alternative moral values:

> These services (also) provide a material resource for labour that mitigates to some extent the exploitative relation of capital and labour, especially for women and ethnic minority groups. The state sector can provide progressive employment and labour relations practices – for instance equal opportunities practices, contract compliance policies, or health and safety procedures – practices which advance the public interest although these may not be the agencies' specific policy objectives.
>
> (Cousins, 1987, p.185)

The move during the 1970s from a political consensus over the provision of state welfare to one which emphasises the rights and obligations of individuals within a market economy is documented by Deakin (1987) and Klein (1983, 1989), and the range of different systems of ideas involved in what has come to be called 'The New Right' is described by Green (1987). In summarising the relationship between markets and morality Green describes a set of beliefs which are almost completely at variance with those set out by Cousins above:

> It is frequently said that markets promote selfishness ... that there can be little doubt that the market fosters personal attributes, such as greed and a lack of concern for one's neighbour ... What truth is there in such claims? The new liberals have typically argued, not that selfishness is a

good thing, but that selfishness exists whether we like it or not, and they have urged that we must therefore strive towards institutions which prevent selfishness from doing too much harm. Competition is said to be the chief safeguard available ... . The case for liberty rests only in part on the value of competition in channelling the efforts of possibly selfish individuals into the service of their fellows. It also rests on the belief that there are any number of alternative ways of meeting human wants – some like charity and mutual aid the very antithesis of profit seeking – and that only in a free society can such alternatives flourish.

(Green, 1987, p.217)

The task of the policy analyst is to tease out the concepts and values which underpin statements such as these, and then to evaluate the consequences of their application for different groups of people involved in the system. Feminists would argue, for example, that charity and mutual aid usually involve the exploitation of women somewhere in the process, while state welfare, too, has depended on the cheap use of women's labour. The latter has had the benefit, however, of providing a sense of identity with health care as a moral enterprise – an identity which is fast becoming alienated as welfare work is transformed into a market economy through contracting out and other mechanisms (Tonkin and Hart, 1989).

Part Two: politics and policy analysis in nursing – some examples from the literature

Thinking about the issues to be discussed in the second part of this chapter began in 1987 when four of the five books on nursing politics cited at the beginning of the introduction had been recently published. Asked at that time to review one of them (White, 1986a) I found myself struggling to identify a conceptual framework which would provide a structure for analysis across the wide range of nursing topics which were being called *political*. It was very difficult. White's two extant publications contained a range of fascinating case study material, but one was hard put to discover a unifying political theme running through them.[8.3] Indeed, while the notion of power was always implicit, the mechanisms through which it is mediated in nursing were rarely discussed. Similarly, Salvage (1985) and Clay (1987), while arguing very strongly for consciousness-raising and political awareness among nurses, seemed to be coming at the problem from different positions.

In examining White's work at that time I tentatively identified five broad categories within which the subject matter of her 1985 and 1986a edited collections could be discussed. These were:

1. the case for unity in nursing: a false premise?
2. the divisive effects on nursing of cost-containment and other contemporary policy initiatives;

3. the marginalisation of nursing arising from the implicit value conflicts in health policy;
4. the structural effects of class and gender on nursing;
5. the power of nurses as oppressors.

In writing this chapter in 1989 I returned to my earlier (unpublished) paper to try to identify how well White's further (1988) collection could be fitted together with Clay's and Salvage's work into the framework provisionally developed for the two earlier volumes. Even with subsequent modification it is still not perfect for conceptual analysis. One particular problem is that there is considerable overlap between the categories. Nevertheless it is a beginning. Setting out the discussion which follows within this modified structure, I am conscious of writing for a textbook on the knowledge base for nursing practice. This seems to be an excellent forum in which to achieve the following important goals: to declare the provisional state of our knowledge on nursing politics; to demonstrate the very different perspectives which are already emanating from this embryonic conceptual debate; to challenge students to continue the process of clarification through their projects and essays; and to plead with them for *publication*, so that our knowledge base can be developed and refined. What follows is no definitive state of the art – it is put forward for challenge and refutation.

The framework in current use

Returning to the analysis referred to above after a two-year breathing space I was struck by the need for a greater sense of balance in the proposed framework. Subjects did not appear as clear-cut as when I had reviewed them earlier. Nurses were putting forward varied perspectives on the same subject. The framework was therefore modified as follows:

1. nursing as a force for challenge and change – the costs and benefits of unity;
2. contemporary health policy initiatives – the potential and the risks for nurses and their clients;
3. the structure of nursing – its constraints and its potential for development;
4. class, gender and race in nursing;
5. nurses as oppressors or enablers – power for or against each other and the client?

The following discussion sets some of the contents of the five books cited in the introduction within the above framework. Surprisingly, given nurses' increasing challenge to the medical model, the five volumes contain relatively little about nursing's relationship with medicine. They do, however, contain rich empirical evidence for nursing's place within different welfare systems. Also strongly implicit is the idea of conflicting values and the pressures to which these subject different groups of nurses. This leads naturally to the issues concerning power and value systems described in Part One. Hopefully this process moves us slowly but closer to an underlying theory, or theories, of politics in nursing.

Nursing as a force for challenge and change: the costs and benefits of unity

Two conflicting issues dominate much of the material in the five books:

- the contribution made to its powerlessness by the historic divisions within nursing;
- nursing as a potential force for challenge and change in health care.

The authors all have very different ideas about how to resolve the first in order to achieve the second. Trevor Clay, writing as General Secretary of the Royal College of Nursing, put forward a powerful argument for unity within one umbrella staff organisation:

> This diversity, currently a weakness, could, if unified, be the profession's greatest strength. Of course, it is the RCN's belief that the profession will be stronger and serve society better if there is only one organisation for nurses called the RCN.
>
> (Clay, 1987, p.29)

He disagrees vehemently with Rosemary White's (1985) account of nursing as a pluralistic society and her argument that 'the enforcement of a unitary policy, of consensus, inhibits change,' (Clay, 1987, p.33). White, in her turn, is equally convinced of the power of diversity – although there is little doubt that her sympathies lie with the professionalist group of nurses who look for their authority to 'higher education and a specialized knowledge base' (White, 1988, p.19). In describing three distinguishable groups White identifies two, the managers and the professionals, who, by virtue of identifying with the value systems of their respective peer groups, are locked within inevitable conflict. The remainder, the 'generalists', are in White's terminology 'the task workers ... content to work within the hierarchy, supervised by the nurse managers' (p.19). It is this third group with whom Jane Salvage, in a book which 'strongly reflects the author's own feminist and socialist beliefs' (Dunn, 1985), apparently identifies. Her belief that the personal is political and that nurses at *all* levels should be aware of, and react to, policy initiatives which constrain their practice also brings its own sharp rebuff from Trevor Clay. He only agrees on one level with Salvage's argument that 'nurses must confront the consequences of political and policy decisions as they affect them in work and in their personal experience of those decisions' (1987, p.2). He supports nurses in 'a little personal confrontation' (with the hierarchy, doctors or general managers), but when it comes to threatening patients' welfare 'there is another way' (p.3). Unsurprisingly, the route lies, in Clay's terms, through organising as a profession and as a trade union.

Here, in simplified terms, we see some of the fundamental roots of disagreement within nursing over ways of overcoming its powerlessness. Each of these highly credited authors puts forward the values derived from his or her system of ideas; we hear the views of the professional trade union, the representative of a professional elite, and the voice of the worker on the ward. It is fascinating to reflect that the third, proletarian, view is expressed by a nurse who entered nursing after a Cambridge degree, and went on after working as a staff nurse to become a highly respected nurse journalist and eventually a supporter of nursing development units – a true grass-roots movement (Salvage, 1990). Already it is possible to see from this brief outline of the different systems expressed that we do not need to look outside nursing in order to begin to appreciate the location and exercise of power. We may guess but do not yet understand how different career patterns may influence individual perceptions of power and change. Hardy in White (1986a) begins to explore the politics of the career histories of senior nurses but there is, as yet, no systematic attempt to explain the relationship between biography and ideology.

It is possible, however, to tease out the importance of historical and cultural contexts to nursing developments from other authors in White's collections. Larsen (1988) in White (1988) argues for nursing leaders to understand the politics of public policy-making and to act appropriately. Unsupported by reference to empirical evidence, her case verges on the polemic. Perhaps in Canada (of which she writes) nurses are more able to become politically assertive, but we should not assume that this form of action is feasible in every culture. Davies (1980b) develops an extremely useful international comparative perspective on nurse education in the UK and the USA up to 1939, which helps us to understand the importance and complexity of cultural variation. She concludes that American nurses had far greater self-confidence than the British. In addition, there were differences in the legislative framework, the educational system and the patterns of employment available to them. Asking why such arrangements were available in the USA and not in the UK, Davies states that the answer would require:

> a consideration of how economic, political and social forms are deeply intertwined. The point of the present argument, however, is to show that a different matrix of institutions gives different experiences and different opportunities for compromise and struggle for an occupational group such as nurses.
>
> (Davies, 1980b, p.115)

Davies' lesson is that the defining and achievement of policy goals cannot be understood divorced from the cultural context in which they are formulated.

Zwanger's (1986) account of Jewish nursing education in Palestine between 1914 and 1948 provides a national comparative perspective. There was, it seems, a striking difference between the content of the syllabi in the British colonial schools of nursing in Palestine and those in Jewish national nursing schools. The British were committed to traditional forms of training, and the Jewish to wider educational values. Regrettably, Zwanger's description excludes any analysis of the respective political ideologies involved. Nevertheless one detects the implicit notion of higher values being placed on nurse education by national interest groups than by the resident colonial power. Is this, we may enquire, characteristic of nationalist movements everywhere and, if so, what part do women play in these drives for self-determination? If, as may be hypothesised, their contribution is more highly valued during periods of intense pro-nationalist activity, does nursing, by association, stand to benefit? Alternatively, are women naturally more assertive during these periods of historical development?

Further international comparisons may be made from White's collections. For example, can a parallel be drawn between the situation described in Palestine and the account of nursing's move to higher education in Australia described by Parkes (1986)? She attributes the successful outcome of the struggle for educational reform in Australia during the 30 years following the Second World War to her belief that the education movement amongst nurses served as a massive consciousness-raising activity and as a focus for unity. This unity, Parkes argues, together with the increased political partici- pation which followed, was both a necessary and a sufficient condition for change. Her analysis in this respect does not ring entirely true. She does not account for *party* political influence in Australia at that time and the national commitment to increase female participation in higher education. This may have been the *sufficient* condition required before nurses' *necessary* activity in campaigning for higher education produced results.

Fondiller (1986) is less idealistic than Parkes about the idea of unity. She describes how, paradoxically, the perceived need for a unified nursing pro- fession led to the policies which had exactly the opposite effect. The American Nurses' Association (ANA) and the National League for Nursing (NLN) were originally created in 1952 in order to function in a complemen- tary fashion. (The ANA functioned as a professional nurses' association; the NLN focused on organised community service and the educational stan- dards and facilities necessary to provide a good nursing service to the public.) The two organisations subsequently found themselves representing different groups and different interests. Concentrated to a large extent on the level, location and entry requirements for nurse education, these con- flicts have a familiar ring. The recently achieved consensus in the USA on the educational preparation of professional baccalaureate nurses and techni- cal nurses, as described by Fondiller, reflected more the proportionate strength of the respective memberships of these two organisations, than the achievement of any substantial unity between them. Fondiller's (1986) detailed account of these political manoeuvrings is an object lesson for anyone who subscribes to the utopian ideal of unity. She is realistic and con- cludes that with the rise of the clinical specialisation movement, nursing groups will continue to evolve and multiply. She strongly advocates, there- fore, the logical development of coalitions, arguing that if nurses are to deliver a collective clout to national policy-making then a common voice on key issues will be essential.

The ways in which nurses have sought, perhaps unwittingly or perhaps deliberately, to strengthen the power of one group to the detriment of others is part of the subject of Campbell's chapter in White (1988), reviewed later for its account of the social construction of nursing documentation. It contains a telling account of how the Canadian Nurses' Association's commitment to an all-graduate profession has worked *against* the career interest of non- graduate nurses. The talk of unity becomes an empty vessel unless nurses are prepared to address the claims of challenging and repressed interest groups within nursing.

It is from examples such as these that nurses may come to realise the crucial importance of cultural context to the presence of nursing issues on a policy agenda in a particular place at a particular moment in time. Furthermore, consensus does not necessarily mean the absence of conflict. Instead, faced with supra-ordinate goals, nurses may have to address the question of internal negotiation more realistically in order for their collective activities to be meaningfully directed.

Contemporary health policy initiatives: the potential and risk for nurses and their clients

Two chapters in White's most recent volume (1988), one from the UK and one from Canada, take up the theme of the effects of wider contemporary health policy initiatives on nursing, which in her two earlier volumes was left to North American nurses to explore. Their chapters centre on cost-containment policies in the USA, and because there are important general political lessons to be learned from the phenomena which they describe, their work will be summarised in some depth.

Gray (1984) points out that the phenomenon of cost-containment in health care is now a matter of international concern and, as a result, particular aspects of the North American health care system are slowly being extrapolated to other cultures. One of these – the introduction of Diagnostic Related Groups (DRGs) and their effects on nursing – is the subject matter of the three chapters from North American authors – Milio on *Nursing within the Ecology of Public Policy: a Case in Point* (White, 1985), Melosh on *Nursing and Reagnomics: Cost Containment in the United States* (White, 1986a) and Beatrice and Philip Kalisch on *Nurses on Strike; Labour Management Conflict in US Hospitals and the Role of the Press* (White, 1985).

Melosh and Milio both argue that DRGs are part and parcel of an overall fiscal policy which aims to reduce a huge government deficit by cutting social programmes. By providing a fixed predetermined payment for the health services given within each of the 467 DRGs, providers are forced to operate within a traditional market economy model. If the service they provide exceeds the allowable cost, then the shortfall must be met by cost-cutting within other sections of their budget. If, on the other hand, the service can be provided for less then providers are given the incentive of keeping at least a proportion of the saving made. Proponents of the system argue that DRGs not only provide essential controls over individual professional (medical) profligacy, but also give those same professionals real motivation in seeking 'value for money'. If they are encouraged to manage their own budgets in this way, then the power to ensure the availability of resources for new developments lies firmly in their hands.

All of this now has a familiar ring in the UK but, nevertheless, in considering the possible extrapolation of these ideas to other cultures, it is critically important to keep in mind the key background to these developments. Health care costs in the USA had rocketed from the 1960s onwards (Gray, 1984). The introduction of state-sponsored Medicare and Medicaid had led to a 'blank cheque' approach to medical care in a system which 'traditionally included little structure or incentive for controlling costs' (Melosh, in White, 1986a, p.146). There was therefore an urgent need to address congressional concern about resultant over-treatment and at the same time to work through the complexities of the American health care billing system. Certainly this *could* mean that DRGs are less appropriate in other settings, but the evidence needs to be systematically assessed. The various implications of this policy for nursing also need to be thought through carefully and the lessons from the American experience noted. All of these three North American authors offer analyses of cost-containment policies which fall into three broad categories:

- the opportunity which they provide for enhancing the professional power and status of some nurses;
- the increased workload which they bring for some nurses, accompanied by the impoverishment of others;
- the possible benefits (and potentially adverse consequences) which can be identified for patients and their families.

Thus they argue that a policy initiative such as cost-containment, introduced through the medium of DRGs, can result in some costs and some benefits for different groups. Not only may certain sections of nursing find their interests at odds with others, but also those same interests may coincide, or conflict, with those of the patients. A summary of their evidence, under the three broad headings, follows.

Opportunities for enhancing nurses' power and status

Melosh (1986) describes the conflicting perspectives on DRGs which can be found from her reading of nursing journals since 1983. Nursing proponents of the system are to be found mainly amongst nurse managers, who display a guarded optimism. The DRG hospital is portrayed as an arena of opportunity, the system is accepted as given and the discussion centres on strategies for negotiating its risks and benefits. She argues that this cautiously optimistic view rests on the hope of using the DRG system as a device to support nursing's historical struggle for professional autonomy – nurses being urged to establish their own productivity measures in order to demonstrate their cost-effectiveness *vis-à-vis* the doctors.

Nurses' major grievance is undoubtedly that nursing costs are merely collapsed into the daily DRG room rate, giving no account of the nursing acuity of individual patients, illustrating in a specific way the general principle outlined in Part One that nursing issues are frequently excluded from the policy agenda. American nurses have therefore challenged the validity of the DRG indicator as an adequate predictor of the *real* costs of patient care. Such challenges call for a major revision of the categories used in calculating DRGs, and offer a variety of instruments for calculating nursing costs. In turn, nurses' claims for a pivotal managerial role for nursing are enhanced and nurses are exhorted to become computer-literate and to learn cost-accounting as an essential management tool. In this context primary nursing is promoted as a cost-effective pattern of practice, but Melosh cautions nurses to consider dangerous historical precedents when extrapolating from this argument to the suggestion that nursing might in future be based on fee-for-service practice. She summarises nursing's optimistic view of DRGs by locating its search for more independent nursing arrangements within the cost-containment system.[84] Nevertheless, in justifying their loosening of dependence on the doctors by pointing to their cost-effectiveness, nurses also have to look to threats emerging from below. In the USA, medical technicians emerge as potential substitutes for higher-paid nurses and Melosh (1986) cites examples where nurses' associations have sought to confine the activities of these lower-paid competitors.

The increased workload and impoverishment of some nurses

Milio (1985) summarises a variety of hospital administrative strategies which were introduced in order to deal with the economic and competitive problems exacerbated by the attempts of Congress to contain Medicare and Medicaid, which included the introduction of DRGs. She suggests that the overall effects on hospital services were likely to include:

- computerisation of jobs;
- reduction in the lesser-reimbursed services, for example, maternity care;
- increase in admissions and intensity of care;
- increase in too early discharges, of the long-term and severely ill;
- avoidance of the severely ill who do not have maximum private insurance or payment capacity.

(Milio, 1985, p.92)

Milio describes this as the language of 'skim and dump'. The system skims the least risky, paying patients like cream from the milk. The rest, the low payers and the high-risk patients are either refused, transferred, or released into public sector hospitals.

The effects on nursing are several-fold. First, for hospital-employed nurses, nurse managers match patient 'case-mix' with nursing 'skills-mix'. The results include:

- reducing the proportion of registered nurses;
- hiring nurses on a seasonal or part-time basis, avoiding fringe benefits and job security;
- increasing the intensity of workload with nurses caring for sicker patients with shorter hospital stays.

Secondly, and hypothetically, nurses working in community-based care are likely to be more involved with a sickness-remedial perspective than with a wellness-preventive point of view. In addition, nurses are called upon to try to remedy the adverse effects of premature discharge upon sick patients sent home without adequate informal systems of care.

The Kalischs (1985), in their turn, describe the impact of such policies on *industrial relations* in nursing. Closures and lower utilisation rates were one consequence of attempts to minimise hospital expenditure. When hospitals in Minneapolis found themselves in competition for patients they turned to cutting labour costs, their biggest item of financial outlay. Nurses being the largest labour group took the worst toll (in 1984, 30 per cent of Registered Nurses (RNs) were employed full time, compared with 50 per cent in 1980). Senior, more expensive, nurses were laid off in preference to cheaper, junior staff. Part-time positions became obligatory, and working hours were cut. This situation led, in 1984, to the largest strike of nurses in the history of the USA. The Kalischs' case study thus provides empirical support for Melosh's (1986) analysis of nursing in a DRG future:

> Hospitals are likely to work their staffs harder, retain fewer full-time workers and rely on temporaries to cover the busiest times … . In this unfavourable climate, nurses will not easily be able to defend or extend improvements in wages and working conditions. Already hospitals are economizing by cutting health benefits and resisting pay rises.
>
> (Melosh, 1985, pp.160–1)

The consequences for patients and their families

Milio (1985) describes the effect of cost-containment policies in health care alongside broader cuts in income maintenance, food stamps, subsidies for heating fuel and housing and in the enforcement of environmental and health standards. She cites evidence that up to 10 per cent more people were impoverished in 1983 than in 1979, and claims that this became a particularly acute economic and health-threatening problem for children. She concludes:

> Thus the accumulating weight of recession, the withdrawal of supportive Federal social policies and the DRG-induced pressures on already-limited public health services carry high risks to the health of those who are already most vulnerable: the poor, who are disproportionately children, elders, women and racial minorities.
>
> (Milio, 1985, p.95)

Thus, in describing the effects of specific health policy within the overall context of public policy, she highlights the probable long-term health consequences for the sick and especially the sick poor. She argues that there will be an increase in preventable health problems which will bring in train an unintended *increase* in total health care costs. Her arguments bear a close resemblance to those of the British Black Report (Department of Health and Social Security, Research Working Group, 1980) and The Health Divide (Whitehead, 1987).

These three studies of the effects of cost-containment policies in the USA illustrate the complexity of the relationship between the values of a dominant political ideology and the policy initiatives which it generates. Nursing, in reacting to the costs and/or benefits of such policies, becomes divided as the various sub-groups within it identify with either dominant, challenging or repressed interests. At the time when they were written, these case studies described the impact of a policy on nursing which functioned within a very different health and welfare system to that of many other countries. The extrapolation of similar ideologies to other cultures has led nurses in other countries to begin to examine their implications for nursing although not specifically within cost-containment policies. The two authors in White's most recent volume (1988) explore the following contemporary issues: Campbell on *Accounting for care: a framework for analysing change in Canadian nursing*; and MacGuire on *Dependency matters: an issue in the care of elderly people*.

They describe various ways in which nurses are attempting to improve nursing practice through the development of scientific or quasi-scientific methods for delivering or auditing nursing care. Their observations, in line with many of the analyses referred to in this review, demonstrate that for every apparently rational human act there are unintended consequences which carry costs and benefits.

Campbell's (1988) Canadian account of the social organisation of nursing documentation demonstrates how the development of tools such as Care Plans, Patient Classification Systems and Nursing Audits tends to lead to their taking precedence over nurses' primary task – that of caring for people. The production of information becomes the focus around which nurses' work is oriented. She observes:

> What I have described is not an aberration, but the contemporary method of knowing objectively, designed for efficient and effective management of an enterprise.
>
> (Campbell, 1988, p.65)

This outcome conflicts with the original intention of documentation, which is to account for nursing's 'ideal representations' of their work through various models for practice. Instead, the paperwork not only assumes a life of its own, but also becomes recruited into the service of management as a tool for implementing budget cuts and justifying efficiency drives. Nurses find themselves in this situation struggling to maintain their own levels of excellence under difficult conditions. Campbell sees the problem of how nursing can *shape* its practice without being coerced into *adapting* practice to the corporatisation of health care as the major challenge facing nurses today.

MacGuire's (1988) detailed review of the concept of dependency contains similar challenges. She suggests, amongst a wealth of other information, that major shifts in the definition of the category of old age are taking place, with

a postponement of entry into official old age. She concludes that it is tempt-
ing to suggest that 'a restructuring of reality' is taking place 'akin to the bases
for redefining the unemployed' (MacGuire, 1988, p.73). Geriatric beds in the
NHS have declined and the rate of provision per 1000 members of the population in local authorities has gone down sharply; meanwhile the number of
beds in private nursing homes has doubled. MacGuire argues, in the light of
all these changes, that dependency is a crucial variable on which information
is essential when assessing admission and discharge policies, nurse staffing
establishments and quality assurance issues. Hence she sees the *proper* management of documentation on dependency as vital to the success of auditing
both individual patient care *and* organisational performance over time.
Dependency information can give nursing staff the power to argue for
changes in policy relating to patient admissions and length of stay, including
the provision of adequate discharge facilities, and for staffing levels appropriate to identified, real-time, patient needs. Here we see the crucial role of
nursing information in order to argue a proper case in the face of cost-containment issues. Yet MacGuire (1988) observes that dependency data are
rarely collected routinely and that many nurses are either unaware that such
systems exist or, alternatively, believe that they run 'counter to the principle
that every patient is unique and care must be tailored to meet his specific
requirements' (p.79). Meanwhile, the statistical indicator of patients per occupied bed is widely utilised whilst ignoring the fact that the patients in the
beds may be getting sicker and that the numbers of nursing staff may be
going into relative decline.

Both of these authors highlight the crucial importance to the policy
agenda of how social reality is constructed, defined and documented. Nurses
are encouraged to participate in the development of scientific management
techniques by various inducements, such as greater autonomy for nursing or
a more rational basis for planning staffing in relation to patient need. Whilst
the benefits of such strategies appear to be undeniable, the North American
experience of cost-containment policies suggests that a whole range of
hidden costs may be incurred. Perhaps one answer is for nurses to insist that
they must retain the control and ownership of the data, and that its utility
must be demonstrated in routine formal audits on the quality of care. This
may be just a pious hope unless the ideological positions subscribed to by
nurses in various organisational positions and the divisions within nursing
which result are seriously addressed.

The structure of nursing: its constraints and potential for development

This section summarises the work of six authors (five chapters) each of
whom attempts to encapsulate the effects on nursing of more diffuse and
less explicit ideologies. It may not be coincidental that three – McIntosh on
District Nursing: a case of political marginality, Robinson on *Health visiting and
health* (White, 1985) and Hennessy on *The restrictive and wanting policies affecting health visitors' work in the field of emotional health* (White, 1986a) – write

about community nursing within the UK NHS, while Storch and Stinson on *Concepts of deprofessionalization with applications to nursing* (White, 1988) work in a University Department of Community Medicine in Canada. It is in non-institutional care that the broader, inter-sectoral aspects of welfare policy are most apparent and often the most difficult to address. Keyzer (White, 1988) is something of an exception to this rule. His chapter on *Challenging role boundaries: conceptual frameworks for understanding the conflict arising from implementation of the nursing process in practice* is based on empirical research in a community hospital, geriatric, psychogeriatric and psychiatric rehabilitation units – areas which are nevertheless marginal in many debates about nursing power and politics (see Chapter 1).

McIntosh (1985) describes the marginalisation of district nursing during the historic process of change in the years following the introduction of the NHS in 1948. She claims that this was an effect of 'policy drift' which arises because health policy is determined as much by interest groups outside parliament as by governmental dictat. In describing groups contending for power amongst themselves and who, as a result, successfully block government initiatives for resource reallocation, McIntosh, like White herself, subscribes implicitly to the theory of a power élite in health care. She believes that the inability of district nursing to compete successfully for the status which would ensure a greater share of resources originates from a number of historical events. First, in 1948, district nursing was catapulted from the arena of voluntary sector provision into the statutory framework of the NHS. The requirement at that time that local health authorities should provide home nursing care resulted in the nursing voice being suppressed by the managerial authority of the Medical Oficer of Health. This had long-term implications for district nurse training which reverberate today.

Secondly, the ultimate managerial control of community nursing by nurses recommended by the Mayston Report (Department of Health and Social Security, Scottish Home and Health Department and the Welsh Office, 1969) proved a mixed blessing. On the one hand, divisions in which several groups of community nurses were managed under one head tended to have a health visitor as director of nursing services. On the other hand, these managerial changes also coincided with the 1974 reorganisation of the NHS, which not only abolished the former local authority control but also introduced a 'centrally controlled techno-bureaucracy' (McIntosh, 1985, p.49). One outcome was that community nursing divisions were integrated into hospital management structures, with the further loss of district nursing input into crucial policy-making groups. McIntosh argues, in familiar terms, that a second outcome of this change was for district nurse managers to identify with managerial instead of nursing reference groups. However the most crucial implication of all of these managerial changes for district nursing was its distancing from any direct influence over the total budget. Thus despite government policies intended during the 1970s to bring about a reallocation of resources to the district nursing service, and to the priority groups which formed a large part of its clientele, other powerful forces were able successfully to obstruct their implementation. This was particularly true of the attempt to redistribute any substantial amount of resources from the hospital to the community sectors. Two decades later, community nurses in the UK fear that this situation may worsen following the implementation of two White Papers on health and welfare service provision (Department of Health, 1989a, 1989b).

Thirdly, policies for the attachment of district nurses to primary health care teams, which were being implemented concurrently with the 1970s managerial change, often proved divisive in terms of leadership, authority and control of district nursing. The empirical evidence of district nurses being perceived to be merely handmaidens of the doctors contrasted vividly with the rhetoric of egalitarianism in team relationships. This not only reinforced district nurses' subservient position, but also prevented their managers from organising and allocating their scarce resources in order to meet wider needs than a general practice population might require.

McIntosh (1985) does not subscribe explicitly to any specific welfare ideology. Yet she clearly feels strongly that district nursing has been marginalised along with the needs of those groups, such as the elderly, disabled and chronic sick, who form its focus of concern. This outcome can be usefully compared with the results of cost-containment policies described above, MacGuire's (1988) work on dependency in the elderly and Hennessy's (1986) account of policies affecting health visitors' work in emotional health which follows. It appears that the power to exclude nursing issues from policy agendas is exercised in many and subtle ways. Nurses, it seems, can often be the victims of the *rhetoric* of policy change. On the one hand, they are encouraged to believe that if they comply with certain policy initiatives then their concerns will become more dominant. On the other, nothing changes because of the failure of policy-makers to address underlying power and resource issues.

Hennessy describes the ambiguous nature of the policy objectives and guidelines for health visitors when working in the field of maternal emotional health. She states:

> Health visitors have to be flexible. In one situation they must respond to health needs defined by the family and, in the next, they must note health needs of the family, as defined by professionals, the district health authority, local social service policies and national guidelines. Health visitors are therefore in a very difficult situation with conflicting guidelines and policies. The result of a health visitor not searching for the professionally defined needs of an abused child leads to public criticism, whereas the impact is not quite the same when health visitors do not search for those needs that the patient identifies, such as the depressed mother. This does not help the health visitor's dilemma.
>
> (Hennessy, 1986, p.89)

Hennessy claims that, despite their growing awareness of emotional problems, health visitors do not recognise all postnatally depressed mothers. She suggests a number of factors which may account for this failure. First, many women who are distressed in the postnatal period do not experience sufficiently severe symptoms to need referral to a psychiatrist. As a result, health visitors are searching for a set of criteria which do not merit a *medical* diagnostic label. Indeed, the diagnosis of moderate distress depends on how the mother says she feels as compared with how she felt before she had her baby.

Secondly, individual general practitioners react idiosyncratically to post-natal depression. Many will not be interested if the syndrome is not deemed to be worthy of the 'medical' label. This places the health visitor in an invidi-ous position if she has identified a need but can find no collaborative profes-sional network in which a care strategy could be planned.

Thirdly, the situation may be exacerbated by the organisation of commu-nity psychiatric care. Many community psychiatric nurses, considered to be a outreach of institutional psychiatric care, only accept referrals from a consul-tant psychiatrist. Hence the one nursing colleague with whom the health vis-itor might confer is frequently out of reach.

Fourthly, professional help for moderately distressed postnatal mothers usually involves the provision of a 'listening ear', and possibly the organisa-tion of community support systems. Hennessy (1986) points, however, to the anomalous organisational position in which health visitors find themselves: despite exhortations to work with the whole family, the health visitor's workload is defined statistically only in terms of the children; 'listening' is not deemed officially to constitute skilled professional work, especially if no medical diagnosis is involved; and finally, community development work by health visitors is frequently discouraged by their own nurse managers.

Thus from the point of view of both district nursing and health visiting, those client needs and issues which appeal to concepts of health and sickness outside the frame of reference of the dominant medical model, with associ-ated lower priority ratings in a needs hierarchy, tend to be excluded from the day-to-day policy agenda. They may feature grandiloquently in strategic plans, but nurses may find their actions obliquely diverted when they make serious attempts to address the needs in practice. These are examples of the repressed issues described by Alford (1975) and Lukes (1986), cited in Part One. The nursing care which is performed in relation to these client needs lacks status as important 'work', and may be dismissed as 'work' at all, partly on the grounds that it is carried out invisibly in the home, and partly because it defies evaluation and quantification.

The two remaining chapters in this group of four describe policy concerns in more abstract, conceptual terms. Robinson (1985) focuses on an analysis of the vulnerable basis which the abstract ideal of 'health as a value' provides for legitimated health visiting activity, and touches on several of the philosophical and ideological questions which underpin some of these issues. She argues in line with Stacey's (1976) position that the generalisation of value subscription to *one* concept of health throughout society is a highly questionable proposi-tion. Health in western society is conceived along several dimensions:

- individual or collective;
- functional fitness or welfare (care);
- preventive or curative or ameliorative.

Robinson (1985) notes that the dominant interests of medicine have ensured that the predominant model in health care is based on the concept of individual functional fitness, and curative service objectives. This marginalises on the one hand the concerns of district nurses who are likely to be more concerned with care and amelioration than with cure and, on the other, health visitors who are educated to see their role as involving collective as well as individual prevention.

Robinson believes that many health visitors, faced with the ideological dilemmas which underpin these different conceptual approaches, rationalise their claims to effectiveness through the use of quasi-scientific evaluation techniques. In the process they ignore some of the fundamental distinctions between positivist and interpretive paradigms for understanding and interpreting the behaviour of both health care providers and their clients. Nursing, although she does not describe the phenomenon in these terms, is once again divided into those who seek to identify with the values of the dominant interest groups, a challenging minority, and a repressed majority.

Storch and Stinson's (1988) Canadian perspective on concepts of deprofessionalisation might equally be included in the preceding section on contemporary health policy initiatives. It is discussed here only because their conceptual analysis relates to the more abstract idea of structure rather than to concrete examples drawn from empirical research, although they relate their observations to 'real world' situations currently affecting mental health professionals. Deprofessionalisation, they argue, is a contemporary phenomenon in many health care occupations which previously sought full professional status. However, the concept itself has been described in the literature in three different ways: as deskilling, as proletarianisation, and as the erosion of professional knowledge and trust. Their clarification of these perspectives is invaluable.

Deprofessionalisation as *de-skilling* arises from a combination of circumstances which include a general anti-professional bias and management pressures for increased efficiency. This 'attack on two fronts' is related to Braverman's (1974) thesis that the labour process is shaped by the accumulation of capital and that a dominant goal in profit-making is to purchase labour as cheaply as possible. As a result, workers who aspired to professional status by the possession of unique knowledge and skills and autonomy of action become subjected to the principles of 'scientific management'. Job analysis leads to its break-up into component parts, the sum of which becomes divorced from the whole. The worker becomes divorced from control of the totality of the labour process. Storch and Stinson believe that nursing is faced with increased pressure to comply with scientific management. The measurement of patient acuity levels, nursing workload, etc. (all commendable activities if they enhance decision-making) can, if used as a means to the end of cost-containment, lead to 'cheaper and less effective levels of care, and become instruments of the deskilling of nurses because the craft and creativity of nursing is destroyed' (Storch and Stinson, 1988, p.36). Deprofessionalisation as *proletarianisation* occurs when applied to professional occupations. First, advances in technology lead to huge capital investment in complex machines rather than in people; the control of this investment is centralised by various means. Secondly, although certain professional services may expand in order to meet the needs of large numbers of clients, the professionals themselves tend to become controlled by a central administration. Thirdly, professional markets for clients are invaded by public and private capital. The result is that professionals have become subordinate employees within the control of centralised bureaucracies.[8.5]

It may be argued that nurses in the NHS have always been subjected to bureaucratic control and that nursing has therefore always been proletarian by nature. The arguments put forward by Storch and Stinson (1988) suggest, however, that full proletarianisation may not yet have run its full course. For example, the progressive fragmentation of work leads to a situation in which knowledge about the *whole* task is separated from the execution of its component parts. Indeed, the tasks may be allocated to different groups of workers outside the control of nursing – a form of *technical* proletarianisation. There is another form, however, – *ideological* proletarianisation – where the very values, goals and social purposes of the work are taken over by others. If nurses cannot maintain control of a nursing system which defines nursing work in acceptable terms for them, then they are rendered truly powerless by the process of alienation.

Storch and Stinson's summary of this situation is very telling:

> The proletarianization of professionals has commonly been discussed in the context of unionization and the use of union tactics by professionals. Perhaps a better understanding of the proletarianization theses can sensitize us to the frustrations many nurses experience when they feel they have lost control over the social purpose of their work (ideological proletarianization) and when they are denied the satisfaction of conceptualizing their nursing tasks but are instead directed to execute their tasks as prescribed by management (technical proletarianization).
>
> (Storch and Stinson, 1988, p.7)

Deprofessionalisation as *erosion of professional knowledge and trust* is an extension of the consequences of the two former categories. As tasks are fragmented and controlled by others, the whole notion of a coherent, professional, public service ethos becomes dissipated and demystified. In terms of meeting client need in non-hierarchical ways this may indeed represent a beneficial and humanising process rather than the reverse, but only if occupational disintegration can be prevented. Otherwise, nursing as a *human* service agency will be denied its own coherent value system, and nursing tasks will merely exist as isolated interventions in a vacuum created by the principles of scientific management.

Keyzer's (1988) chapter on the conflicts arising from implementing the nursing process represents an intriguing analysis of the structural constraints on implementing change. Just as McIntosh observes in the case of district nursing, so the official rhetoric of policy objectives appeared to support overtly a change in nursing practice. The reality was somewhat different. The power of entrenched interest groups was so great that, whether deliberately or by default, the *real* process of changing nursing practice was continually obstructed. For, as Keyzer explains in detail, the introduction of the nursing process implies a revolution in power structures and attitudes to practice:

> A true patient-centred model for nursing practice, which imbues the client with the power over decision-making, would be a direct challenge to the tightly controlled boundaries ... between the roles of the doctor, the nurse and the woman in her own home ... It is unlikely that such a model for practice would be welcomed by those whose power it seeks to remove.
>
> (Keyzer, 1988, p.105)

Keyzer sees nursing's structural relationship with medicine as the key obstacle to reform in clinical nursing practice. All other structural constraints are seen as secondary to this – the emphasis on nurses as the managers rather than autonomous clinical practitioners, and the denial of adequate continuing education in order to assume that the clinical role merely serves to confirm the status quo.

Each of the five chapters discussed in this section has illustrated the constraining power of existing structures in society against which nurses have to struggle if they are serious about effecting change. All of them, at their root, express concerns about nurses' powerlessness to help their clients *effectively* because of these constraints. It is at once both depressing and exciting to realise just how many nurses are beginning to identify the relatively obscure sources of power in society. (But then, if you have the power there isn't any need to publicise the fact.) It is depressing because challenging the status quo is extraordinarily difficult. Those in existing positions of authority can isolate, ignore, ridicule and make those challenging them feel guilty and unworthy. It is not surprising that many nurses give up in the attempt. It is also exciting because the published evidence now demonstrates that nurses are coming of age politically. What is needed now is the will to take the issues forward.

Class, gender and race in nursing

In the earlier version of this paper I commented that it was disappointing that relatively little empirical evidence on class and gender emerged from the first two volumes on *Political Issues in Nursing*. Once again it is encouraging to note that White's more recent volume redresses the balance. In addition to the two exceptions in White (1986a) – Hardy in *Career politics: the case of career histories of selected leading female and male nurses in England and Scotland*, and Simnett in *The pursuit of respectability: women and the nursing profession, 1860–1900*, Orr and Thompson in White (1988) address, respectively, women as receivers of care and nursing in South Africa.

Hardy (1986) documents the great dissimilarities between the career histories of 36 female and 13 male nursing leaders. The women in the group were older, and came from middle-class backgrounds, while the men were younger and had working-class origins. Most of the women, unlike their brothers, and despite their social advantage and scholastic ability, had not been encouraged to think seriously about a career. Nursing embodied the notion of 'worthwhile work', but even so most of the women, like the men, entered nursing by accident.

Once in nursing, striking differences emerged. The women made more horizontal career moves between different specialisms, whereas the men demonstrated an orderly swift move up the vertical nursing hierarchy. The women therefore took much longer to reach senior positions. This pattern appeared to stem partly from different career aspirations – the men had longer-term ambitions – and partly from irrational expectations within nursing. The women felt that gaining other certificates was expected, and every change of direction brought a return to the bottom of the career ladder. Hence they achieved an average of 5 qualifications, compared with 3.5 for the men, who were more concerned in any case with higher educational achievements than with nursing certificates. (This observation was not supported in a recent national survey of Chief Nurses at District Health Authority level (Robinson et al., 1989), in which the female nurses had more general education.)

Hardy (1986) found that the availability of mentors was an important factor in helping both men and women to break out of traditional career patterns. Even so, the men experienced more help of this kind, and earlier in their careers. She concludes that the domination of top posts in nursing by men arises from the complex and different socialisation process which men and women experience. It is partly the product of self-image, with women expecting to serve others, not themselves, and partly the effect of direct influence by others. Both aspects intermesh and illustrate how gender, even in a predominantly female profession, can still substantially determine who enters its dominant interest groups.

Simnett (1986), using a relatively rare historical perspective, examines the social origins of women entering nursing in Billericay Poor Law Union Workhouse and St Bartholomew's Hospital between 1860–1900. She concludes that, despite the apparent differences in these institutions' ability to recruit in the first place, nursing during the early part of the period was not a solidly middle-class occupation even in the London hospital. The middle-class women who did enter St Bartholomew's often appear to have been driven by the economic necessity of family circumstances into making provision for themselves.

Nevertheless, the status of nursing as an occupation was raised, albeit relatively, in both institutions during the period studied. The policy of the Local Government Board eventually forced the Boards of Guardians to employ trained nurses as supervisors, whilst the propaganda effects of the 'lady' probationer image led to improved recruitment and attempts to improve standards in the London teaching hospital. The situation in the workhouse was nevertheless, by contrast, bleak. Most of the nursing care during the early part of the period was carried out by the able-bodied paupers themselves.

Both of these accounts are interesting vignettes of the impact of class and gender on nursing in different contexts and at different times. Gender works in two ways in nursing. It is usually women who *deliver* care, but women are also frequently the *recipients* of care, and discrimination can work so that both categories are divided against each other (Robinson, 1989). In a chapter which takes a sophisticated view of the mediation of power in health care, Orr (1988), writing on *Women's health: a nursing perspective*, describes four main themes. First, the medicalisation of life experiences from birth to death ensures that neither women as patients nor as nurses find it possible to challenge doctors' claims to intervention. By defining situations as pathological, any other interpretation is ruled out. Hence women's mental health problems get treated with tranquillisers and their social origins become relegated as unimportant. Thus the power of governments, drug companies and doctors goes unchallenged.

Secondly, the increased use of technology alienates people from their bodies and conveys a sense of mystery and power to those in control of the machines. Hence the progressive medicalisation of childbearing has resulted in pregnancy and birth being treated as disease processes instead of as altered states of health. Women's knowledge and experience of their bodies is discounted.

Thirdly, the division in health care labour reflects the sexual division of labour in all other areas of life. Thus doctors are male and identified with high-status 'scientific' knowledge, and nurses are female and concerned with 'caring' which is considered low-status, women's work (see Chapter 7).

Finally feminists, at least, see that the existing ways in which health care is provided perpetuate the structure of power in society and act as a powerful mechanism of social control. Nurses as doctors' handmaidens are often seen in this context as oppressors rather than supporters of other women. (In this sense Orr's chapter could have been included in the final section.)

All of the issues described in this section illustrate Lukes' (1986) third face of power. The socialisation of women into 'knowing their place' is achieved through the sheer weight of institutions – family, education, nursing careers, the prevailing definition of 'Science' – shaping their expectations and leading them to adopt certain attitudes and roles. Orr (1988) does see a way out of the impasse through her experience of the women's health movement. However, this involves an enormous shift in attitudes and challenge to the status quo. If nurses are to play a key role in influencing health care policies for women, they will first need to become aware of the structures which oppress *all* women. Only then can they work *with* women as equal partners, helping them to define their problems and solutions for themselves. In doing this it is inevitable that nurses will find themselves challenging existing value systems, something which does not come easily to a group for whom the unequal experience of power is so deeply entrenched.

The final part of this section touches on the structural issue of race, although Thompson's *The development of nursing in South Africa* in White (1988) refers only obliquely to the subject. Race, in general, remains a sadly neglected area in the study of the politics of nursing. One concludes that

Thompson's chapter was written with the constraints of the South African political regime very much in mind, for although it contains a wealth of statistical information on demography and the labour force participation in nursing by different racial groups, the reader is left very much to draw his or her own conclusions about the practical effects. Hence we are told that with a population in which 72.2 per cent is black, just 0.23 per cent of that population received a university or college education in 1985.

The black population has a high birth rate and high mortality rates at all ages, resulting in a population pyramid characteristic of an underdeveloped country. The white population pyramid, by contrast, resembles the developed world, with a low birth rate and a large proportion of elderly people. Yet Thompson shows that in 1985 the blacks had a ratio of one qualified nurse to 721 total black population, compared to 1:157 for whites. Commenting on the World Health Organisation's recommendation that a ratio of one registered nurse to 500 members of the population is required to deliver a basic comprehensive health service in a Third World Country, Thompson (1988) claims that the number of black nurses admitted to the profession would need almost to double in order to achieve this ratio by the year 2000. Economic factors make this an enormous task. There are shortages of teaching posts *and* shortages of teaching staff. Yet the blacks experience patterns of disease which are most amenable to basic primary and secondary health care – infective and nutritional diseases predominate.

Compared with accounts of nurse education elsewhere, South Africa appears historically to have been remarkably progressive in some areas. South Africa was the first country in the world to achieve state registration for nurses and midwives in 1891, and university diploma courses for nurse tutors began in 1937. The first Chair of Nursing was established in 1967, although a degree programme had been established in 1956. Nevertheless Thompson is clear that progress has been limited to very small numbers, and that much remains to be done. Not least, one concludes, for the black nurses who must experience multiple forms of discrimination through race, gender and class, and yet are so desperately needed. The experience of apartheid leads us to conclude that meeting the nursing needs of the different populations within that country remained as two separate and unequal agendas for action.

Nurses as oppressors or enablers: power for or against the client?

Discussion until now has concentrated upon the diverse ways in which nursing issues may be affected by policy and politics. By extension, it is claimed that the concerns of the patient, client or consumer become sucked into the consequences of the power to define certain issues in certain ways. Only Orr (1988), of the authors considered so far, has openly claimed that nurses are ever anything but on the same side as the patient. Several other chapters contain the suggestion that nurses, in pursuing certain policy objectives, may indeed work against the interests of their clients. On the whole, however, nurses are portrayed as being 'on the side of the angels'. Only Hawker (1985), in *Gatekeeping: a traditional and contemporary function of the nurse* (cf. White, 1985), has the temerity to make this dark aspect of nursing policy the central focus of her enquiry. She does so by describing a historical role for nurses – that of keeping patients' visitors at bay. Admittedly it may be argued that nurses merely carried out the rules. Yet Hawker shows that over a period of years many policy initiatives designed to open access for the families of patients have been successfully obstructed by nurses and by doctors (see Chapter 6).

Some nurses, it seems, while becoming more aware of their own power-lessness in the policy arena, have in addition begun to systematically evaluate the even greater powerlessness of their clients, and their own potential contribution to this situation. The World Health Organisation's current initiatives in seeking Health for All by the year 2000 emphasise not only the crucial role that nurses can play, but also stress that success will be dependent upon enabling customers actively to control the factors which contribute to their health (see Chapter 3). It is encouraging that many of the authors reviewed in these collections have begun to analyse the powerlessness of patients from a variety of perspectives. Nevertheless, it is essential that in raising their own awareness nurses remain conscious of their considerable power to act against the best interest of their clients. Future analyses of nursing policy and politics must keep the relationship of nurses' to consumers' power firmly on the agenda.

Conclusion

The contents of the second part of this chapter reveal a heightened awareness among nurses (and other authors) of the relevance of understanding the nature of politics and power to the practice of nursing. They also demonstrate how elusive in general terms these concepts can sometimes prove to be, and that teasing them out of a mass of empirical data is no easy matter. Five provisional categories have been suggested within which most of the subject matter reviewed could be subsumed: problems of unity in nursing, and nursing as a force for challenge and change; the potential and the risks for nurses and clients of contemporary health policy initiatives; the structure of nursing – its constraints and its potential for development; class, gender and race in nursing; and nurses as oppressors or enablers – power for or against the client. What this analysis has begun to show is how different systems of value and belief can impinge in different ways upon a range of health policy issues which have important bearings on nursing practice. As a result, different groups of nurses and clients frequently find themselves subjected to conflicting pressures. Unpacking the various dimensions of any one situation requires first and foremost a crucial awareness of the social, political and economic culture within which particular health policy initiatives take place. There is then a need to establish whether any common themes can be traced across the diverse subject areas and cultures in order to identify where general principles pertaining to power and politics can be applied to nursing.

What then, if any, are the general lessons that we can learn from this exercise? First, on the basis of the evidence reviewed it appears that nursing is virtually never primary in policy terms. This reinforces the messages from the first part of the chapter regarding the hidden face of power – the power to keep issues *off* the policy agenda, or the power to ensure that issues are defined only in certain ways. It appears that policy in relation to nursing almost invariably develops second-hand as a consequence of other actors' responses to health and welfare initiatives which, in turn, are developed elsewhere. Secondly, in the process of trying to adapt to various initiatives, nursing becomes subdivided as certain sub-groups seek to gain the maximum advantage from policy change. Nursing is almost always, therefore, an example of a divided issue only parts of which succeed in obtaining a place on the public policy agenda. Claims for reform in the delivery of nursing care, for developing methods of providing a more cost-effective service, and for paying attention to people's *real* health needs (as opposed to medically defined areas) almost invariably fall on deaf ears. Why should this be? Presumably because suggesting to those who currently hold the power to determine the nature of health care and the way in which it is provided that there could be a better, cheaper or more effective way of delivering a service is to admit to the real power of a challenge to the status quo. As nurses struggle to gain a hearing for their claims, there are a great many losers who may or may not be aware of their experience of oppression. The effects of class, race and gender on this unequal state of affairs have been touched upon but, as yet, these are imperfectly explored in relation to nursing. The fact that nurses are not agreed on a way to move forward is exemplified by the different positions adopted by Clay (1987), Salvage (1985) and White (1985, 1986a, 1986b, 1988), all key authors on the subject of nursing and politics.

Understanding this oppressive state of affairs could nevertheless be a liberating experience for nurses. If gaining an advantage invariably means the exploitation of someone else in the system, then nurses everywhere could begin to see that their real power lies in solidarity with their weaker members and, above all, with their client groups. Nurses have to ask 'if I gain a benefit, who stands to lose, and am I content with that state of affairs?' If the answer is 'No', then they have to decide what they are prepared to do about the situation.

In this review of the available evidence an attempt has been made to push the debate along, to begin to identify the issues which could be used in order to develop some, broader generalisations. It is one small step in what must be an enormous and continuing task.

Endnotes

8.1 I am indebted to Culyer (1983) for his discussion of the development of the study of Health Indicators and, in particular, for clarification of concepts such as 'area, topic of study' and 'mode of thinking'.

8.2 Other authors who have produced categorisations within health policy and management research include Hunter (1986) and Pettigrew *et al.* (1987).

8.3 White's idea of pluralism is open to debate. The system she describes as pluralistic could more accurately be termed élitist, for it consists of nurse managers who identify with the values of a dominant, managerial class, a challenging but small minority intelligentsia and a repressed proletariat. Pluralism in political theory describes a concept which embodies inbuilt societal checks and balances (usually through a democratic voting system) which then ensure a consensus where the majority view prevails. Clearly this rarely happens in nursing (and, according to Lukes' thesis, does occur in reality anywhere else).

8.4 Melosh differs from the Kalischs' analysis of the effects of cost-containment on RNs. She claims that it was Licensed Practical Nurses (LPNs) who lost their jobs, leaving RNs as a greater proportion of the labour force.

8.5 Carpenter first described the proletarianisation of nurses at the same time as the 1974 reorganisation of the NHS, with its emphasis on managerial values (Carpenter, 1977). In a more recent study he finds that however militant they may have been in 1972, by 1984/85 a new realism had taken its toll. Their attitudes to unions and professional associations had become less to do with their perceived potential for collective action than with their role of protection and indemnity against the risk of making mistakes (Carpenter *et al.*, 1987).

References

Alford, R. R. 1975 *Health care politics: ideological and interest group barriers to reform.* Chicago: University of Chicago Press.

Bachrach, P. and Baratz, M. S. 1962 The two faces of power. *American Political Science Review* **56**, 947–52.

Braverman, H. 1974 *Labor and monopoly capital: the degradation of work in the twentieth century.* New York: Monthly Review Press.

Campbell, M. L. 1988 Accounting for care: a framework for analysing change in Canadian nursing. In White, R. (ed.), *Political issues in nursing: past, present and future.* Vol. 3. Chichester: Wiley, 45–70.

Carpenter, M. 1977 The new managerialism and professionalism in nursing. In Stacey, M., Reid, M., Heath, C. and Dingwall, R. (eds), *Health and the division of labour.* London: Croom Helm, 165–93.

Carpenter, M., Elkan, R., Leonard, P. and Munro, A. 1987 *Professionalism and unionism in nursing and social work.* Coventry: Department of Applied Social Studies, University of Warwick.

Clay, T. 1987 *Nurses: power and politics.* London: Heinemann.

Cousins, C. 1987 *Controlling social welfare: a sociology of state welfare and work organisations.* Brighton: Wheatsheaf.

Crenson, M. A. 1971 *The unpolitics of air pollution.* Baltimore, MD: Johns Hopkins University Press.

Culyer, A. J. 1983 *Health indicators*. Oxford: Martin Robertson.

Davies, C. (ed.) 1980a *Rewriting nursing history*. London: Croom Helm.

Davies, C. 1980b A constant casualty: nurse education in Britain and the USA to 1939. In Davies, C. (ed.), *Rewriting nursing history*. London: Croom Helm, 102–22.

Deakin, N. 1987 *The politics of welfare*. London: Methuen.

Department of Health 1989a *Working for patients: the Health Service: caring for the 1990s*. London: HMSO (Cmnd 555).

Department of Health 1989b *Caring for people: community care in the next decade and beyond*. London: HMSO (Cmnd 849).

Department of Health and Social Security, Scottish Home and Health Department and the Welsh Office 1969 *Report of the Working party on management structures in the local authority nursing services*. London: DHSS.

Department of Health and Social Security, Research Working Group 1980 *Inequalities in health: report*. London: DHSS (Chairman D. Black).

Dingwall, R. and McIntosh, J. (eds) 1978 *Readings in the sociology of nursing*. Edinburgh: Churchill Livingstone.

Dunn, A. 1985 Foreword. In Salvage, J., *The politics of nursing*. London: Heinemann, vii–viii.

Fondiller, S. H. 1986 The American Nurses' Association and National League for Nursing: political relationships and realities. In White, R. (ed.), *Political issues in nursing: past, present and future. Vol. 2*. Chichester: Wiley, 119–43.

Gray, A. 1984 European health care costs. *Social Policy and Administration* **18**, 213–28.

Green, D. G. 1987 *The new right: the counter revolution in political, economic and social thought*. Brighton: Wheatsheaf.

Ham, C. and Hill, M. 1986 *The policy process in the modern capitalist state*. Brighton: Wheatsheaf.

Hardy, L. K. 1986 Career politics: the case of career histories of selected leading female and male nurses in England and Scotland. In White, R. (ed.), *Political issues in nursing: past, present and future. Vol. 2*. Chichester: Wiley, 69–82.

Hawker, R. J. 1985 Gatekeeping: a traditional and contemporary function of the nurse. In White, R. (ed.), *Political issues in nursing: past, present and future. Vol. 1*. Chichester: Wiley, 1–17.

Hennessy, D. A. 1986 The restrictive and wanting policies affecting health visitors' work in the field of emotional health. In White, R. (ed.), *Political issues in nursing: past, present and future. Vol. 2*. Chichester: Wiley, 83–100.

Hunter, D. J. 1986 *Managing the National Health Service in Scotland: review and assessment of research methods*. Scottish Health Service Studies 45. Edinburgh: Scottish Home and Health Department.

Jolley, M. and Allan, P. (eds) 1989 *Current issues in nursing*. London: Chapman and Hall.

Kalisch, B. and Kalisch, P. 1985 Nurses on strike: labour-management conflict in US hospitals and the role of the press. In White, R. (ed.), *Political issues in nursing: past, present and future. Vol. 1*. Chichester: Wiley, 105–51.

Keyzer, D. M. 1988 Challenging role boundaries: conceptual frameworks for understanding the conflict arising from the implementation of the nursing process in practice. In White, R. (ed.), *Political issues in nursing: past, present and future. Vol. 3*. Chichester: Wiley, 95–119.

Klein, R. 1983 *The politics of the National Health Service*. London: Longman.

Klein, R. 1989 *The politics of the National Health Service*, 2nd edn. Harlow: Longman.

Larsen, J. 1988 Being powerful: from talk into action. In White, R. (ed.), *Political issues in nursing: past, present and future. Vol. 3.* Chichester: Wiley, 1–13.

Lukes, S. 1974 *Power: a radical view.* London: British Sociological Association.

Lukes, S. 1986 *Power: a radical view.* London: Macmillan (first published in 1974 by the British Sociological Association).

MacGuire, J. M. 1988 Dependency matters: an issue in the care of elderly people. In White, R. (ed.), *Political issues in nursing: past, present and future. Vol. 3.* Chichester: Wiley, 71–94.

McIntosh, J. B. 1985 District nursing: a case of political marginality. In White, R. (ed.), *Political issues in nursing: past, present and future. Vol. 1.* Chichester: Wiley, 45–66.

Melosh, B. 1986 Nursing and Reaganomics: cost containment in the United States. In White, R. (ed.), *Political issues in nursing: past, present and future. Vol. 2.* Chichester: Wiley, 145–70.

Milio, N. B. 1985 Nursing within the ecology of public policy: a case in point. In White, R. (ed.), *Political issues in nursing: past, present and future. Vol. 1.* Chichester: Wiley, 87–104.

Millett, K. 1977 *Sexual politics.* London: Virago.

NHS Management Inquiry Team 1983 *NHS management inquiry.* London: NHS Management Inquiry Team (Team leader E. R. Griffiths).

Nursing Times and Nursing Mirror 1989 Regional CNO resigns. *Nursing Times and Nursing Mirror* **85**, 5.

Orr, J. 1988 Women's health: a nursing perspective. In White, R. (ed.), *Political issues in nursing: past, present and future. Vol. 3.* Chichester: Wiley, 121–37.

Parkes, M. E. 1986 Through politics to professionalism. In White, R. (ed.), *Political issues in nursing: past, present and future. Vol. 2.* Chichester: Wiley, 101–18.

Pettigrew, A., McKee, L. and Ferlie, E. 1987 *Understanding change in the NHS: a review and research agenda.* Coventry: Centre for Corporate Strategy and Change, University of Warwick.

Pollitt, C., Lewis, L., Negro, J. and Patten, J. (eds) 1979 *Public policy in theory and practice.* London: Hodder and Stoughton.

Rein, M. 1976 *Social science and public policy.* Harmondsworth: Penguin.

Robinson, J. 1985 Health visiting and health. In White, R. (ed.), *Political issues in nursing: past, present and future. Vol. 1.* Chichester: Wiley, 67–86.

Robinson, J. 1989 Nursing in the future: a cause for concern. In Jolley, M. and Allan, P. (eds), *Current issues in nursing.* London: Chapman and Hall, 151–78.

Robinson, J. and Strong, P. 1987 *Professional nursing advice after Griffiths: an interim report.* Nursing Policy Studies 1. Coventry: Nursing Policy Studies Centre, University of Warwick.

Robinson, J., Strong, P. and Elkan, R. 1989 *Griffiths and the nurses: a national survey of CNAs.* Nursing Policy Studies 4. Coventry: Nursing Policy Studies Centre, University of Warwick.

Salvage, J. 1985 *The politics of nursing.* London: Heinemann.

Salvage, J. 1990 The theory and practice of the 'new' nursing. *Nursing Times* **86**, 42–5.

Simnett, A. 1986 The pursuit of respectability: women and the nursing profession, 1860–1900. In White, R. (ed.), *Political issues in nursing: past, present and future. Vol. 2.* Chichester: Wiley, 1–23.

Skevington, S. (ed.) 1984 *Understanding nurses: the social psychology of nursing.* Chichester: Wiley.

Stacey, M. 1976 *Concepts of health and illness: a working paper on the concepts and their relevance for research.* Coventry: Department of Sociology, University of Warwick

(Paper produced for the Health and Health Policy Panel of the Social Sciences Research Council).

Storch, J. L. and Stinson, S. M. 1988 Concepts of deprofessionalisation with applications to nursing. In White, R. (ed.), *Political issues in nursing: past, present and future. Vol. 3.* Chichester: Wiley, 33–44.

Strong, P. and Robinson, J. 1988 *New model management: Griffiths and the NHS.* Nursing Policy Studies 3. Coventry: Nursing Policy Studies Centre, University of Warwick.

Strong, P. and Robinson, J. 1990 *The NHS under new management.* Milton Keynes: Open University Press.

Thompson, R. 1988 The development of nursing in South Africa. In White, R. (ed.), *Political issues in nursing: past, present and future. Vol. 3.* Chichester: Wiley, 163–202.

Tonkin, E. and Hart, E. 1989 *I love my work, I hate my job: a study of hospital domestics.* Birmingham: Department of Sociology, University of Birmingham (Report prepared for the Economic and Social Research Council).

White, R. (ed.) 1985 *Political issues in nursing: past, present and future. Vol. 1.* Chichester: Wiley.

White, R. (ed.) 1986a *Political issues in nursing: past, present and future. Vol. 2.* Chichester: Wiley.

White R. 1986b From matron to manager: the political construction of reality. In White, R. (ed.), *Political issues in nursing: past, present and future. Vol. 2.* Chichester: Wiley, 45–68.

White, R. (ed.) 1988 *Political issues in nursing: past, present and future. Vol. 3.* Chichester: Wiley.

Whitehead, M. 1987 *The health divide.* London: Health Education Authority.

Zwanger, L. 1986 Jewish nursing education in Palestine 1918–1948. In White, R. (ed.), *Political issues in nursing: past, present and future. Vol. 2.* Chichester: Wiley, 25–44.

9 Principles and practice of curriculum development – towards the year 2000

Alan Myles

Introduction
General aspects of the education provider and proposed curriculum
Philosophy
Scheme of study
Modes of teaching/learning
Schemes of assessment
Curriculum validation
Summary
References

Introduction

This chapter focuses on key issues in curriculum development and innovation in the context of moving towards the year 2000. The major and long sought after reforms are now well under way, with significant changes to both pre- and post-registration nursing education impacting on the higher education sector. Colleges of nursing and midwifery have a variety of affiliation links with institutions of higher education based on different forms of partnership agreement. Pre-registration nursing education is taught to at least diploma level, and most post-registration courses are 'nested' within a higher education framework with pathways leading towards an honours degree. Staff in colleges of nursing and midwifery education and institutions of higher education have gained considerable experience in developing long and short courses for health care professionals over the past quinquennium. They have been indefatigable in responding to the demands from the profession for a range of flexible learning opportunities, including taught courses and distance education. They have had to do this in the context of complex funding arrangements and in the face of increasing competition from other providers. This has not been without institutional and personal cost. Education providers have had to extend their provision with demands for enhanced quality, often within a thinner resource 'envelope'.

In this chapter, the principles and practice of curriculum development will be revisited within the current context of health care education and demands for high quality provision. A number of examples will be used to illustrate the principles, and a range of relevant issues will be addressed, including a focus on modularisation. As a conceptual framework for the chapter, an adaptation of the Further Education Curriculum Review and Development Unit's model will be used (Further Education Curriculum Review and Development Unit, 1982). The model is based on four phases, namely the *initiation, development, implementation* and *evaluation* phases, which are suitable when considering higher as well as further education. To some extent, there is overlap between the phases, but each will be addressed successively for ease and clarity of presentation. A brief description of each phase will be followed by a range of 'worked examples' to illustrate curriculum development in action.

Initiation phase

During this phase, curriculum development groups or course planning teams need to identify and articulate priorities for course development. This has become increasingly important within the current purchaser–provider context and the increased competitiveness of the market place, with different higher education institutions bidding for student numbers. The rationale for new courses and their broad educational intentions are normally identified during this phase, although their translation into more precise statements of intent usually occurs later. During this phase, institutions need to determine whether they are *demand-led* or *resource-led*. The former is characterised by responding to market demand without necessarily having the resources in place to support a new programme. The latter is characterised by only moving forward if there are resources in place to support the initiative. The latter approach is 'safer' in many ways, but institutions may 'miss the boat' and not take advantage of gaps in the market. The writer advises a prudent approach based on a synthesis of the two approaches.

Development phase

This is the phase during which new modules and courses are developed. Important decisions made during this phase are concerned with the precise educational intentions of the course, the selection/rejection of content for the scheme of study, the modes of teaching and learning, and the scheme of assessment. Within the context of contemporary education for health care professionals, this phase is characterised by intensive work on the production of course documentation for validation purposes which are now invariably of a conjoint nature, e.g. involving a higher education institution and one of the National Boards. It is acknowledged that this is often a difficult aspect of curriculum development because of the deadlines for first and second stage validation events. The fact that education staff are now more experienced in the production of course documentation, coupled with the premise that many staff have enhanced their skills in computer literacy, may have ameliorated the trials and tribulations of this phase. However, as there are invariably a number of other pressures competing for quality time, the amelioration may be a false perception rather than a reality!

Implementation phase

Implementation refers to the curriculum and associated materials in action. However, the curriculum in action may differ significantly from the formal curriculum, i.e. the actual experiences of students and teachers may be quite different from that described in the definitive course document. This situation is most likely to occur when the consultation process between stakeholders has been less than satisfactory. There is likely to be a higher degree of congruity between the actual and the formal curriculum when dialogue between course-planning teams and stakeholders has taken place regularly during the developmental process. The importance of first and second stage validation events cannot be overemphasised at this point, and will be addressed in more detail later in the chapter.

Evaluation phase

It is recognised that evaluation should be ongoing. Wells (1987) defines evaluation as a judgemental process whereby people attempt to ascribe a degree of worth or value to a curriculum. The demand for more rigorous approaches to curriculum evaluation has grown significantly across the further and higher education sector, as reflected in a number of publications from the Higher Education Quality Council (HEQC), e.g. Higher Education Quality Council (1994). Current issues pertaining to this phase will be explored later in the chapter.

Having outlined the four phases of curriculum innovation, the following key areas of course development will be addressed within the Further Education Curriculum Review and Development Unit (1982) framework:

- general aspects of an education provider and proposed curriculum;
- rationale and philosophy;
- scheme of study;
- modes of teaching/learning;
- scheme of assessment;
- course approval.

General aspects of the education provider and proposed curriculum

When seeking approval for a new course, an institution is asked to provide information on its history and its current and future curricular activities. This provides a context within which any new proposal can be considered. Such information is normally available from a range of documentation, e.g. in the institution's annual quality assurance report. Information is required on the institution's normal source of students, i.e. local and regional catchment areas. Most importantly, information is sought regarding the institution's quality assurance systems. Institutions need to be explicit about their mission and overall objectives which should include cycles of review and strategies for improvement (Higher Education Quality Council, 1994). Validating panels normally explore the general aspects of the education provider early on in the validation process.

When seeking to develop a new course, it needs to be justified on a number of fronts, both political and ideological. The rationale for a course is its *raison d'être*. The reasons for developing a new course are likely to include market demand and the emergence of a developing field of study, e.g. courses in complementary therapies. The demand for programmes preparing nurse practitioners for their roles in different settings is a prime example. It is also now more common for 'hard' evidence to be required to substantiate development plans for new courses. This makes sense, given the points made earlier about institutional mission and resource management.

It is good practice to have a well-developed *Approval in Principle* process. Approvals in principle are normally submitted to the institution's academic board (or other appropriate structure). The documentation at this stage is relatively brief and succinct. It mainly consists of an outline of the proposed course, including briefs of course units, and the resource implications for offering the programme.

Philosophy

The place of an educational philosophy in course submission documents has been a more prominent feature over the past decade, and rightly so. It is important for stakeholders to gain insights into the values and beliefs of the course team, and to gain some feel as to what the curriculum in action is likely to be in practice.

Schofield (1972) describes three terms which are frequently used in the context of educational philosophy, i.e. philosophical, linguistic and concept analysis, respectively (see Chapter 10). He states that linguistic and concept analysis are really more precise expressions of philosophical analysis. The importance of this in the context of curriculum development is for writers of course documents to clarify what they mean by key terms, e.g. the meaning of key concepts such as *health*, and the values and beliefs held by the course team about the concepts central to the course. This leads on to the next task, which is how to go about articulating an educational philosophy for a course. An adaptation of Torres and Stanton's (1982) procedure can be used to good effect. It consists of the following steps:

1. Identify the key concepts of a course.
2. Conduct a values clarification exercise concerning those key concepts.
3. Identify relationships and ordering among the concepts.
4. Prepare a draft philosophical statement.
5. Circulate the draft statement to the course team for critical comment to facilitate ownership.
6. Revise the statement following feedback.

Each step will now be discussed with reference to a pre-registration diploma in higher education. Step 1 one can be achieved by brainstorming or by a modified nominal group technique. Brainstorming is a very useful procedure for generating many ideas quickly. One person usually writes the group's ideas on a flip-chart or overhead projector transparency. The inputs are usually collected without censure in order to ensure a free flow of ideas. If a nominal group is used, the following steps are usually adopted:

a) group members write down in private the concepts that they consider to be key;
b) ideas are pooled without discussion to reveal the whole list;
c) open discussion follows in order to clarify meaning and to produce a definitive list.

Step 2 of Torres and Stanton's (1982) process is likely to be quite lengthy, and sufficient time should be allowed for the values clarification exercise (see Chapter 1). This step often has several benefits in that thoughts and feelings are clarified and shared, respectively. Values and beliefs about education are likely to be articulated in most course submissions. However, as Peters (1966) suggests, defining the concept *education* is problematic. Rather than attempting to define education, Peters considers the following three criteria instead:

(a) education implies the transmission of what is worthwhile to those who become committed to it;
(b) education must involve knowledge and understanding and some sort of 'cognitive perspective' which is not inert;
(c) education at least rules out some procedures of transmission on the grounds that they lack willingness on the part of the learner.

In course documents, one often finds Peters' (1966) criteria for education reflected in belief statements such as: 'The course team believes that knowledge informs practice and vice versa' [Peters' criteria (a) and (b)] and 'The course team believes that students should participate in decision-making about the content and process of the course [Peters' criterion (c)].

For step 3 of the modified procedure of Torres and Stanton (1982), readers are referred to Figure 9.1, which depicts the ordering and relationships between eight key concepts from a pre-registration Diploma in Higher Education course (Project 2000).

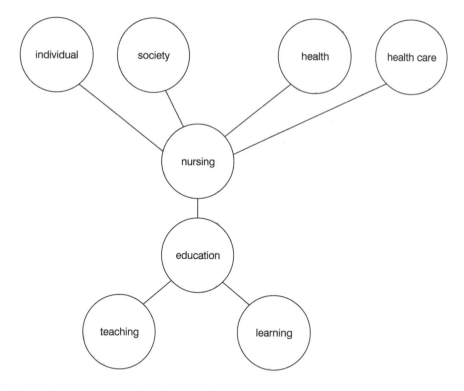

Figure 9.1   Key concepts for a Diploma in Higher Education (Nursing) (English National Board for Nursing, Midwifery and Health Visiting, 1989, p.178)

After this step, a member of the course team usually 'volunteers' to write a draft statement of philosophy. In the writer's experience, this individual is often the course leader. Steps 5 and 6 follow sequentially, the end-result being a statement of philosophy owned by the course team.

It is also important that there is a relationship between an institution's philosophy and the philosophies of the courses under its aegis, as illustrated in Figure 9.2.

Philosophical statements for different courses may well have their own individual characters. At the same time, different courses will have different philosophies, but each should reflect the philosophy of the parent institution.

Scheme of study

The scheme of study is a term which encompasses the aims and broad learning outcomes of a course and the course units/modules that make up that course. Course aims can be described as general statements of purpose (Myles, 1995), e.g. for a course preparing nurse teachers, one of the aims is likely to be: 'To prepare participants for their roles as teachers of nursing'.

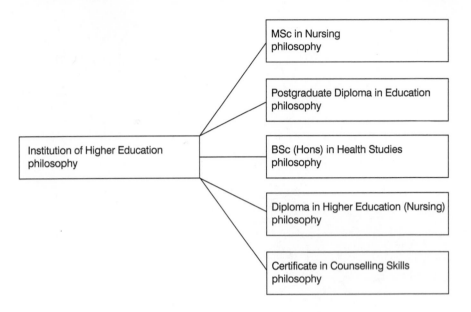

Figure 9.2   Relationship between institutional and course philosophies

Learning outcomes are statements describing what course participants will be expected to achieve. These are written at the course and modular level, the latter having a higher degree of specificity than the former. An example of the former within the context of a teacher preparation course might be as follows: 'Students will be able to demonstrate skills in facilitating learning using a broad repertoire of methods.' An example of the latter might be as follows: 'Students will be expected to compare and contrast product and process models of curriculum development.'

Since the advent of Credit Accumulation and Transfer Schemes (CATS), the number of modular programmes of study has increased sharply. These programmes consist of a number of compulsory and optional course units. Students are required to choose appropriate pathways which lead to a named award. A pathway can be defined as 'an acceptable route through a modularised course' (Myles, 1995, p.44).

A module can be defined as: 'a relatively discrete unit of learning which comprises its own title, credit rating, aims, learning outcomes, indicative content, teaching/learning methods, scheme of assessment, and indicative reading' (Myles, 1995, p. 44).

Modular schemes of study confer a number of advantages for students, teachers and organisations. There are also a number of disadvantages. A summary of the relative merits of modular schemes and modularised courses will be presented later. Prior to that, a distinction needs to be made between a modular scheme and a modular course. The former can be regarded as being at the *macro*-level, and the latter as being at the *micro*-level. This can be seen from the following brief descriptions.

A *modular scheme* can be regarded as the framework within which an institution operates its modular programme, e.g. a scheme based on a full-time student taking three 20-credit-point modules in each of two 15-week semesters. This is a common model for full-time students studying for an honours degree based on 360 credit points. Students are normally required to study 120 credit points in one full-time academic year.

A *modular course* is constructed from a range of modules. As indicated earlier, this construction is not random, and there should be a balance between core, specialist and elective modules. The course experience must be coherent. This coherence is ensured by having pathway rules and sound principles and procedures for the management of advanced standing. Advanced standing can be defined as: 'The sum total of general/specific credit awarded against a specific pathway' (Myles, 1995, p.44).

Advanced standing is based on the assessment and accreditation of prior achievements, consisting of credit for certificated and/or non-certificated learning. This is often referred to as *accreditation of prior learning (APL)* and *accreditation for prior experiential learning (APEL)*, respectively.

The progress of students through a modular scheme is prefaced by the assessment of their advanced standing, usually through the verification of certificates for prior learning (APL) and/or the scrutiny of a portfolio (a folder of evidence) for experiential learning (APEL). An early assessment of advanced standing enables course teachers to advise students on their pathway selection. For example, a student who wishes to enrol for a Master's Degree in Nursing based on 10 modules may elect for the following pathway if she has been awarded two M-level module exemptions for study at another institution of higher education:

semester 1 (year one)	two core units
semester 2 (year one)	two specialist units
semesters 1 and 2 (year two)	research project (four units)

As indicated earlier, modular schemes and modularised courses have relative advantages and disadvantages for the various stakeholders, which are summarised in Figure 9.3.

There is no doubt that modularisation has been one of the most significant changes in post-compulsory education, if not the most significant one. The implications for stakeholders are now being felt to a significant degree, but the writer asserts that most would agree that the change to modularity has been both necessary and welcome. Modularity has also had an influence on methods of teaching/learning, which will be the subject of the next part of this chapter.

Modes of teaching/learning

Much has been written about teaching methods in nursing education over the past few years (English National Board for Nursing, Midwifery and Health Visiting, 1987, 1989; Ewan and White, 1984; Kenworthy and Nicklin,

ADVANTAGES	DISADVANTAGES
For students • shorter course of study • acknowledgment of prior learning • reduced cost • shared learning with other students • 'tailor-made' courses	• more demanding material at level 2/3 to learn early on in a pathway • missing out on learning opportunities afforded by taking more modules • potential 'dilution' of degree studies • cost in terms of time/money processing APEL claims • missing out on culture associated with a proscribed programme of study • dilemmas over choice!
For teachers • job satisfaction associated with students' advantages • opportunity to develop credibility and subject expertise further	• time spent in advising students on advanced standing and pathway selection • repeating teaching on modules and potentially losing enthusiasm if it is the third repeat of that day!
For organisations • recognition for offering a wide range of continuing education • increased funding for offering more opportunities for more students • flexible entry/transfer of students based on multiple entry and exit points	• can be difficult to plan and resource • resource-intensive • large complex schemes can be difficult to manage (e.g. the examinations and assessments)

Figure 9.3   Relative merits of modularity (Myles, 1995, pp.49–50)

1989; Quinn, 1988). It is not the intention of this chapter to reproduce well-documented coverage of the principles and practice of different teaching methods, but to reinforce the assertion that nurse teachers need to be skilled in the use of a wide range of teaching methods if they are to provide stimulating and challenging experiences for their students. The English National Board for Nursing, Midwifery and Health Visiting (1989) suggested that experiential learning was likely to be a major feature of Common Foundation and Branch Programmes. It is now acknowledged that formal lectures given to large groups are also a major feature of such programmes. However, the writer would like to remind readers that models of experiential learning can and should be used to good effect whenever appropriate. This is demonstrated in the following example. In the English National Board for Nursing, Midwifery and Health Visiting (1989) Project 2000 Guidelines, it is suggested that the nature and implications of client empowerment be addressed. Steinaker and Bell's (1979) experiential learning taxonomy could be adapted to enable students to learn about client empowerment as shown in Table 9.1.

It is interesting to note how the role of the teacher alters commensurate with the changing role of the student as the taxonomy is ascended. This conceptual framework has much to recommend it, since there is scope for the use of a diverse range of teaching methods which are predominantly student-centred. This may be in the form of a *learning agreement*, the next subject for consideration. A learning agreement (which in the past was called a learning contract) can be defined as a teaching/learning strategy in which a

Table. 9.1   Experiential taxonomy adapted from Steinaker and Bell (1979)

Level	Role of teacher	Role of student
Exposure	Motivator	Learns about populist models of health
Participation	Catalyst	Involves a client under her care in conjoint care planning with supervision
Identification	Moderator	Develops confidence in fostering client self-help
Internalisation	Sustainer	Promoting client empowerment is a characteristic of her nursing care
Dissemination	Critic/evaluator	Teaches other students ways of fostering client empowerment

student (or students) negotiates with her facilitator the outcomes, methods for achieving these *and* the criteria for evaluating her achievement of these outcomes (Myles, 1991). They can range from informal verbal to formal written agreements, and it is suggested that each type is appropriate for a range of courses, including Common Foundation and Branch Programmes. The more formal agreements are appropriate when the outcomes reflect competency statements. Before discussing examples and the practical aspects of facilitating learning agreements, justification for their increased use will be made with reference to the concept of social need as defined by Bradshaw (1972). According to Bradshaw, social service is based on need, and in that context he identifies four types: normative, felt, expressed and comparative. In the English National Board for Nursing, Midwifery and Health Visiting (1989), the writer describes each type.

1. Normative need is what the expert or professional defines as need in any given context. The pre-registration learning outcomes (Project 2000 Guidelines) outlined by the English National Board for Nursing, Midwifery and Health Visiting (1989) can be regarded as normative in that they suggest the 'desirable standard' to be reached by students to enable them to be admitted to the register of the United Kingdom Central Council for Nursing, Midwifery and Health Visiting and to assume the responsibilities and accountability that nursing registration confers. Teacher-designed curriculum objectives can also be regarded as normative in that they are based on professional expertise. Normative needs change as the body of knowledge increases through research, and as societal values change. With reference to the fourfold curriculum (Beattie, 1987), maps of key subjects and schedules of basic skills can be further defended on normative grounds in that their selection is usually based on professional expertise and research. However, the potential problems of a teaching session based predominantly on normative need are those of paternalism and parochialism, i.e. a 'we know what's best for you' approach.

2. Felt need is equated with wants and is influenced by individual perceptions. An example of felt need in the context of a Common Foundation Programme might be a student who wishes to develop her assertion skills. In terms of the fourfold curriculum, portfolios of meaningful experiences are likely to generate felt need. The main advantage of teaching sessions based on felt need lies in the fact that those sessions are very student-centred. One potential disadvantage for teachers is that they may not feel adequately prepared for such sessions. Felt need may also be deemed an inadequate measure of 'real' need in that vital curricular areas could be overlooked.
3. Expressed need is felt need turned into action. The merit of expressed need is the realisation of felt need, and this can be achieved by a learning agreement.
4. Comparative need is a measure of need found by studying the characteristics of those receiving a service. For example, if the learning agreements of students on an Adult Nursing Branch Programme were based mainly on felt need, whereas the learning agreements for students on other Branch Programmes were based on normative need, it could be said that the latter groups are 'in need' of learning agreements based on felt need. One of the advantages of teaching sessions based on comparative need is that perspectives can be broadened by considering what happens with other groups. However, in a Diploma in Higher Education context, a disadvantage could be that cross-curricular norms are established and ritualised. This could stifle creativity at both the macro-level of curriculum development and at the more micro-level of teaching/learning. Figure 9.4 illustrates the balance of social need which could underpin two learning agreements, each with a different philosophical basis.

Learning Agreement 1 is strongly based on professional judgement and on what happens on other Branch Programmes, with little acknowledgment of the student's felt and expressed needs. It appears to be based on an empirical-rational strategy for changing the student's behaviour. Conversely,

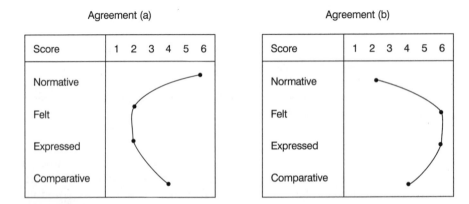

Figure 9.4 Social need and learning agreements

Learning Agreement 2 is more student-centred, and appears to be based on a normative re-educative approach to facilitating learning.

With reference to social need, readers are asked to reflect on the appropriateness of 'concave' and 'convex' learning agreements (Figure 9.4, models (1) and (2), respectively). It is suggested that 'convex' learning agreements reflect the notion of the curriculum as a 'trading post' on the cultural boundary between students and teachers, to which ideas and artefacts are brought, exchanged and taken away (Jenkins and Shipman, 1976). They should enable the felt needs that students bring to the 'trading post' to be articulated as expressed needs and subsequently realised through the learning agreement. Before the term 'learning agreements' came into use, it was more common to find reference to the term 'learning contract'. The term 'contract' proved problematic because of the legal ramifications associated with that term.

Knowles (1984) identifies eight stages of a learning contract which can be condensed to five as follows:

1. Assess learning needs with reference to a competency scale.
2. Formulate appropriate objectives.
3. Identify the resources available with related actions and time frames.
4. Carry out the contract.
5. Evaluate learning outcomes against the objectives of the contract.

These five stages are equally applicable to learning agreements.

One of the pre-registration learning outcomes of a Diploma in Higher Education course is that students will be able to use relevant literature and research to inform the practice of nursing. A student in the early period of a Common Foundation Programme is unlikely to be familiar with a range of literature on nursing practice and research. However, as she progresses through the course, it would be expected that she would always base her care on appropriate research findings if these were available. Therefore, a competency scale for that nurse might be scored as follows.

Absent	Low (awareness)		Moderate (understanding)		High (expert)
0	1	2	3	4	5
	(P)		(R)		

'P' denotes the student's present competency and 'R' denotes her required competency. As she progresses through the course, her competency scale should change as follows.

Absent	Low (awareness)		Moderate (understanding)		High (expert)
0	1	2	3	4	5
			(P)		(R)

The next stage of the process is to articulate more specific learning outcomes which, if achieved, will reduce the 'P'–'R' interval. Table 9.2 provides an example of the key stages of a learning agreement that might be appropriate for a student who is in the early days of her course and who wishes to develop her skills in the use of relevant literature and research.

The framework for the learning agreement outlined in Table 9.2 has been adapted from one described by Keyzer (1985). Further examples of this particular framework in use in continuing professional education can be found in Keyzer (1985) and English National Board for Nursing, Midwifery and Health Visiting (1989). These references also give examples of other formats.

The use of learning agreements provides the opportunity for both teachers and students to individualise teaching and learning. However, their use can initially be very time-consuming and demanding for both parties. Once teachers and students are used to the process, the time constraints become less of a concern. It is worth stressing that the outcomes of a learning agreement often differ from what was originally envisaged. This situation has to be judged by all parties on individual merit. After all, Peters (1966) did suggest that education is not so much about reaching a destination as about travelling with a different point of view!

Following this discussion about the use of Steinaker and Bell's (1979) experiential taxonomy and the theory and practice of learning agreements, attention will now be turned to some of the issues pertaining to student assessment.

Schemes of assessment

Much has been written about the nature and purpose of student assessment (Rowntree, 1987). It is neither the intention nor the remit of this chapter to revisit prior debate, but rather to identify some of the key issues surrounding assessment within the current context of continuing professional development. The main principle is that schemes of

Table. 9.2   A sample learning agreement

Learning outcomes	Resources	Actions	Time	Criteria for evaluation
1. I will have developed my information retrieval skills	1. library 2. librarian 3. personal tutor	1. I will contact the librarian to undertake a supervised search	3 days	1. I will produce a book/journal list on a selected topic
2. I will understand more about how to use research findings on my current placement	1. ward manager 2. personal tutor 3, journal club	1. I will look up three research articles related to pre-operative preparation	7 days	1. I will present a resumé of each of the articles to my personal tutor during the next study day

assessment should reflect their respective schemes of study. This is sound educational practice, since incongruity is illogical and unfair on the students. The methods of assessment should be valid, reliable, fair and economical, to enable students to learn from the experience. In the case of modular programmes, each course unit will have its own assessment. A higher education sector norm appears to be in the region of 2000 to 2500 words per 10 CATS points. For example, 20-credit-point modules are likely to have either a single 4000- to 5000-word assignment, or two shorter pieces of work. Three-hour examinations when used are often seen as the equivalent of a 5000-word assignment. The weighting in terms of words is the same between levels 1, 2 and 3, but the demands on the students become increasingly challenging as the levels increase. More is expected of the students in terms of synthesis and critical evaluation, which are two of the hallmarks of level 3 study.

Modular schemes commonly have a combination of *en route* assignments and end-of-module examinations. This has raised a number of issues for teachers and support staff, e.g. the scheduling of submission dates for assignments in modularised schemes and the turnaround time between internal and external examiners in order to meet for examination board meetings. The burden on both internal and external examiners has inevitably increased with the growth in post-compulsory education.

The Higher Education Quality Council (HEQC) has recently consulted the sector on the need for a fundamental reform of the external examiner system (Higher Education Quality Council, 1994). The HEQC argues that the reform is vital if the external examiner system, which is one of the key foundations on which quality assurance is based, is to be of continuing value in the future. Silver *et al.* (1995), in their report on the external examiner system, discuss the extension of the role of external examiners beyond the 'additional' role of a second marker with specific subject expertise, to include a responsibility for ensuring that examination processes are internally fair and also equitable with other comparable programmes across the higher education sector. One of the main influences here is the growing concern in the sector about the need to conceptualise and articulate the essence of *graduateness* reflected in debates about threshold standards and core outcomes which should be achieved by graduates. The report makes a number of recommendations concerning the external examiner system, which include the following:

- the need for an extension of the available reservoir of suitable external examiners and the need to include national and local measures to prepare them for their changing and complex roles;
- the need for more overt recognition of the demands of the role in terms of release time and status, and recognition of the role for the purposes of career development;
- the role of the external examiner as an additional marker should be abandoned in favour of sampling and other inputs to verify the fair operation of procedures resulting in awards to students;

- institutions should consider ways of enabling their external examiners, and their staff who are external examiners, to meet and share their experiences.

The writer supports all of the above recommendations and all of the other recommendations made in the report. In addition, opportunities should be created for external examiners to meet with internal examiners (who may not necessarily be external examiners) outside formal examination board settings. This can be in the form of an annual seminar based on an agenda of mutually relevant issues. Following this brief coverage of key issues regarding schemes of assessment, attention will now be focused on matters concerning the approval and reapproval of courses.

Curriculum validation

So far, issues apposite to the initiation, development and implementation phases of curriculum development have been addressed. The final part of this chapter will address issues of central concern to the evaluation phase, particularly with regard to validation. Practical guidelines for those involved in curriculum evaluation will be suggested following a clarification of some of the related terminology. Evaluation is a judgemental process in which an attempt is made to ascribe a degree of worth or value to a curriculum (Wells, 1987). Validation is the process whereby judgement is reached by a group including external peers as to whether a course designed to lead to an award meets the requirements of that award (Council for National Academic Awards, 1988). In the context of professional education, validation ensures that a course adequately prepares participants for their professional roles. Validation nowadays is mainly of a conjoint nature, carried out by two or more duly authorised bodies working in equal partnership, e.g. an institution of higher education and the English National Board for Nursing, Midwifery and Health Visiting. Validation is concerned with 'threshold adequacy', which is based on criterion rather than norm referencing. In other words, if a course falls below threshold adequacy, it will not be validated.

Nixon (1989) considers how styles of validation have shifted from a central to a peripheral approach over the last two and a half decades. From 1964 until the early 1970s validation was based on an inquisitorial/adversarial model. This approach is characterised by intermittent face-to-face encounters with the validators, e.g. General Nursing Council (GNC) Inspectors, who passed judgement (the optimum 'sentence' being a quinquennial reprieve before they returned). During the later 1970s and early 1980s, the emphasis shifted to institutional self-monitoring, quality enhancement and quality maintenance. The change from GNC Inspectors to ENB Education Officers was intended to foster more collaborative links between training institutions and the statutory bodies through more frequent contact at both formal and informal levels. The 1980s, particularly the latter part of the decade, saw further shifts towards institutional self-regulation linked to systems of peer review. During the 1990s, this shift has continued, with an emphasis on

first- and second-stage validation events. Walker (1989) identifies two important aims of validation:

- to ensure value for the students;
- to ensure value for the community in general.

Walker describes five different types of validation judgement: academic,
professional, economic, institutional, and judgements about team performance. A brief account of each type of validation judgement related to nursing education follows.

- Academic validation is concerned with the overall coherence of the
scheme of study and scheme of assessment. In the context of a Diploma in
Higher Education, this would relate to the organisation and relationships
between Common Foundation and Branch Programmes.
- Professional validation asks the question 'Can course members do the job
that the course is supposed to prepare them for?' This type of validation
appears to be synonymous with professional accreditation, and in the context of a Diploma in Higher Education would pose questions regarding
the 12 pre-registration learning outcomes.
- Economic validation is concerned with the management of financial, technical and human resources. In the context of a Diploma in Higher
Education this would be concerned with education budgets, resources
such as computers and open-learning materials, and staff-student ratios.
- Institutional validation is concerned with how a course fits into an institution's academic plan. For example, the relationship between pre- and post-
basic education would be a topic for discussion in the context of
institutional validation.
- The fifth type of validation judgement is concerned with team performance, and in the context of a Diploma in Higher Education would focus
on the teaching cadre and practice-based staff concerned with the education of pre-registration students.

The writer believes that Walker's (1989) classification brings the process of
validation more sharply into focus. As identified in ENB Pack 2 (English
National Board for Nursing, Midwifery and Health Visiting, 1989), Tyler's
(1949) four basic questions could be used by curriculum development groups
to evaluate their courses. The questions could also be used by members of a
validation panel to set the agenda for an approval visit. The questions,
adapted from Pendleton (1988), are as follows.

1. *What educational purposes should the institution seek to attain?*
   (a) Is the course framework clearly described and justified?
   (b) Is the course philosophy clearly articulated with reference to key
       concepts?
   (c) Is the philosophy reflected throughout each aspect of the course?
   (d) Are the learning intentions/outcomes comprehensive enough to facili-
       tate the development of a competent practitioner?
   (e) Is the course content related to the key concepts and course
       intentions?

(f) Is the content appropriately balanced and are there any notable omissions?

2. *What educational experiences can be provided that are likely to attain these purposes?*
   (a) Have you decided on the sequencing of placements in the practice settings, using as your yardstick the educational needs of the students?
   (b) What consideration has been given to the fostering of an effective learning environment in order that achievable learning outcomes may be realised?

3. *How can these experiences be effectively organised?*
   (a) How is integration between theory and practice achieved?
   (b) Does the course structure facilitate a progressive broadening and deepening of the students' knowledge and experience?
   (c) Are teaching methods related to the scheme of study and based on the tenets of adult learning?
   (d) Has the level and quality of qualified supervision been established?

4. *How can we determine whether these purposes are being attained?*
   (a) Is there an appropriate balance between formative and summative assessment?
   (b) Are the assessment methods of a sufficient variety?
   (c) Are the submission dates for coursework realistic? For example, will the students have had sufficient time to complete assignments?
   (d) Is there an appropriate balance between formative and summative modes of curriculum evaluation, addressing both the processes and the outcomes of the course?
   (e) Is there evidence to suggest that curriculum development arises from curriculum evaluation?

If the above questions can be answered with confidence, validation should be granted.

Summary

In a recent survey of higher education institutions in the UK (Higher Education Quality Council, 1994), it was found that the management of quality across institutions was variable. While several areas of good practice were identified, a number of deficiencies were also highlighted. In the search for excellence in education, a number of new challenges must be faced and addressed. These include a critical review of the modules and courses that institutions of higher education currently provide. This is needed in order to keep pace with market demand for cost-effective programmes of a high quality based on flexible modes of teaching/learning. All of this is likely to be undertaken within the context of major organisational reviews and development. To this end, higher education institutions are creating new alliances built around different models of partnership. The number of franchised programmes has proliferated and this has widened provision. In addition, the demand for nurse teachers to ensure that their teaching is more closely related to practice has never been stronger, and this exhortation is taking place within the context of debates about clinical competence and clinical credibility. These challenges merit a comprehensive coverage which is beyond the remit of the present chapter.

This chapter, however, has focused on several key issues which need to be addressed when developing courses to meet the needs of tomorrow's pre- and post-registration students. The conceptual framework chosen for discussion of the issues consisted of the initiation, development, implementation and evaluation phases of curriculum development. The issues discussed reflect a number of key agendas for education providers. If the content of this chapter is able to inform that debate in any way, it will have achieved its purpose.

References

Beattie, A. 1987 Making a curriculum work. In Allan, P. and Jolley, M. (eds) *The curriculum in nursing education*. London: Croom Helm, 15–34.

Bradshaw, G. 1972 The concept of social need. *New Society* **19**, 640–43.

Council for National Academic Awards (CNAA) 1988 *Handbook*. London: CNAA.

English National Board for Nursing, Midwifery and Health Visiting (ENB) 1987 *Managing change in nursing education. Pack One: Preparing for change*. London: ENB.

English National Board for Nursing, Midwifery and Health Visiting (ENB) 1989 *Managing change in nursing education. Pack Two: Workshop materials for action*. London: ENB.

Ewan, C. and White, R. 1984 *Teaching nursing: a self-instructional handbook*. London: Croom Helm.

Further Education Curriculum Review and Development Unit (FEU) 1982 *Curriculum styles and strategies*. London: FEU.

Higher Education Quality Council (HEQC) 1994 *Guidelines on quality assurance*. London: HEQC.

Jenkins, D. and Shipman, M. D. 1976 *Curriculum: an introduction*. London: Open Books.

Kenworthy, N. and Nicklin, P. J. 1989 *Teaching and assessing in nursing practice: an experiential approach*. Harrow: Scutari.

Keyzer, D.M. 1985 *Learning contracts: the trained nurse and the implementation of the nursing process*. Unpublished PhD Thesis, University of London, Institute of Education, London.

Knowles, M. 1984 *The adult learner: a neglected species*, 3rd edn. Houston, TX: Gulf.

Myles, A. P. 1991 Independent studies and the curriculum in nursing education. In Pendleton, S. M. and Myles, A. P. (eds), *Curriculum planning in nursing education*. London: Edward Arnold, 116–84.

Myles, A. P. 1995 New wine in old bottles. In Jolley, M. and Brykczynska, G. (eds), *Nursing: beyond tradition and conflict*. London: Mosby, 29–54.

Nixon, N. 1989 *'Validation in nursing' Conference*, July 1989, unpublished seminar notes. London: South Bank Polytechnic.

Pendleton, S. M. 1988 *Guidelines for internal validation* (unpublished). London: Institute of Advanced Nursing Education.

Peters, R. S. 1966 *Ethics and education.* London: Allen and Unwin.

Quinn, F. M. 1988 *The principles and practice of nurse education,* 2nd edn. London: Croom Helm.

Rowntree, D. 1987 *Assessing students: how shall we know them?* London: Kogan Page.

Schofield, H. 1972 *The philosophy of education: an introduction.* London: Allen and Unwin.

Silver, H., Stennet, A. and Williams, R. 1995 The external examiner system: possible futures. *Report of a Project commissioned by the Higher Education Quality Council.* London: Quality Support Centre.

Steinaker, N. W. and Bell, M. R. 1979 *The experiential taxonomy: a new approach to teaching and learning.* New York: Academic Press.

Torres, G. and Stanton, M. 1982 *Curriculum process in nursing.* Englewood Cliffs: Prentice-Hall.

Tyler, R. 1949 *Basic principles of curriculum and instruction.* Chicago: University of Chicago Press.

Walker, A. 1989 *Validation in nursing Conference,* July 1989, unpublished seminar notes. London: South Bank Polytechnic.

Wells, J. A. C. 1987 Curriculum evaluation. In Allan, P. and Jolley, M. (eds), *The curriculum in nursing education.* London: Croom Helm, 176–208.

Knowledge for nursing practice

Kim Manley

Introduction

'The definition of a knowledge base for a discipline begins with the separation of that knowledge which is important to the discipline and that which is not' (Visintainer, 1986). But what is meant by *knowledge*, who should judge the relevance of that knowledge, and what *knowledge base* is important to nursing? This book provides insights into the knowledge considered relevant to nursing by its various authors. However, it is the aim of this chapter that the nature of knowledge itself be examined, and that certain themes pertinent to the practice of nursing be considered in relation to knowledge, namely *theory, philosophy, power, professionalism* and finally *accountability*. Just as nursing is growing and developing, so our ideas and understanding are being refined and developed. Many writers on nursing theory quoted in the earlier edition of this chapter have further evolved their ideas, and these developments are acknowledged here.

Knowledge and knowing

According to Walker and Avant (1995), knowledge is the product of knowing. It is both *experiential* and *summative*. However, knowing something does not necessarily mean that what is known is understood. For example, one can know that it is necessary to monitor for sugar in the urine of patients who are taking steroids, but this is quite different from knowing why an increased level of urine sugar can occur, knowing how to recognise its signs, and knowing how to measure it.

Knowledge itself can be defined in different ways:

- familiarity gained by experience of a person, thing or fact (Concise Oxford Dictionary, 1976);
- theoretical or practical understanding of a subject (Concise Oxford Dictionary, 1976);
- the sum or range of that which can be perceived or learned (Walker and Avant, 1995);
- philosophically – certain understanding as opposed to opinion (Concise Oxford Dictionary, 1976), or a justified true belief (Runkle, 1985).

From these definitions it can be seen that even in lay terms knowledge does not just consist of facts and information, but also includes experience and understanding. Thus the knowledge base of anything, be it a discipline, profession or any activity, encompasses experience and understanding in addition to facts.

There are therefore two different dimensions to understanding the nature of knowledge: knowledge as *product* and knowledge as *process*. Parallel to this perspective is knowledge as *objective* and knowledge as *subjective*. Knowledge as product equates with knowledge as facts and information. The knowledge base of nursing so frequently referred to takes the perspective of knowledge as product; such knowledge is also frequently referred to as objective. Knowledge as process similarly equates with the view that knowledge is about experience and understanding, and is therefore of a subjective nature. Further parallels include Schon's (1983) concepts of *knowledge-for-action* and *knowledge-in-action*, the former relating to knowledge as product, and the latter to knowledge as process – only to be revealed in action. From this perspective, knowledge is now being linked with its purpose – a further dimension associating it with action and decision-making, an area that will be returned to later (under the headings of *Carper's patterns of knowing* and *Generating theory in the interpretive approach*).

Know-how and know-that

The above discussion suggests that there are different kinds of knowledge: there is a difference between knowing that and knowing how, and knowing why, and knowing what. Several philosophers differentiate between *know-how* and *know-that* (Kuhn, 1970; Polanyi, 1962; Ryle, 1949). Know-how consists of practical expertise and skills. Examples include knowing when a surgical patient is deteriorating, how to give an injection, how to identify a patient's strengths and weaknesses, how mutually to agree upon goals with patients, or how to build up a therapeutic relationship with clients. All of these examples demonstrate the practical knowledge that is used daily in practice settings. Benner (1984) considers that such clinical expertise has not been adequately described (see Chapter 1).

In contrast, know-that knowledge encompasses theoretical knowledge, i.e. that found in textbooks, and includes formal statements about interactional and causal relationships between events (Benner, 1984). Examples in nursing would include the following: knowledge that the most important need of relatives of acutely ill patients is the need for hope (Norris and Grove, 1986); knowledge that there is a relationship between life events, their perceived significance, and physical and psychiatric illness (Brown and Harris, 1989); or knowledge that various stages can be observed in individuals who have experienced or anticipate bereavement (Kübler-Ross, 1970; Parkes, 1986). This type of knowledge is probably what most of us accept as the lay meaning of the word 'knowledge'. It can be defined more precisely as that which is systematically organised into general laws and theories (Carper, 1978). This kind of knowledge is considered in more detail under the heading *Knowledge and theory* (cf. p. 309). Know-how knowledge is usually acquired through practice and experience, and often cannot be theoretically accounted for by know-that knowledge, which is synonymous with practical knowledge.

Practical knowledge

Benner (1984) considers that practical knowledge is gained over time. She has identified six areas of practical knowledge that can be observed in nursing experts, derived from her study of intensive-care nurses. These areas are described below.

1. *Graded qualitative distinctions* are made on the basis of perceptual recognition. They cannot be reduced to minute variables, and are not context-free. Examples given by Benner include judgements of muscle tone in the premature infant, or the degree of cyanosis or respiratory distress. Another more sophisticated example would be the perception that a patient is not responding positively to an intervention. This practical knowledge depends on nurses knowing their patient as a person, and his or her normal and unique response patterns. The concept of *knowing the patient* is now well defined (Tanner *et al.*, 1993), and has obvious implications for how nurses organise their care, to enable them to be in the best position to achieve this.
2. *Common meanings* are developed by nurses working with common issues. Meanings are developed over time and shared.
3. *Assumptions, expectations and sets* relate to practical situations in which nurses have learnt to expect a certain course of events. For example, nurses may recognise the early signs of sleep deprivation in patients who

have been seriously ill, when the patient begins to hallucinate, say strange things and show early signs of psychosis.

4. *Paradigm cases and personal knowledge* are particular situations that stand out in the practitioner's mind and which alter his or her subsequent understanding and perception of clinical situations. An example of this may be the practitioner who has learned always to validate particular messages conveyed by the patient, following a previous false assumption that such behaviour meant something else.

5. *Maxims* are cryptic instructions which only make sense if there is already a deep understanding of the situation. The cryptic instruction encompasses the patient's condition, the outcomes to be striven for and the appropriate interventions. These are all implicit within the maxim, and would be understood by other expert nurses in the same context.

6. *Unplanned practices* are those which nurses may have been delegated, and have taken on because they are constantly at the bedside, and have as a result become highly skilled in these practices. Benner calls this unplanned delegation or *delegation by default*. She provides as an example the intensive-care nurse who has become highly skilled in the titration and weaning of vasodilator and anti-arrhythmic drugs. Although such drugs may be prescribed by doctors, the nurse has developed expertise in titrating them in relation to a range of cues from the patient. Similar expertise is seen in Macmillan nurses in their fine-tuning of pain control for patients who are terminally ill.

Benner (1984) argues that the expert nurse perceives the situation as a whole, and that expertise is based on experience and many hours of direct patient observation and care. She also states that the knowledge embedded in this clinical expertise is central to the advancement and development of nursing science. This practical knowledge she considers would have much to offer the development of nursing theory, if it was described and studied (see Chapter 1).

Two main camps, know-how and know-that knowledge, have been identified. A third, contemporary view, namely practical knowledge, has been alluded to – one that links it to its purpose. Knowledge from this perspective provides enlightenment and subsequently empowerment to take action, is viewed as emancipatory (Habermas, 1965) because it facilitates action. This is a powerful concept that is relevant not only to nursing but also to other practice disciplines such as teaching and social work, as represented by the growing movements of action research, action learning and reflective practice. *Praxis* is the term often used to describe this type of knowledge at a personal level – knowledge that informs action. This may be defined as reflection and action upon the world in order to transform it (Freire, 1972). Such knowledge is constantly under review – it is dynamic, not static. Both knowledge and action are subject to change. Praxis in turn is similar to Schon's (1983) concept of *reflection-in-action*. In Table 10.1 the range of words and ideas used to describe different kinds of knowledge is collated.

Table. 10.1 Key ideas and words associated with different views about the nature of knowledge

Knowledge as facts and information	Knowledge as experience and understanding	Knowledge linked to its purpose/action
Knowledge as product	Knowledge as process	Praxis
Knowledge as objective	Knowledge as subjective	Knowledge as emancipatory
Know-that knowledge	Know-how knowledge	
Theoretical knowledge	Practical knowledge	
Knowledge for action	Knowledge in action	Reflection in action

Tacit knowledge and intuition

Linked to the nature of knowledge is the question 'how do we know'? In relation to practical knowledge, the ways that we know may be explained by the concepts of *intuition* and *tacit knowledge*. These concepts have been the subject of much philosophical discussion outside nursing, and latterly within nursing. Tacit knowledge was the term coined by Polanyi, a contemporary philosopher who defined it as 'knowing more than we can say or articulate' (Polanyi, 1967). There are problems in defining, describing and making explicit such knowledge.

The same could be said of intuition, defined as 'understanding without rationale' (Benner and Tanner, 1987), and linked to expert human judgement. It is presented as a legitimate activity with six interdependent key elements, not as an irrational act or guesswork. Benner and Tanner (1987) provide examples of intuitive judgement in expert nurses using Drefus' six key aspects as a framework (Table 10.2).

The concept of practical knowledge is also promoted by contemporary writers, such as Schon (1983, 1987), who have tried to elucidate the nature of knowledge in practice disciplines other than nursing. Schon (1987) acknowledges that in explaining expert professional practice, outstanding practitioners are not said to have more professional knowledge than others, but more wisdom, talent, intuition or artistry. He also recognises that unfortunately these names are seen as 'junk categories, attaching names to phenomena that elude conventional strategies of explanation' (Schon, 1987).

In the past, professional or clinical judgements have been equated with intuition, and explained by more traditional scientific rationales such as the information-processing view, or by the statistical weighting of information to make judgements (Elstein and Bordage, 1988). It is interesting to note the possible links with gender of such terms as 'intuition' and 'professional judgement'. Intuition is often associated culturally with women's ways of knowing, whereas professional judgement is likely to be a term associated

Table. 10.2 Six key aspects of intuitive judgement (adapted from Benner and Tanner, 1987; see also Leddy and Pepper, 1993)

Pattern recognition
Perceptual ability to recognise relationships without pre-specifying components of the situation

Similarity recognition
The ability to see similarities and parallels among patient situations, even when there are marked dissimilarities in objective features

Common-sense understanding
A deep grasp of the culture and language, so that flexible understanding in diverse situations is possible. A grasp or understanding of the patient's lived experience of illness which enables the nurse to 'tune in' to the patient

Skilled know-how
Based on a combination of 'know-how' and 'know-that', permitting flexibility in actions and judgement in differing situations

A sense of salience
Deciding what is of most significance in a situation

Deliberate rationality
The use of analysis and past experience to consider alternative interpretations of the clinical situation

with men. Within nursing, Carper (1978) has undertaken the foundation work of bringing together all of the ways of knowing that are pertinent to nursing, integrating both practical and theoretical knowledge.

Carper's 'patterns of knowing'

Carper (1978) was one of the first nurses to consider the nature of knowledge in nursing by focusing on the questions 'What does it mean to know?' and 'What kinds of knowledge are held to be of most value in the discipline of nursing?' She identified four patterns of knowing from the nursing literature:

- empirics – the science of nursing;
- aesthetics – the art of nursing;
- personal knowing;
- ethical knowing.

EMPIRICS

Scientific knowledge or, as Carper describes it, empirics, concerns the science of nursing. Such knowledge is organised systematically into general laws and theories, the purpose being to describe, explain and predict phenomena. However, Chinn and Kramer (1995) suggest that the science of nursing has broadened to include evidence that does not strictly fall within the realms of hypothesis testing, such as phenomenological descriptions or inductive (grounded) means of hypothesis generation. Empirics equates well in this context with the concept of theoretical knowledge and know-that knowledge mentioned earlier. It is important to note that underlying assumptions about the nature of reality and human beings are fundamentally different in *empiricism* and *phenomenology*.

Pure empiricism is an influential theory, central to science, that is concerned with how knowledge is obtained. It can be described as the process whereby evidence rooted in objective reality and gathered through the human senses is used as the basis for generating knowledge through the scientific approach (Polit and Hungler, 1991). 'Scientific approach' in this sense means a set of orderly, systematic and controlled procedures for acquiring dependable empirical information (Polit and Hungler, 1991). This view of traditional science is often termed *logical positivism* after a group of Viennese philosophers who believed that this approach was as valid for explaining human behaviour as it was for explaining the natural world. Any statement, then, whose truth can be confirmed by observation of the world is an empirical statement (Hospers, 1990). However, the source of such statements may be theories from the creative imagination, or a rational logical argument from preceding laws and propositions.

Empiricism provides one way of justifying how we know, remembering the philosophical definition of knowledge discussed earlier as 'a justified true belief'. Hypotheses are therefore generated, and these are tested by observation and experiment, as is the case in the core empirical sciences of biology, chemistry, physics and even psychology (see Chapters 4 and 5).

Empiricism itself is only one theory, yet a powerful one, of how knowledge can be justified and therefore generated. Such theories are encompassed by *epistemology*, a key branch of philosophy. Other major theories that have been developed to explain how we know include, *rationalism* and *pragmatism*. Each has different underlying assumptions about the nature of truth and reality. To the empiricist there exists an objective reality waiting to be discovered; such reality is independent of the observer. To the rationalist, truth is evidenced through logical processes, and knowledge can only be gained through the exercise of reason independent of the senses. To the pragmatist, truth is linked to usefulness as determined by its users.

Empirical knowledge is equated with scientific knowledge, which is in turn often considered to be synonymous with knowledge itself. It is this type of knowledge that currently holds much power within society. For example, advertising strategies often capitalise on this by promoting their products as 'scientifically tested'. However, this approach has been severely challenged because of its underlying assumption that reality is objective and that human beings can be understood by reducing them to their constituent parts. In contrast, phenomenology focuses on subjective experience and multiple realities – human beings are considered to be complex, and multi-faceted; we cannot understand people by reducing them to parts. Such approaches have been used to make sense of expert practical knowledge in nursing (Benner and Wrubel, 1989), and also to understand patients' experiences (Benner, 1994; see also Chapter 6).

AESTHETICS

Aesthetic knowing is the art of nursing expressed by individual nurses in their actions and interactions with patients in unique situations. Chinn and Kramer (1995) consider art to 'exist at the moment'; 'art is not expressed in language but artistically in the moment of the experience-action.' They identify three linked creative processes as follows:

- *engaging* – the direct involvement of the self within a situation, which leads to the experience of the moment;
- *intuiting* – the subsequent meaning of the moment and its understanding which comes from deep within the subjective experience. It is intuited from the context of the individual's experience through being in the situation at that moment. It leads directly to;
- *envisioning* – a creative response to the unique moment and the envisioning of new creative possibilities.

Intuition is therefore integral to aesthetic ways of knowing. Benner and Tanner (1987) reinforce this view: art in nursing is unique, creative, and falls outside what can be taught. They consider that intuitive judgement involves both complex skilled performance and artistry. Hampton (1994) argues that intuition and expertise are closely related and, furthermore, that they are at their most highly developed in expert nurses, where expertise is more closely related to art than to empirical aspects of nursing.

However, Johnson (1994) considers that there is much diversity in what is meant by art in nursing. She aims at conceptual clarity by using discourse analysis of nursing literature over a century as part of her examination of nursing art. Five exclusive *senses of nursing art* are identified, each relating to the nurse's ability to:

- grasp meaning in the patient's encounters;
- establish a meaningful connection with the patient;
- perform nursing activities skilfully;
- determine a course of nursing action rationally;
- conduct his or her nursing practice morally.

The first three senses encapsulate the more contemporary views of Benner and Tanner (1987) and Chinn and Kramer (1995). The fourth sense of nursing art derives predominantly from the more historical literature on the subject for the century up to the mid-1980s. The fifth sense, in contrast, seems to equate well with Carper's (1978) concept of *ethical knowing*.

PERSONAL KNOWING

Personal knowing relates to the way in which nurses view themselves and the client, and is about knowing one's self. Personal knowing is essential for the 'therapeutic use of self' (Carper, 1978) within client–carer relationships (see Chapter 5). This type of knowledge is the most difficult to teach and master. Examples demonstrating the need to develop this type of knowledge can be seen in the work of Barber (1986) and in Chapter 6 of this volume, and in the work of Burnard (1988). In Sweeney's (1994) concept analysis of personal knowledge, Carper's view equates with self-knowledge. On the other hand, Polanyi's (1962) view is seen to be more global – to include linking the knower to the known, recognising the energy and activity involved in developing personal knowing. Smith (1992) concludes that personal knowing is fundamental to all other ways of knowing.

ETHICAL KNOWING

Finally, ethical knowing encompasses 'the understanding of different philosophical positions about what is good, right and wrong' (Carper, 1978). This type of knowledge develops from a consideration of areas of ethical enquiry and analysis of moral decision-making, e.g. from the perspectives of Jeremy Bentham's (1748–1832) utilitarianism, or from Immanuel Kant's (1724–1804) idealism. It also focuses on values and a consideration of harmful effects and benefits. However, within nursing, ethical knowing is more than ethical theories. It concerns the making of ethical judgements that often involve conflicting values, norms, interests and principles (Chinn and Kramer, 1995). The three expressive processes associated with this are considered to be clarifying, valuing and advocating (Chinn and Kramer, 1995).

Carper considers each pattern of knowing to be fundamentally distinct, yet interrelated and interdependent with the other ways of knowing.

Knowledge and theory

Theory provides a method for generating knowledge. The word 'theory' is often used loosely by lay people to mean 'the content covered in the classroom, as opposed to the actual practice of performing nursing activities' (Polit and Hungler, 1991); it may be used in lay terms to indicate the opposite of the practical or useful (Chinn and Kramer, 1995). If this is how theory is viewed by practising nurses, it is not surprising that so much concern and confusion exists about the nature and purpose of nursing theory and theory in nursing. Theories are often misconstrued because they are considered to be the product of academic theorising in academic institutions that are far removed from practice settings. In fact, theories represent 'a scientist's best efforts to describe and explain phenomena' (Polit and Hungler, 1991). Theories do, therefore, serve some purpose, as they help us to make sense of what we observe and perceive by suggesting relationships between concepts. Such statements of relationships between variables are termed propositions in traditional science. All of these characteristics are nicely brought together in Riehl and Roy's (1980) definition of a theory as 'a logically inter-connected set of propositions used to *describe, explain,* and *predict* a part of the empirical world'.

However, this definition is a very traditional one in terms of our earlier discussion about the nature of knowledge and reality. It is congruent with a view of knowledge as being objective. The purpose of theory in this context, then, is to describe, explain and predict the empirical world. The underlying assumption is that such theories can be generalised to all situations because there is only one reality.

This definition of theory would therefore be appropriate for the genera-tion of knowledge in traditional science, because it brings together a logical and rational set of propositions together with a view of reality that is objec-tive. This is often termed *logical empiricism* or *logical positivism.* However, it would not be an appropriate definition for theories that describe subjective experience or individual interpretation, as these experiences cannot be gen-eralised to every person or situation – multiple realities are very much accepted. Such multiple realities may still share areas of common ground. Nonetheless, descriptions of such experiences can still generate theory, but they proceed no further than descriptions. Chinn and Kramer's (1995) defini-tion is more representative of theory encompassing both approaches: theory is a 'systematic abstraction of reality that serves some purpose'. However, Watson (1985) considers that the purpose of theory is to understand and illu-minate. This, it could be argued, is more congruent with nursing's purpose, and encompasses all ways of knowing that are relevant to nursing.

If nursing acknowledges the value of ways of knowing (discussed above), it is logical and essential for nurses to understand how theory is generated for all ways of knowing. This is not only to articulate nursing's contribution to health care, but also to understand the directions that other members of the multidisciplinary team, with whom we collaborate, may be coming from.

Theory generation will now be considered from the three perspectives of traditional science/logical positivism, interpretative approaches and *critical theory.*

Theory generation in traditional science/logical positivism

Returning to the traditional scientific or logical positivist sense of the word theory, the following example illustrates how theories may be developed from their descriptive purpose to their predictive purpose. A theory about the swallowing difficulties of people with Alzheimer's disease may *describe* the swallowing problems and the context in which they occur, *explain* the relationships between factors (e.g. eating alone may be linked to the swal-lowing problems) and finally, in its most sophisticated form, allow us to pre-scribe nursing actions which we can confidently *predict* will reduce swallowing problems in response to specific interventions.

Assessment tools developed in nursing often integrate descriptive, explanatory and predictive theory. These tools are derived from a description of the factors that are commonly associated with a particular phenomenon, e.g. pain, incontinence or decubitus ulcers. These factors may then be weighted due to more positive correlations between some factors than between others, as is found, for example, in the Glasgow coma scale (Teasdale and Jennett, 1974) or various pressure sore tools (Waterlow, 1985). These tools may be predictive in the way that they identify particular high-risk groups, such as possible victims of child abuse, depression or alcoholism.

Benner and Tanner (1987) link the use of assessment tools to nurse performance at competence level and to a check-list mentality (see Chapter 1). They warn against the slavish use of prescribed assessment tools, which can limit the development of more flexible ways of knowing. Expert practice is characterised and developed by active enquiry and skilled pattern recognition. This is achieved by focusing on the whole situation, rather than by dissecting the situation into elemental parts (Benner and Tanner, 1987). The moral here is that there is a place for assessment tools in assisting novice nurses to become competent, but that their underlying assumptions must always be acknowledged. These assumptions relate not only to the nature of reality, but also to the way in which expert practitioners rather than competent practitioners perceive situations.

When generating and refining theory while adopting this approach, Dickoff and James (1968) reiterate the importance of the purpose of theory, in that nursing must generate theory which will serve to achieve its purposes and goals. Consequently, this determines how Dickoff and James propose that theory is generated. They suggest four levels of theory generation whereby the fourth level, entitled 'situation-producing' theory, is the most sophisticated. This level of theory is practice-orientated because it involves the prescription of nursing actions to achieve desired outcomes. For this reason, Walker and Avant (1995) suggest that fourth-level theory is really therefore 'practice' theory. Each of the lower levels of theory acts as a basis for the next, so contributing to the development of theory with prescriptive status. Walker and Avant (1995) considered that these four levels 'roughly paralleled the acts of description, explanation, prediction and control'. However, before 'practice' theory can be developed, Dickoff and James (1968) state that the other three levels of theory must be passed through. Table 10.3 links the four levels of theory to Walker and Avant's terms, using the example of swallowing difficulties.

First-level theory (factor-isolating) is concerned with the identification of factors and variables, and their subsequent definition. Dickoff *et al.* (1968) consider that the generation of first-level theory, i.e. that of isolating and naming factors, is one which is so basic that it is often overlooked. Johnson (cited in Adam, 1985) also supports the view that nurses may be neglecting the first levels of theory development. Fawcett (1978), too, considers that basic descriptive studies which could provide 'the baseline data crucial for theory-building' have been neglected in favour of experimental studies, which have predominantly been preferred as a research approach for theory-testing, even though they lack a firm theoretical foundation. Describing the concepts that are central to nursing practice is therefore both

Table. 10.3 Four levels of theory (Dickoff and James, 1968) and their corresponding description (Walker and Avant, 1995), applied to the example of difficulty in swallowing

Level 1 Factor-isolating DESCRIPTION	Patients with Alzheimer's, particularly those with the most limited short-term memories, appear to forget to swallow when they are eating alone.
Clarifying phenomena	The swallowing difficulties may be described as the person appearing to forget that there is food in their mouth. They then start choking as they continue to breathe normally, as if there was no food in their mouth.
Level 2 Factor-relating EXPLANATION	The swallowing problems may be explained by the fact that the patient forgets that the food is in their mouth.
Correlating or associating factors	Eating alone also means that there are no visual cues from other people to remind the patient to chew and swallow.
Level 3 Situation-isolating PREDICTION *Explaining and predicting how situations are related*	It may be predicted that by enabling patients with these swallowing difficulties to eat their meals with others, the number of swallowing problems may be reduced.
Level 4 Situation-producing CONTROL	Nurses may specifically prescribe an intervention on the care plan, to enable their patients to eat meals with others, with the specific purpose of reducing identified swallowing problems.

appropriate and important as a place to start in theory-building, as concepts are the building blocks of theory.

The directory and classification of nursing diagnosis (Gordon, 1982) provides useful insights into concepts considered important to nursing both in the past and in the present. Increasingly common, however, within the UK literature is the use of concept analysis, a philosophical approach to describing and clarifying the nature of concepts (Allan, 1993; McCormack, 1993; Masterson, 1993). Yet even within concept analysis there are different approaches which relate to different views of reality. Walker and Avant's (1995) approach, used by many writers, applies a traditional positivist approach to concepts. If used strictly, concepts exist independently in reality, and they can be operationally defined in ways that allow them to be identified empirically. Criticisms are made by Rodgers (1993), among others, concerning this point. Rodgers suggests a much less rigid approach which focuses on the common use of the concept rather than how it is physically defined. Both approaches are useful in developing and clarifying common meanings if their underlying assumptions and/or limitations are acknowledged.

Second-level theory attempts to explain the situation by identifying possible relationships between factors, and several other propositions could be developed in relation to the example shown in Table 10.3. *Third-level theory* predicts what may occur if factors are varied or manipulated. In *fourth-level theory*, control of the situation can be achieved where nursing intervention has a high probability of accomplishing desired goals. This approach, although congruent with traditional views of theory generation, has been strongly criticised for the underlying assumption that human beings can be manipulated and reduced to a number of variables, which can in turn be separated from their context and wholeness.

It is Dickoff and James's (1968) major contention that 'all theory exists finally for the sake of practice (since in a sense every lower level of theory exists for the next higher level, and the highest level exists for practice ...)'. If Dickoff and James's view of theory is to be accepted, then nursing knowledge development will commence with the generation of theory at first level where various phenomena need to be described and defined. However, support for higher levels of theory may depend upon underlying values in relation to the philosophy of science. Such an approach is consistent with the traditional scientific approach which suggests that there are variables which can be manipulated within a controlled environment, rather than recognising that phenomena are complex and context dependent. It is these very criticisms that have led to different approaches to theory development in a number of disciplines, including nursing.

Generating theory in the interpretive approach

Theories from an interpretive perspective would describe and make sense of phenomena from the *emic* perspective, that is, from the perspective of the person undergoing the experience, rather than from the researcher's *etic* viewpoint. The interest of this approach is in understanding the subjective experience and reality as perceived by individuals. If nursing is about helping people to make sense of their experiences and to make informed choices about health care-related issues and the implications of these choices, then an understanding of how this is experienced by patients is vital knowledge for nursing. For example, patients who undergo surgery to reduce intra-optic pressures for glaucoma may not realise that their sight may be considerably worse afterwards, that this visual impairment may continue for months, that they may develop a cataract as a side-effect of such surgery, that their lifestyle may be dramatically changed if they cannot drive and they live in an inaccessible area, and that hobbies involving close visual work would become impossible to pursue. Understanding how such experiences are lived can therefore assist nurses in preparing patients to have realistic expectations and subsequently to engage in more informed decision-making.

Approaches to theory development in this area then draw on research methodologies that enable such experiences to be described and their meanings understood from the patient's point of view. Phenomenology and ethnography are two such examples. Such approaches are underpinned by the view that reality is subjective and that multiple realities can and do exist. These approaches are being used to begin to make sense of both the patient's and the nurse's experiences in caring (Benner and Wrubel, 1989) and in knowing the patient (Tanner *et al.*, 1993).

The research methods used within such methodologies would need to ensure consistency with the underlying assumptions about the nature of reality within this approach. Such methods generate rich data, which then has to be verified at various stages of analysis with the informants, in order to ensure that the informant's interpretation rather than the researcher's view is being represented. Approaches to ensure the trustworthiness of the resulting theory are identified by such writers as Lincoln and Guba (1985). The theory resulting from these approaches would convey descriptions and meaning to informants about their experiences. This in turn can help nurses to understand the nature of such experiences, to connect with others undergoing similar experiences, or to gain insights into how nursing practice can be improved in the future.

Like positivism, this approach also has its critics, and these criticisms mainly relate to the context or social reality in which the individual acts being described as neutral (Carr and Kemmis, 1986). The influence of the social context on the individual is not therefore acknowledged. Indeed, Carr and Kemmis believe that positivism itself has created the illusion of an objective reality over which the individual has no control, and hence to a decline in the capacity of individuals to reflect upon their situations and change them through their own actions. It is this situation that is addressed by critical theory.

Theory generation and critical theory

Critical theory is the label given to a view of theory that has the central task of emancipating people from the positivist 'domination of thought' through their own understandings and actions (Carr and Kemmis, 1986). Habermas (1965) is the most prominent of modern critical theorists. He considered that knowledge was the outcome of human activity motivated by natural needs and interests, and his analysis suggested three types of interest:

- *technical*, such as scientific explanations, as with traditional science;
- *practical*, which clarifies meanings in communication, as in the interpretive view;
- *emancipatory*, which goes beyond a concern for subjective meaning in order to understand the context in which social action takes place. This is the focus of critical social science.

Critical social science provides the kind of self-reflective understanding that will permit individuals to explain why the conditions under which they operate are frustrating (see Chapters 3 and 5 to 8). In turn, this also suggests 'the sort of action that is required if the sources of these frustrations are to be eliminated' (Carr and Kemmis, 1986). Reflection is, therefore, inextricably linked to action. Reflective practice and praxis (reflection and action) are the key ways of developing theory within this approach (Emden, 1991). Such theory may be of a personal rather than a public nature. Theory from reflection both influences practitioners in their everyday practice and is itself derived from reflection on their practice and actions.

Tools that facilitate and guide reflective practice through mechanisms such as clinical supervision (Johns, 1995) assist the practitioner in uncovering the influences within their practice situations, and in helping them to become more effective in their practice through the provision of challenge and support. Such tools facilitate practitioners' learning by helping them to make sense of real situations by transforming nursing's body of knowledge and integrating it with their own personal knowledge and experience (Johns, 1995). Fundamental to this knowledge and experience are the values and beliefs held by the practitioner.

A range of tools exists to facilitate reflection, such as those proposed by Boud *et al.* (1985), Johns (1994) and Mezirow (1981). In Johns' view, reflection should always be guided, a view that is held by both Habermas (1974) and Boud *et al.* (1985), who identify the danger of self-deception in self-reflection.

Developing theory and knowledge from practice through reflection must be one of the most important challenges to contemporary nursing today. This approach will not only enable nurses to make explicit what they do, and the complexities of their situations, but will also allow professional situations to be changed in a direction that will enable future challenges in health care to be met. In addition, it will be a powerful strategy for enabling patients and their families to become enlightened and therefore emancipated to change their circumstances.

The scope of theory in nursing

Nursing theories are often equated with nursing models but nursing models are only one type of theory, namely grand theory. Theory types can be classified according to their scope, i.e. their degree of *generalisability*. Walker and Avant (1995) identify four types of theory;

- meta-theory;
- grand theory (sometimes called macro or molar theory);
- middle-range theory;
- practice theory.

Meta-theory is concerned with philosophical and methodological aspects of theory-building in nursing, e.g. philosophical issues about the relationships between nursing theory, the philosophy of science and nursing knowledge. Examples include the work of Dickoff and James (1968) and Suppe and Jacox (1985). It is 'the designated theory about theory and the processes for developing theory' (Chinn and Kramer, 1995). Some would say that it is theorising about theory! Nevertheless, it is because of meta-theory that nursing is in a much stronger position today in being able to state what knowledge is important for nursing, and how such knowledge should be generated.

Grand theories are those known as models in nursing. They define nursing broadly and abstractly from a global perspective, describing 'the whole of nursing's concern' (Chinn and Kramer, 1995). Fawcett (1995) defines such nursing theories as conceptual frameworks, and differentiates them from grand theories, conceptual frameworks being broader in scope. Such grand theories, according to Walker and Avant (1995), have made an important contribution, conceptually distinguishing nursing from the practice of medicine by demonstrating the presence of distinct nursing perspectives. However, because of the vague terminology used and the lack of clear interrelationships between concepts at this stage in their development, most of these theories are untestable (Suppe and Jacox, 1985; Walker and Avant, 1995). They cannot be generated or tested empirically, but are generated through thoughtful and insightful appraisal of existing ideas (Fawcett, 1995).

Middle-range theories, although still abstract, contain elements of grand theories but have less scope and fewer variables, so are therefore more suitable for testing (Walker and Avant, 1995). Fawcett (1995) considers that they are composed of concepts and propositions that are empirically measurable. Some middle-range theories have been developed from grand theories with which they are congruent, e.g. King's (1981) *theory of goal attainment* and Orem's *self-care deficit theory* (1985). These theories do include propositions which could be empirically tested.

Finally, the last level identified by Walker and Avant is *practice theory*, which was initially described by Dickoff and James (1968) as situation-relating theory. This view of practice theory is very narrow and has a more traditional scientific focus, as interventions are linked causally to the achievement of specific goals. However, practice theory today is viewed in a completely different light, and has a different meaning. It is much more along the lines of praxis and accessing the knowledge embedded in practice through reflection (Gray and Forsstrom, 1991). This view of practice theory captures the uniqueness of nursing in practice situations, and relates to the nature of intuition and artistry.

Classifications of nursing models (grand theories) in nursing

Most nursing models or theories can be classified as grand theory because they are abstract. They 'give some broad perspective to the goals and structure of nursing practice' (Walker and Avant, 1995). Nursing theories, according to Chinn and Kramer (1995), 'ought to guide practice, generate new ideas, and differentiate the focus of nursing from other professions'. All nursing models or theories state something about the following four concepts (see Chapter 4), which Fawcett (1995) collectively referred to as the *metaparadigm of nursing*:

- *person* – the recipient of nursing;
- *environment* – includes the person's significant others as well as the physical setting;

- *health*;
- *nursing* – its nature and role.

The metaparadigm of a discipline outlines global concepts that identify the phenomena of interest to a discipline (Kuhn, 1977). In fact, these four global concepts, or 'constructs' to be more correct (constructs being more abstract and including a number of concepts), are fundamental to nursing's knowledge base, and therefore form the building blocks of the Project 2000 curriculum (see Chapters 3 and 9).

As previously stated, nursing models are not designed to be tested. Instead, they are representations of the values and beliefs held by the theorists about what nursing is, and its central concepts. The values espoused also tell us something about the world-view in which theorists operate, and how they view reality. They are abstract, and are not intended to be practical. Many early nursing models were augmented and supported by theories from other disciplines, and were often presented as ripe for testing and transfer into practice. It is this image that provokes the criticism that models are prescriptive and represent the 'nursing as it should be' view, rather than 'nursing as it is'. Modern nurses are generally making more informed choices about the models that they use based on their own or common values and beliefs, which are first clarified before selecting a model that has the most congruent value system (Manley 1992; Warfield and Manley, 1990).

Theories from other disciplines have been used to augment many nursing theories. They have also been used extensively in nursing in the past to describe and explain phenomena observed in practice, e.g. Engel's (1962) middle-range theory from psychology which relates psychosocial stressors to the physiological state of 'fight and flight' (see Chapter 5). This theory may be used in nursing to prescribe nursing care in, for example, the patient who has recently suffered a myocardial infarction. Such a person may be particularly vulnerable to cardiac arrhythmias as a result of increased circulating adrenaline, secondary to sympathetic arousal. Such arousal could, according to Engel's theory, also result from exposure to psychosocial stressors. If the person is of a highly independent nature, then it may be more stressful psychologically if dependence in activities of living is enforced, rather than allowing the person to continue with his own self-care. From this example alone the values underlying such theories about the nature of the individual person could be extrapolated, and today would not possibly be considered consistent with contemporary views. In the past these assumptions were not challenged, and the appropriateness of transferring such theories to nursing situations was automatically accepted. This author is not arguing that all theories developed outside nursing are inappropriate, but that they be considered carefully in relation to their relevance to nursing practice and their underlying values. A further example is the use of adult-learning theory. Such theory was developed in well people, but how appropriate is it for developing educational strategies with sick people?

Similarly, theories from social science such as *symbolic interactionism* (grand theory) have been used by nurse theorists such as Orlando (1961), Riehl-Sisca

(1989) and Wiedenbach (1964) to suggest how the interaction between client and nurse can be understood. Symbolic interaction is a grand theory which shares similar values and beliefs to the interpretive approach mentioned earlier, where knowledge is understood to be subjective. The use of nursing models based on these theories may be congruent with such organisational approaches as primary nursing, where the focus is on developing a therapeutic relationship (Manley, 1990). In Chapters 5, 6 and 7, psychological and sociological theories are considered in more detail as a source of nursing knowledge.

Several classifications of nursing theory exist. Riehl and Roy (1980) classify nursing models according to the origin of their underpinning theories as follows: those underpinning theories that originate in disciplines outside nursing, namely *developmental theories*, e.g. Kohlberg's (1981) moral reasoning developmental theory and Maslow's (1968) psychosocial theory; *systems theories*, e.g. von Bertalanffy's (1968) general systems theory; and *theories of interaction*, e.g. those based within symbolic interactionism.

Understanding nursing from the perspective of these nursing models would then dictate the knowledge basis for nursing. For example, if one uses models based on systems theory, then within the nurse–patient relationship both patient and nurse would be mutually affected by any change – changes in one partner of that relationship will have an effect on the other, and vice versa. This supports the value of aesthetic knowledge and knowledge of self as proposed by Carper (1978). Models based on growth and development imply that nurses, depending on the setting, would need to assess and recognise where clients were placed in their psychological, social, psychosexual, moral, cognitive and interpersonal development, before they could help the client to move forward. It is often assumed that clients, relatives and students can grasp complex moral issues without considering what stage they are at with regard to their moral reasoning, using either Gilligan's (1982) or Kohlberg's (1981) moral reasoning and developmental stages.

Although all theories can be criticised, it is important to remember the previous point made about the nature of theory, that it is the theorist's best tool for describing and explaining observed phenomena (Polit and Hungler, 1991). For the individual practitioner, theories may or may not be helpful for making sense of individual situations. Often theories act as heuristic devices by providing guidelines so that practitioners may find out things for themselves.

There are other classifications, and before leaving this topic we should mention the classification proposed by Meleis (1991), as it conveys an evolutionary view of nursing's development. Meleis classified nursing models into schools of thought which relate to some extent to their chronology, to the backgrounds of the theorists, and to the social context at the time of their development. Each school of thought is associated with a particular question which determines the main focus of the model. These questions, if considered carefully, can also throw some light on the knowledge important to nursing. The three schools of thought are termed *needs*, *interaction* and *outcome* theories. According to Meleis, needs theorists asked the question 'what do nurses do?', interaction theorists asked the question 'how do nurses do whatever it is they do?' and outcome theorists asked the question 'why?', although they did not ignore the aspects 'what?' and 'how?'

Needs theorists based their models on theories by Maslow (1968) and the developmental theorist Erikson (1995). Further examples of needs theorists are Henderson (1966) and Orem (1985). The focus of this school of thought is on problems, deficits and needs, with nursing fulfilling the role of meeting needs. Although distinct from the medical model, the focus is still very much on illness, without perceptions of the client or environmental influences.

The *interactionist* school of thought represented by theorists such as King (1981) and Peplau (1952) developed from the needs school, and was influenced by the social and cultural changes of the 1950s and 1960s, which are described more fully by Meleis (1991). The characteristics of the interactionists are that nursing is seen to be an interaction process which is deliberate, and involves helping and caring (see Chapter 1). Caring is considered to be humanistic rather than mechanistic. The nurse–patient relationship is considered to be therapeutic, which means that the nurse would use herself in a therapeutic way (see Chapter 6). To achieve this, she needs to consider, clarify and evaluate her own values (personal knowledge). Illness is considered an 'inevitable human experience' (Meleis, 1991), one from which the individual can grow and learn. The theories underpinning this school relate to humanism, interactionism and phenomenology (where experiences of the world are central) and existential philosophies (where individuals are considered to be unique beings who are able to make choices).

Theorists of the *outcome school*, including Rogers (1970) and Roy (1984), are concerned with the outcome of care. Building on the 'what?' and 'how?', they focus on the recipient of care and his or her harmony with the environment. The goal of nursing care is therefore to bring back 'some balance, stability, and preservation of energy, or [enhance] the individual and the environment' (Meleis, 1991).

So what are the issues for the future in relation to nursing models? Have models passed their 'sell by' date? As nurses become more able to promote and articulate their philosophy, do we actually need them? How far is it provocative to suggest that perhaps we could manage equally well with clear statements of values and beliefs about our purpose, complemented by individualised strategies of care and assessment tools congruent with our philosophies? This is of course a controversial view. However, this author believes that nursing models fulfil three important purposes. First, models are *heuristic devices*, that is, they are tools which can assist practitioners so long as their underlying assumptions are acknowledged. This is a purpose they have in common with all theories. Secondly, models provide general direction and guidance which can facilitate a common purpose. Thirdly, models represent a set of values and beliefs which may best represent the values and beliefs held by a group of nurses in the absence of devising their own model.

In relation to the last point, nurses in the UK have now developed the skills and maturity to develop their own models, e.g. the 'Burford Model'

(Salvage, 1990). However, nurses are also more able to articulate values and beliefs about nursing's nature and purpose. Thus, the heyday of nursing models may have passed, as they have served their purpose and now need to take their place as one type of theory that is complementary to other types – practice theory and nursing concepts. Nursing concepts by their very nature are much more concrete, and practice theory relates to the practice issues that practitioners address daily. This is not a new direction; the need to address the substance and practice of nursing has been a message frequently directed at the nursing theorist in the past.

Knowledge and philosophy

Many aspects of philosophy have already been referred to, e.g. *metaphysics* (the nature of reality), *epistemology* (the nature of truth, how knowledge is justified and generated), *axiology* (ethics and aesthetics, values and beliefs) and *logic* (deductive and inductive thinking). Such concepts are fundamental to philosophy, and should rightly be the starting point for considering the knowledge appropriate for nursing. Silva (1977) historically notes that 'ultimately all nursing theory and research is derived from or leads to philosophy' and 'if nurse researchers are to study the structure of nursing knowledge, they must first understand the relationships among philosophy, science and theory'. So what is philosophy? 'Philosophy provides a point of view: it is a belief construct, a speculation about the nature and value of things' (Bevis, 1982).

Philosophy is the 'seeking after wisdom or knowledge, especially that which deals with ultimate reality, or with the most general causes and principles of things and ideas and human perception and knowledge of them, physical phenomena and ethics' (Concise Oxford Dictionary, 1976). It is the first discipline, existing for hundreds of years before more specialised fields of enquiry, such as politics and psychology, branched out from under its umbrella. Many philosophers do not agree as to what the components of philosophy are, but in an effort to make philosophy more understandable, and at risk of over-simplifing it, the outline in Figure 10.1 may provide the reader with some boundaries within which to work.

All branches of philosophy are interdependent. For example, views on the nature of reality (ontology) will influence what is knowledge (epistemology) and also what is valuable (aesthetics). However, this chapter, through focusing on knowledge, has emphasised epistemology, but in doing so we hope it has also alerted the reader to issues relating to the other aspects of philosophy which are closely linked to it. Examples of epistemological questions are 'how does one come to know?' or 'what is knowledge?' In most other disciplines, and in nursing until recently, the most valued approach to developing knowledge has been the *scientific–empirical* approach, although this is rapidly changing as alternative ways of knowing are being recognised as important. Each area of knowledge should be analysed both for what it is

PHILOSOPHY

METAPHYSICS	AXIOLOGY	EPISTEMOLOGY	LOGIC
The theory of being	Theory of values What is valuable?	Theory of knowledge What is true?	Theory of reasoning Laws of thought and forms of argument

Ontology
- Nature of ultimate reality
- Nature of god and being
- Nature of mankind e.g. free will and determinism

Ethics
Theory of morality

- Morals and beliefs

- Nature of knowledge and justification of belief Origins, nature, methods, limits of knowledge

- Deduction
- Induction

Cosmology
- Nature of the world e.g. origin and structure of the world

Aesthetics
Theory of beauty
- Study of art and beauty

Truth
Reason
Science

PRACTICAL PHILOSOPHY
Application of philosophical theory to the study of other subjects

Philosophy of religion
Philosophy of the mind,
freedom of the will and
immortality

Politics

Philosophy of science
Philosophy of psychology
Philosophy of law
Philosophy of language

Figure 10.1   Branches of philosophy

and for its purpose by considering the following questions formulated by Chalmers (1982): first, 'what is the aim of knowledge?', which could differ from what the aim is commonly thought to be or presented as being; secondly, 'what methods are used to accomplish the aims?'; thirdly, 'to what degree have the aims been successfully accomplished?'

This line of thought focuses on knowledge itself, rather than on whether or not knowledge can be claimed to be scientific. There have been many criticisms, initially from outside nursing (Chalmers, 1982) and latterly from inside nursing (Suppe and Jacox, 1985), about the traditional approach to science, and views of the nature of scientific knowledge (i.e. the philosophy of science). Before these changes can be examined in more detail, it is important to differentiate between philosophy and science. Table 10.4 indicates more clearly how philosophy differs from empirical science.

Such words as 'knowledge' and 'science' are not well defined, and they are often considered to be basically the same. Furthermore, science is seen to be 'true' knowledge, i.e. knowledge in its supreme form. However, science can be thought of in two ways, first as a body of knowledge such as empirical knowledge which is the outcome of methods used to generate knowledge, and secondly as a process which relates to the logical and systematic methods used to generate knowledge. The problem central to the philosophy of science (Suppe and Jacox, 1985) is understanding the nature of scientific knowledge. It is hoped that the following brief review will illustrate how this has changed over time.

Table. 10.4   Differing characteristics of philosophy and empirical science

Philosophy	Empirical science
(after Bevis, 1982)	
Explores values	Describes facts
Looks at wholes and relationships with other wholes	Reduces phenomena to component parts to study, describe and explain how they operate
Answers 'why?' questions and queries the worth of experience	Answers 'how?', 'when?' and 'where?'
Provides a value system for ordering priorities and selecting from various data	
(after Sarter, 1988)	
Unlimited totality: 'the entire universe'	Domain delineated and definite

Historical aspects of the philosophy of science

Aristotle, Greek philosopher and a pupil of Plato, lived in the ancient world (see Table 10.6). He studied the whole field of knowledge, and considered that knowledge was derived from *deductive logic*. In this view, the scientist was considered to be primarily a passive observer of what was. This view about knowledge continued until the sixteenth century when Francis Bacon, English philosopher and a founder of modern science, rejected Aristotle's view of knowledge generation in favour of the *inductive method*. Bacon considered that the purpose of science was to improve 'man's lot on earth' and 'if we wanted to understand nature then we must consult nature and not the writings of Aristotle' (quoted in Chalmers, 1982). This could only be achieved by inductive methods. Such methods involve producing universal statements by generalising from a series of organised and careful observations of specific situations or phenomena. Whereas induction is concerned with producing generalisations from specific situations, deduction is the reverse – the application of general principles to specific situations through the use of logical argument. In order to clarify the difference between these conceptual approaches, the reader is referred to Table 10.5, which illustrates examples of both, as well as identifying their limitations.

Empiricism (discussed previously) considers all knowledge to be derived from experience via pure observation and the collection of facts through the senses, a position strongly supported by the English philosopher John Locke in the seventeenth century. *Rationalism*, an opposing view of how knowledge about the world is generated, defined as the generation of knowledge through the application of reason, was pioneered by the French mathematician René Descartes in the seventeenth century.

Table. 10.5   Examples to illustrate inductive and deductive approaches in nursing

Induction	Logical argument from the specific observation to the general
Example	Statement of observations made: 'I have observed that all patients that I have admitted for elective surgery have appeared anxious' Generalisation by induction: 'all patients admitted for elective surgery will be anxious'.
Limitations	Although the initial observation may be true, the conclusion may not be true because it may not apply to all patients everywhere.
Deduction	Logical argument from general principles applied to the specific situation
Example	General theory: 'Stressors, be they biological, psychological or social, produce specific physiological changes'.
	Logical deduction: John has stated that he is in constant pain, and he is worried about his wife visiting him after dark. John is experiencing multiple stressors. John will exhibit specific physiological changes.
Limitations	If the initial statement is true, then the conclusion will always be true. However, if the initial statement is false, then the conclusion will be false, even though the statements may be internally logical.

Auguste Comte founded positivism in the nineteenth century. Positivists considered that only data obtained by experiment and objective observation was 'positive' truth. Empirical methods for generating knowledge involve the collection of 'facts' by means of careful observation and experiment and the subsequent derivation of laws and theories from those facts by some logical progression (as quoted in Chalmers, 1982). From the 1920s until the 1960s the philosophy of science was dominated by logical positivism (later renamed logical empiricism). This approach is considered to be an extreme form of empiricism, and was postulated by a group of philosophers subsequently named the 'Vienna Circle'. This view is encapsulated in the 'scientific method', and the focus of this view of science was the 'justification' of discovery, and it resulted from 'an amalgamation of logic with the goals of empiricism in the development of scientific theories' (Meleis, 1991). The key features of logical positivism are as follows:

- only statements confirmed by sensory data through sensory experience are valid;
- true statements are only those based on experience and known through experience;
- there is rejection of abstraction as a method of generating theory, and any ethical considerations;
- science is value-free and scientific method is the only method for generating knowledge;
- scientific method is characterised by reductionism, quantifiability, objectivity and operationalisation.

This approach has been criticised (Watson, 1981) because it takes causal factors for granted and rejects the effects of context on discovery. As a result, the use of the scientific method is no longer seen to be the predominant approach to knowledge generation by many disciplines. However, nursing based much of its early theory-building efforts on this approach, even though such reductionist ideas are incompatible with the holistic values embodied in nursing models. Problems in developing nursing's knowledge base according to Meleis (1991) have occurred because nursing has used this approach to develop knowledge about aspects of nursing which are not reducible, quantifiable or objective. Benner (1984) and Rogers (1989), too, purport that nursing cannot be separated from the context of care; many aspects of nursing cannot be reduced to the minutest detail and examined. Indeed, it is Meleis' view that nurse theorists have not followed the traditional scientific approach, but that they have generated their conceptual frameworks from their experiences, to include ideas that are subjective, intuitive, humanistic, integrative and, in many instances, not based on sense data (Meleis, 1991).

Since the 1950s, Popper, philosopher of science, has rejected the doctrine that all knowledge starts from perception and sensation (Popper, 1968). He proposes instead that it is developed through guesswork and refutation, and he suggests that propositions are only valid if they have repeatedly survived attempts to falsify them. It has been pointed out that it is as difficult to falsify theories as it is to confirm them (Suppe and Jacox, 1985).

Pragmatism is an American school of philosophy concerned with the usefulness of knowledge. It was first proposed by Peirce and James, but was not properly acknowledged until later this century. Pragmatists consider that truth (and therefore knowledge) is validated according to whether it can be put to good use, rather than whether there is evidence to support it. In the 1960s and 1970s, philosophers such as Habermas (1965, 1974) from the Frankfurt School and Kuhn (1970) turned ideas within the philosophy of science upside-down. Table 10.6 provides an approximate chronology to accompany this section.

During the past 30 years there have been constant changes in the way in which philosophers of science describe knowledge. Although the positivists have been discredited, there is no one view that has displaced positivism. The main concern in nursing is identified by Suppe and Jacox (1985), who state that the nursing literature continues to reflect the discredited ideas of the logical positivists, and that nurses who are interested in developing and testing theory must become more aware of issues within the philosophy of science. These authors identify the need for greater diversity and tolerance in theory-testing than has previously been permitted by the logical empiricists. They conclude that multiple approaches to theory development and testing should be encouraged, and that 'debates about inductive versus deductive and qualitative versus quantitative approaches to theory development and testing are useful in so far as they make clear that alternatives exist' (Suppe and Jacox, 1985).

Table. 10.6   The philosophy of science: a chronological table

Date	Founder/theorists	Ideas/theories
BC 429–347	Plato	The world of ordinary experience is illusory; the intellect alone gives access to reality and genuine knowledge
384–322	Aristotle	DEDUCTIVE LOGIC: rationalism as heavily influenced by the teacher Plato, although some tendency towards empiricism
AD 1561–1626	Bacon	INDUCTIVE METHOD (empiricism): experience as a source of knowledge
1596–1650	Descartes	RATIONALISM
1632–1704	Locke	Founder of modern EMPIRICISM
1798–1857	Comte	POSITIVISM
1920s	'Vienna Circle' of philosophers	LOGICAL POSITIVISM: an extreme form of empiricism
1930s	Peirce and James	PRAGMATISM
1950s	Popper	FALSIFICATION
1960s	Habermas	CRITICAL SOCIAL THEORY
1970s	Kuhn	SCIENTIFIC REVOLUTIONS

Knowledge and power

One may ask, 'what is the relationship between knowledge and power?' Power is often regarded as a rather unpleasant characteristic with cynical connotations. Although there may be a grain of truth in such a view, there are in fact many positive aspects of power as well. The amount of power in society has been described by the sociologist Weber as being constant, and therefore power held by one group implies less power for other groups.

Many sociologists consider the concept of power from a macro-perspective, i.e. one concerned with whole populations and societies, such as the Marxist view (see Chapter 7). Others, such as Dahl (1974), consider power from a more interpersonal perspective. He argues that power is being exerted when someone's behaviour deviates as a result of influence. Dahl's definition of power states that it is not an attribute but a particular kind of social relationship – it refers to dependence relationships between people. Power and influence go together (see Chapter 8), as can be seen in social-exchange theory (Homans, 1992), which supports the idea that all interactions involve an exchange of something in return for something else. Power may be legitimate in the form of authority (i.e. there is some recognised official backing). For example, a manager has the authority to demand to know what an employee is doing during work time. French and Raven (1953) produced a historical and still valuable classification of power (see Table 10.7).

In nursing, all of these *power types* are in evidence. Many are concerned with knowledge, be it 'know-how' or 'know-that' knowledge. For example, Stein (1968), a psychiatrist, described the doctor–nurse relationship: nurses were seen to possess a great deal of power which they used subtly and skilfully to influence medical decision-making regarding patient management. They achieved this by providing cues to medical colleagues, and hence maintaining medical omnipotence. On analysis of this example, all of the power types appear to be present. The *physical power* source is covert and not necessarily physical, but it does involve the possible threat of coercion. For instance, if the doctor repeatedly ignores the cues given by the nurse about the best course of action in a certain situation, then the nurse may have little hesitation about telephoning the doctor in the middle of the night about an aspect of care which could have waited until the morning. With regard to *resource power,* the nurse does have the power to reward through co-operation and general ability to 'make life easier' for the doctor via various initiatives that she can implement.

Position power resides with the more senior members of the nursing team, who are often more permanent than the medical staff who pass through. In general the medical staff rely on senior nursing staff to 'show them the ropes'. *Expert* and *personal power* can be exerted through persuasion and

Table. 10.7   Types of power (French and Raven, 1953)

PHYSICAL POWER	The threat of abuse or actual abuse
RESOURCE POWER	The power to award something which is desired by the potential recipient
POSITION POWER	Legal and legitimate power associated with a position
EXPERT POWER	An individual may have power because of knowledge which he or she possesses, or he or she conveys the impression that he or she possesses specialised knowledge
PERSONAL POWER	Sometimes called charismatic power, as it is the power associated with the person and his or her personality
NEGATIVE POWER	The power to stop things happening

interpersonal skills. *Negative power* can also be exerted very subtly through non-cooperation or by filtering information.

The way in which nurses control patients' behaviour through language is another illustration of the use of power. Such control may or may not be deliberate, but it often relates to a lack of know-how in interpersonal skills, or a lack of personal knowledge about how the self may affect others. Such behaviour on the nurse's part may also reflect insufficient moral knowledge. Examples of such controlling language are presented in the work of Lanceley (1985), and Table 10.8 shows some of her examples.

According to Dahl (1974), power exists in all relationships between people. As nurses are party to professional relationships with clients and colleagues, it is therefore essential for nurses to know not only about types of knowledge but also what methods of influence are used to perpetuate the power source. Handy (1985) considers that methods of influence fall into two groups, namely the overt and the unseen. These are summarised in Table 10.9.

The benefits of knowing about power and the relationship of such benefits to practice settings are discussed in Potter (1975). For Potter, the 'correct identification of power relationships can be of the greatest practical significance for people attempting to get things done in society'. If nurses want to be influential in achieving positive change within health care settings,

Table. 10.8   Examples of controlling language used by nurses (Lanceley, 1985)

'We're just going to stand you up'
'Come on Anne, take your tablets . . . there's a good girl'
'Now you must stay with us for a while'
'You will have some lunch, won't you?'

Table. 10.9   Methods of influence (after Handy, 1985)

Power source	Influence (overt)	Influence (unseen)
Physical	Force	Ecology (i.e. environment)
Resource	Exchange	Magnetism
Position	Rules and procedures	
Expert	Rules and procedures	
Personal	Persuasion	

knowledge of power dynamics is an essential prerequisite. Power and influence are fundamental concepts to understand in relation to health promotion (see Chapter 3) and politics (see Chapter 8).

Within nursing, interest in the concept of power is represented by a number of writers (Henderson, 1994; Sines, 1994). A concept analysis undertaken by Hawks (1991) divides power into two different perspectives in relation to nursing, namely *power over* and the *power to*. The first approach is associated with power as forcefulness (a negative association), whereas the second is concerned with effectiveness (a positive focus). This concept analysis builds on many of the points raised earlier in the section on theory-building within the traditional scientific approach. It uses the approach outlined by Walker and Avant (1995) to analyse the concept of power so that it can be operationalised. The concept also appears in King's (1981) grand theory of nursing.

Knowledge and professionalism

Chinn and Kramer (1995) define a profession as 'a vocation that requires specialised knowledge, provides a role in society that is valued, and employs some means of internal regulation'. Rogers (1989) considers that professional practice results from the application of knowledge, and that nursing is a learned profession – it is both an art and a science. She defines science as an abstract body of knowledge that is systematically and logically obtained (see Chapter 2). This does not imply that knowledge should be empirical knowledge, but its methods should reflect the process of science. Rogers considers that there is a need for an abstract body of knowledge concerned with the nature of nursing. She states that the knowledge base for a profession differs from examination of the activity of that profession. For example, the study of what biologists do is not the same as the study of biology. Likewise, the study of what nurses do is not the same as the study of nursing. This is how a knowledge base unique to nursing could be explained.

According to Moore (1969), the 'criteria for a profession dictate that there must be a body of knowledge and that this body of knowledge can be communicated by others'. Nurses who develop knowledge purely for the purpose of aspiring to professional status can be diverted from the purpose of knowledge generation which is, as this author sees it, to improve the care that clients are offered. Professionalism may be a secondary benefit of this purpose. However, even professional status in itself can improve the service through the higher status that nursing achieves. The more that nursing is respected by professionals, the more influence it can exert on health care provision. This can only be achieved through increasing nursing's knowledge (expert power), articulating that knowledge, and making that knowledge evident through nurses' position (position power) in society.

Knowledge and accountability

Whether one considers nursing to be a profession or not, *professionalism* is linked to *accountability*. Denyes *et al.* (1989) state that scientific accountability is a characteristic of a profession. Leddy and Pepper (1993), too, consider that the 'concept of the professional includes legal and moral accountability for the individual's own actions'. Accountability is inextricably linked to being a professional. It is also associated with autonomy, responsibility and authority. Bergman (1981) considers accountability to have three prerequisites: personal responsibility, authority, and ability (i.e. knowledge, skills and attitudes). Bergman's model illustrates the relationship between accountability and knowledge. Knowledge, skill and attitude are taken to be the basic prerequisites for accountability. Responsibility is the next prerequisite, followed by authority – both of these are therefore part of accountability. Responsibility must be given or taken, in order to carry out an action. Authority is legitimised power – the formal backing or legal right to carry out the responsibility. The reporting aspect of accountability relates to answerability. The nurse is answerable to the client first and foremost, to professional colleagues for standards of practice, to the employer with whom she has a contract, and, finally, to the law (Hegyvary, 1982).

One aspect not covered by Bergman (1981) is that of autonomy. Autonomy relates to independence of action, meaning that 'one can perform one's total professional function on the basis of one's own knowledge and judgement'(Leddy and Pepper, 1993). It consists of making decisions and acting upon them. To be autonomous, one must be accountable. Accountability and autonomy both assume a sound knowledge basis for practice – one which supports the need to establish clearly and develop the body of knowledge on which practice is based.

Conclusion

Nursing 'depends on the scientific knowledge of human behaviour in health and in illness, the aesthetic perception of significant human experiences, a personal understanding of the unique individuality of the self and the capacity to make choices within concrete situations involving particular moral judgements' (Carper, 1978). This chapter has attempted to provide insights into the nature of knowledge and how it is linked to nursing. The nature of knowledge has been considered in terms of reviews of specific topics related to knowledge. Specific aspects of nursing knowledge in its various forms have been considered in the preceding chapters.

References

Adam, E. 1985 Toward more clarity in terminology: frameworks, theories and models. *Journal of Nursing Education* **24**, 151–5.

Allan, H. 1993 Feminism: a concept analysis. *Journal of Advanced Nursing* **18**, 1547–53.

Barber, P. 1986 The psychiatric nurse's failure therapeutically to nurture. *Nursing Practice* **1**, 138–41.

Benner, P. 1984 *From novice to expert: excellence and power in clinical nursing practice.* Menlo Park, CA: Addison-Wesley.

Benner, P. (ed.) 1994 *Interpretive phenomenology – embodiment, caring and ethics in health and illness.* Thousand Oaks, CA: Sage Publications.

Benner, P. and Tanner, C. 1987 Clinical judgement: how expert nurses use intuition. *American Journal of Nursing* **87**, 23–31.

Benner, P. and Wrubel, J. 1989 *The primacy of caring.* Menlo Park, CA: Addison-Wesley.

Bergman, R. 1981 Accountability – definitions and dimensions. *International Nursing Review* **28**, 53–9.

Bevis, E. M. 1982 *Curriculum building in nursing: a process,* 3rd edn. St. Louis: Mosby.

Boud, D., Keogh, R. and Walker, D. (eds) 1985 *Reflection: turning experience into learning.* London: Kogan Page.

Brown, G. and Harris, T. (eds) 1989 *Life events and illness.* London: Unwin Hyman.

Burnard, P. 1988 Emotional release. *Journal of District Nursing* **6**, 6, 9.

Carper, B. A. 1978 Fundamental patterns of knowing in nursing. *Advances in Nursing Science* **1**, 13–23.

Carr, W. and Kemmis, S. 1986 *Becoming critical; education, knowledge and action research.* London: Falmer Press.

Chalmers, A. F. 1982 *What is this thing called science?* 2nd edn. Milton Keynes: Open University Press.

Chinn, P. L. and Kramer, M. K. 1995 *Theory and nursing: a systematic approach,* 4th edn. St Louis: Mosby.

Concise Oxford Dictionary (ed.) 1976 6th edn. Oxford: Oxford University Press.

Dahl, R. A. 1974 Power. In Potter, D. and Sarre, P. (eds), *Dimensions of society: a reader.* Sevenoaks: Hodder and Stoughton, 446–65.

Denyes, M. J., O'Connor, N. A., Oakley, D. and Ferguson, S. 1989 Integrating nursing theory, practice and research through collaborative research. *Journal of Advanced Nursing* **14**, 141–5.

Dickoff, J. and James, P. 1968 A theory of theories: a position paper. *Nursing Research* **17**, 197–203.

Dickoff, J., James, P. and Wiedenbach, E. 1968 Theory in a practice discipline. Part 1. Practice-oriented theory. *Nursing Research* **17**, 415–35.

Elstein, A. S. and Bordage, G. 1988 Psychology of clinical reasoning. In Dowie, J. and Elstein, A. (eds), *Professional judgement.* Milton Keynes: The Open University, 109–29.

Emden, C. 1991 Ways of knowing in nursing. In Gray, G. and Pratt, R. (eds), *Towards a discipline of nursing.* Melbourne: Churchill Livingstone, 11–30.

Engel, G. 1962 *Psychological development in health and disease.* Philadelphia: Saunders.

Erikson, E. 1995 *Childhood and society.* London: Vintage.

Fawcett, J. 1978 The relationship between theory and research: a double helix. *Advances in Nursing Science* **1**, 49–62.

Fawcett, J. 1995 *Analysis and evaluation of conceptual models of nursing*, 2nd edn. Philadelphia: F. A. Davis.

Freire, P. 1972 *Cultural action for freedom*. Harmondsworth: Penguin.

French, J. and Raven, B. 1953 The bases of social power. In Cartwright, D. and Zander, A. (eds), *Group dynamics: research and theory*. London: Tavistock, 259–69.

Gilligan, C. 1982 *In a different voice*. Cambridge: Harvard University Press.

Gordon, M. 1982 *Nursing diagnosis: process and application*. New York: McGraw–Hill.

Gray, J. and Forsstrom, S. 1991 Generating theory from practice; the reflective technique. In Gray, G. and Pratt, R. (eds), *Towards a discipline of nursing*. Melbourne: Churchill Livingstone, 355–372.

Habermas, J. 1965 *Knowledge and human interests*. Cambridge: Polity Press.

Habermas, J. 1974 *Theory and practice*. London: Heinemann (translated by J. Viertel).

Hampton, D. 1994 Expertise: the true essence of nursing art. *Advances in Nursing Science* 17, 15–24.

Handy, C. B. 1985 *Understanding organizations*, 3rd edn. Harmondsworth: Penguin.

Hawks, J. H. 1991 Power: a concept analysis. *Journal of Advanced Nursing* 16, 754–62.

Hegyvary, S. 1982 *The change to primary nursing*. St Louis: Mosby.

Henderson, V. 1966 *The nature of nursing: a definition and its implications for practice research and education*. New York: Macmillan.

Henderson, A. 1994 Power and knowledge in nursing practice: the contribution of Foucault. *Journal of Advanced Nursing* 20, 935-9.

Homans, G. C. 1992 *The human group*. New Brunswick: Transaction Publishers.

Hospers, J. 1990 *An introduction to philosophical analysis*, 3rd edn. London: Routledge.

Johns, C. 1994 Nuances of reflection. *Journal of Clinical Nursing* 3, 71–4.

Johns, C. 1995 The value of reflective practice for nursing. *Journal of Clinical Nursing* 4, 23–30.

Johnson, J. L. 1994 A dialectical examination of nursing art. *Advances in Nursing Science* 17, 1–14.

King, I. M. 1981 *A theory for nursing*. New York: Wiley.

Kohlberg, L. 1981 *The philosophy of moral development: moral stages and the idea of justice*. San Francisco: Harper and Row.

Kübler-Ross, E. 1970 *On death and dying*. London: Tavistock.

Kuhn, T. S. 1970 *The structure of scientific revolutions*, 2nd edn. Chicago: University of Chicago Press.

Kuhn, T. S. 1977 Second thoughts on paradigms. In Suppe, F. (ed.), *The structure of scientific theories*, 2nd edn. Urbana: University of Illinois Press, 459–82.

Lanceley, A. 1985 Use of controlling language in the rehabilitation of the elderly. *Journal of Advanced Nursing* 10, 125–35.

Leddy, S. and Pepper, J. 1993 *Conceptual bases of professional nursing*, 3rd edn. Philadelphia: Lippincott.

Lincoln, Y. S. and Guba, E. G. 1985 *Naturalistic enquiry*. Newbury Park: Sage Publications.

McCormack, B. 1993 Intuition: concept analysis and application to curriculum development. 2. *Journal of Clinical Nursing* 2, 11–17.

Manley, K. 1990 Intensive caring. *Nursing Times* 86, 67–9.

Manley, K. 1992 Quality assurance – the pathway to excellence. In Jolley, M. and Brykczynska, G. (eds), *Nursing care: the challenge to change*. London: Edward Arnold, 175–224.

Maslow, A. H. 1968 *Toward a psychology of being*, 2nd edn. New York: Van Nostrand Reinhold.

Masterson, A. 1993 Concept analysis of independence. *Surgical Nurse* **6**, 27–30.

Meleis, A. 1991 *Theoretical nursing: development and progress.* 2nd edn. Philadelphia: Lippincott.

Mezirow, J. 1981 A critical theory of adult learning and education. *Adult Education* **32**, 3–24.

Moore, M. A. 1969 The professional practice of nursing: the knowledge and how it is used. *Nursing Forum* **8**, 361–73.

Norris, L. and Grove, S. 1986 Investigation of selected psychosocial needs of family members of critically ill adults. *Heart and Lung* **15**, 194–9.

Orem, D. 1985 *Nursing: concepts of practice*, 3rd edn. New York: McGraw-Hill.

Orlando, I. J. 1961 *The dynamic nurse–patient relationship.* New York: Putnam.

Parkes, C. M. 1986 *Bereavement: studies of grief in adult life*, 2nd edn. Harmondsworth: Penguin.

Peplau, H. E. 1952 *Interpersonal relations in nursing.* New York: Putnam.

Polanyi, M. 1962 *Personal knowledge.* Illinois: University of Chicago Press.

Polanyi, M. 1967 *The tacit dimension.* New York: Doubleday and Co.

Polit, D. and Hungler, P. 1991 *Nursing research: principles and methods*, 4th edn. Philadelphia: Lippincott.

Popper, K. 1968 *The logic of scientific discovery.* London: Hutchinson.

Potter, D. 1975 Power, conflict and integration: a study guide. In *Social sciences: a foundation course. Making sense of society: power (Course D101, Block 8, Units 25–28).* Milton Keynes: Open University Press, 7–51.

Riehl, J. P. and Roy, C. (eds) 1980 *Conceptual models for nursing practice*, 2nd edn. New York: Appleton-Century-Crofts.

Riehl-Sisca, J. P. (ed.) 1989 *Conceptual models for nursing practice*, 3rd edn. Norwalk: Appleton and Lange

Rodgers, B. L. 1993 Concept analysis: an evolutionary view. In Rodgers, B. L. and Knafl, K. A. (eds), *Concept development in nursing: foundations, techniques and applications.* Philadelphia: WB Saunders, 73–92.

Rogers, M. E. 1970 *An introduction to the theoretical basis of nursing.* Philadelphia: Davis.

Rogers, M. E. 1989 Nursing: a science of unitary human beings. In Riehl-Sisca, J.P. (ed.), *Conceptual models for nursing practice.* Norwalk: Appleton and Lange, 181–95.

Roy, C. 1984 *Introduction to nursing: an adaptation model*, 2nd edn. Englewood Cliffs: Prentice-Hall.

Runkle, G. 1985 *Theory and practice: an introduction to philosophy.* New York: Holt, Rinehart and Winston.

Ryle, G. 1949 *The concept of mind.* Harmondsworth: Penguin.

Salvage, J. 1990 The theory and practice of the 'new' nursing. *Nursing Times* **86**, 42–5.

Sarter, B. 1988 Philosophical sources of nursing theory. *Nursing Science Quarterly* **1**, 52–9.

Schon, D. A. 1983 *The reflective practitioner: how professionals think in action.* New York: Basic Books.

Schon, D. A. 1987 *Educating the reflective practitioner: towards a new design for teaching and learning in the profession.* San Francisco: Jossey Bass.

Silva, M. C. 1977 Philosophy, science, theory: interrelationships and implications for nursing research. *Image* **9**, 59–63.

Sines, D. 1994 The arrogance of power: a reflection on contemporary mental health nursing practice. *Journal of Advanced Nursing* **20**, 894–903.

Smith, M. C. 1992 Is all knowing personal knowing? *Nursing Science Quarterly* **5**, 2–3.

Stein, L. I. 1968 The doctor–nurse game. *American Journal of Nursing* **68**, 101–5.

Suppe, F. and Jacox, A. K. 1985 Philosophy of science and the development of nursing theory. *Annual Review of Nursing Research* **3**, 241–67.

Sweeney, N. M. 1994 A concept analysis of personal knowledge: application to nursing education. *Journal of Advanced Nursing* **20**, 917–24.

Tanner, C. A., Benner, P., Chesla, C. and Gordon, D. R. 1993 The phenomenology of knowing the patient. *Image* **25**, 273–80.

Teasdale, G. and Jennett, B. 1974 Assessment of coma and impaired consciousness. *Lancet* **2**, 81–4.

Visintainer, M. 1986 The nature of knowledge and theory in nursing. *Image* **18**, 32–8.

von Bertalanffy, L. 1968 *General system theory*. New York: George Braziller.

Walker, L. O. and Avant, K. C. 1995 *Strategies for theory construction in nursing*, 3rd edn. Norwalk: Appleton and Lange

Warfield, C. and Manley, K. 1990 Developing a new philosophy in the NDU. *Nursing Standard* **4**, 27–30.

Waterlow, J. A. 1985 A risk assessment card. *Nursing Times* **81**, 49–51, 55.

Watson, J. 1981 Nursing's scientific quest. *Nursing Outlook* **29**, 413–16.

Watson, J. 1985 *Nursing: human science and human care*. Norwalk: Appleton-Century-Crofts.

Wiedenbach, E. 1964 *Clinical nursing: a helping art*. New York: Springer.

Index

Page numbers printed in **bold** type refer to figures: those in *italic* to tables